HIGH FIBER
COOKBOOK

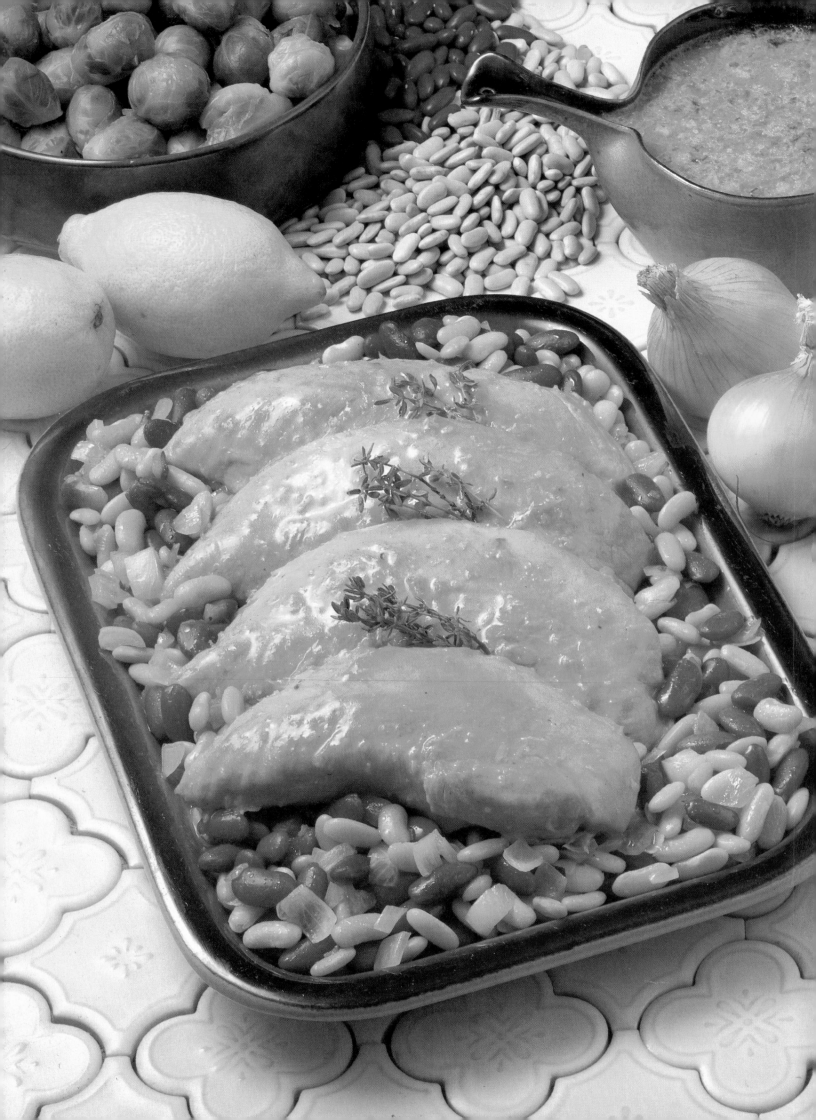

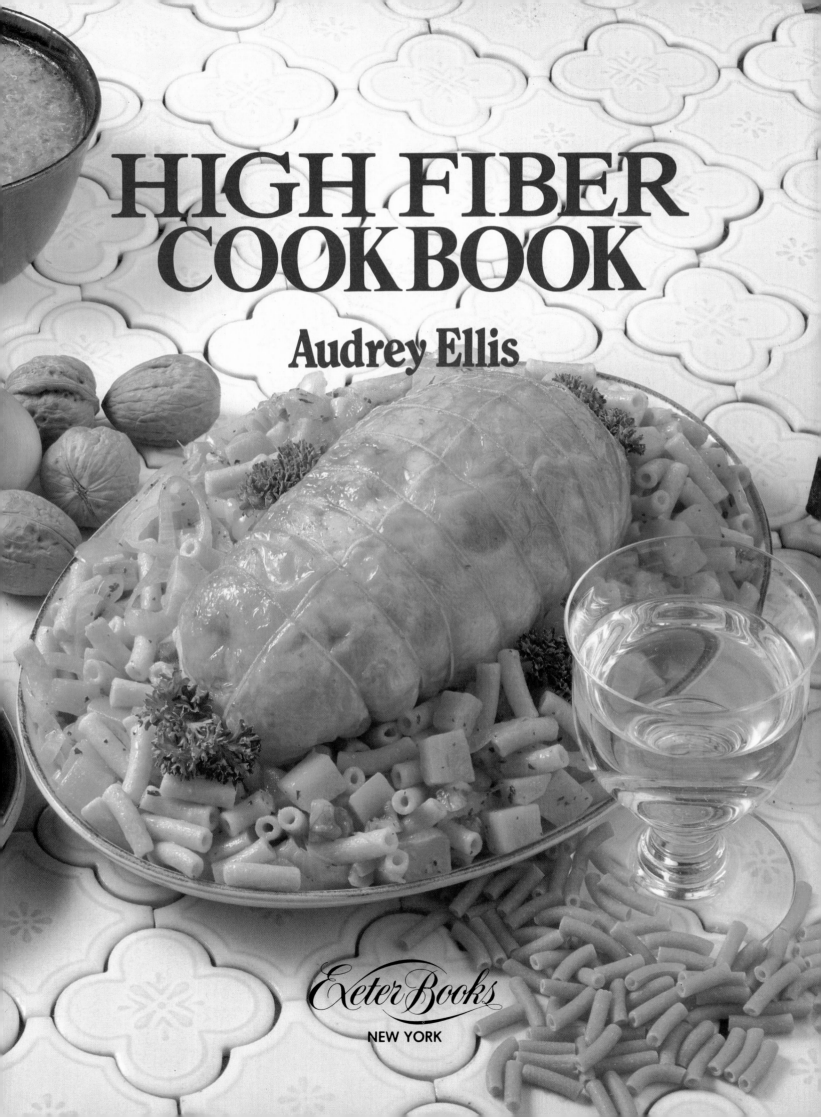

HIGH FIBER COOKBOOK

Audrey Ellis

Exeter Books

NEW YORK

Acknowledgments

The author and publishers would like to thank the following companies for their help in supplying some of the photographs for this book:

Allinson (pages 31, 128, 134, 135)

Apple and Pear Development Council (pages 93, 146/147, 170)

Bacon Suppliers to the UK (pages 23, 185)

Bakewell Non Stick Baking Parchment (page 177)

Batchelors Foods (pages 59, 65, 70, 78/79, 89, 90, 141)

Baxters of Speyside (pages 52, 182/183)

Billingtons Sugars (pages 13, 133, 136)

Blue Band (pages 130/131)

British Meat (page 82)

British Sugar PLC (page 180)

British Turkey Federation (page 2/3)

Cadbury Typhoo Advisory Service (pages 143, 157, 178)

Campbell's Soups Limited (pages 36/37, 66/67, 69)

Carmel (pages 46, 96/97, 101, 117, 119)

Colman's of Norwich (pages 111, 187)

Danish Agricultural Producers (pages 20, 21, 83, 86, 100)

Dupont, Manufacturer of 'SilverStone' nonstick coating (page 42)

Dutch Dairy Bureau (pages 58, 114/115, 118, 126)

Flour Advisory Bureau (pages 149, 158)

Force wheat flakes (pages 146/147)

Gale's Honey and Curds (pages 72/73, 127, 138/139, 142, 144, 154/155)

H J Heinz Company Limited (pages 24, 26/27, 29, 49, 57, 110)

Jordan (Cereals) Limited (pages 122/123)

Kellog Company of Great Britain Limited (pages 16/17)

Libby's Canned Fruit (pages 30, 33)

McVities (page 176)

Mushroom Growers' Association (page 92)

The Nestlé Company Limited (page 39)

New Zealand Lamb Information Bureau (pages 47, 62/63, 74/75, 77)

Ocean Spray Cranberries (pages 172/173)

Pasta Foods Limited (pages 44/45, 104/105, 160)

Pasta Information Centre (pages 60, 99)

Pyrex by Corning (pages 150, 151, 162/163)

Quaker Oats (page 152)

Seafish Industry Authority (pages 34, 41, 55)

Spillers Homepride Limited (page 125)

Summer Oranges (pages 6, 84, 94, 107, 112, 120, 165, 171)

Wall's Carte d'Or Ice Creams (page 175)

Whitworths Holdings Limited (pages 14, 19, 51, 102, 108, 166, 169)

Photographed on title page – Left: Turkey fillets with mixed beans (recipe page 95). Right: Turkey roast with walnut macaroni (recipe page 64)

First published in the USA 1985
by Exeter Books
Distributed by Bookthrift
Exeter is a trademark of Simon & Schuster, Inc
Bookthrift is a registered trademark of Simon & Schuster, Inc
New York, New York

Prepared by
Deans International Publishing
52-54 Southwark Street, London SE1 1UA
A division of The Hamlyn Publishing Group Limited
London·New York·Sydney·Toronto

ISBN 0-671-07720-1

Printed in Italy

Contents

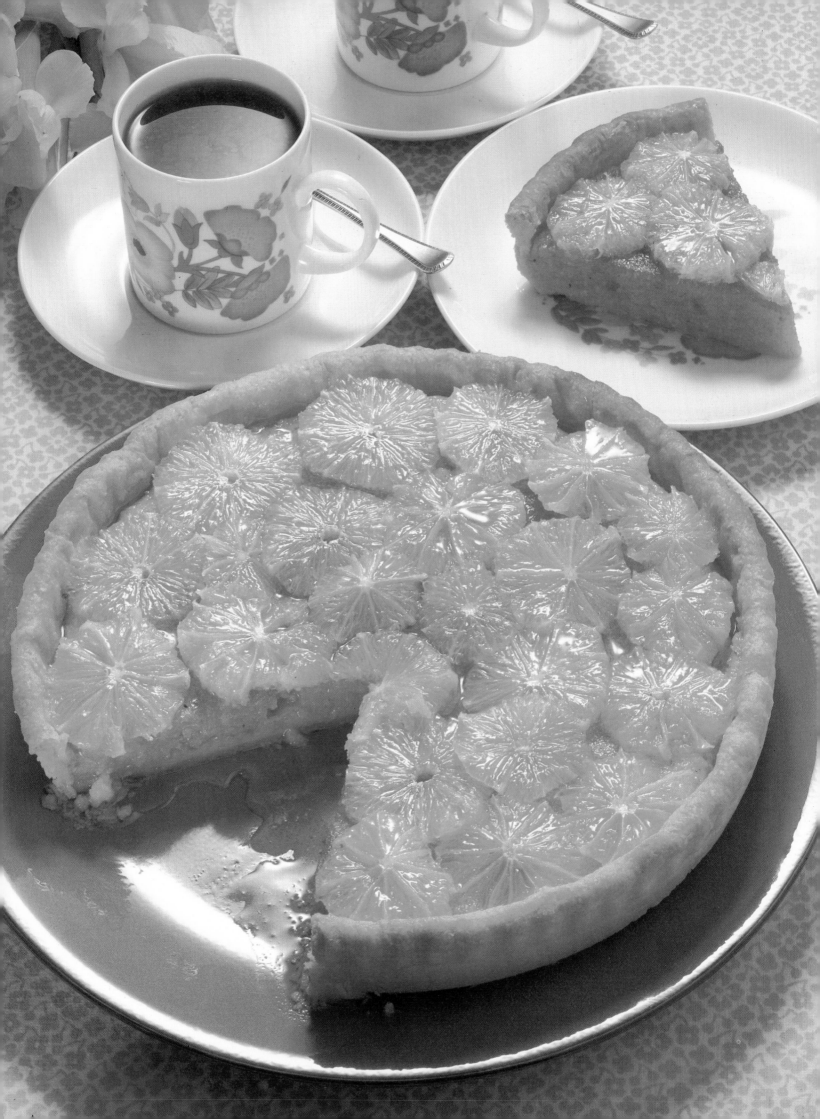

Useful Facts and Figures

Notes on metrication

In this book quantities are given in metric and Imperial measures. Exact conversion from Imperial to metric measures does not usually give very convenient working quantities and so the metric measures have been rounded off into units of 25 grams. The table below shows the recommended equivalents.

Ounces	Approx g to nearest whole figure	Recommended conversion to nearest unit of 25
1	28	25
2	57	50
3	85	75
4	113	100
5	142	150
6	170	175
7	198	200
8	227	225
9	255	250
10	283	275
11	312	300
12	340	350
13	368	375
14	396	400
15	425	425
16 (1 lb)	454	450
17	482	475
18	510	500
19	539	550
20 (1¼ lb)	567	575

Note: When converting quantities over 20 oz first add the appropriate figures in the centre column, then adjust to the nearest unit of 25. As a general guide, 1 kg (1000 g) equals 2.2 lb or about 2 lb 3 oz. This method of conversion gives good results in nearly all cases, although in certain pastry and cake recipes a more accurate conversion is necessary to produce a balanced recipe.

Liquid measures The millilitre has been used in this book and the following table gives a few examples.

Imperial	Approx ml to nearest whole figure	Recommended ml
¼ pint	142	150 ml
½ pint	283	300 ml
¾ pint	425	450 ml
1 pint	567	600 ml
1½ pints	851	900 ml
1¾ pints	992	1000 ml (1 litre)

Spoon measures All spoon measures given in this book are level unless otherwise stated.

Can sizes At present, cans are marked with the exact (usually to the nearest whole number) metric equivalent of the Imperial weight of the contents, so we have followed this practice when giving can sizes.

Lemon and almond flan (recipe page 130)

Notes for American and Australian users

In America the 8-oz measuring cup is used. In Australia metric measures are now used in conjunction with the standard 250-ml measuring cup. The Imperial pint, used in Britain and Australia, is 20 fl oz, while the American pint is 16 fl oz. It is important to remember that the Australian tablespoon differs from both the British and American tablespoons; the table below gives a comparison. The British standard tablespoon, which has been used throughout this book, holds 17.7 ml, the American 14.2 ml, and the Australian 20 ml. A teaspoon holds approximately 5 ml in all three countries.

British	American	Australian
1 teaspoon	1 teaspoon	1 teaspoon
1 tablespoon	1 tablespoon	1 tablespoon
2 tablespoons	3 tablespoons	2 tablespoons
3½ tablespoons	4 tablespoons	3 tablespoons
4 tablespoons	6 tablespoons	3½ tablespoons

An Imperial/American guide to solid and liquid measures

Imperial Solid measures	American	Imperial Liquid measures	American
1 lb butter or margarine	2 cups	¼ pint liquid	⅔ cup liquid
		½ pint	1¼ cups
1 lb flour	4 cups	¾ pint	2 cups
1 lb granulated or caster sugar	2 cups	1 pint	2½ cups
		1½ pints	3¾ cups
1 lb icing sugar	3 cups	2 pints	5 cups (2½ pints)
8 oz rice	1 cup		

American terms

The list below gives some American equivalents or substitutes for terms and ingredients used in this book.

British/American
Equipment and terms
cling film/plastic wrap
deep cake tin/spring form pan
double saucepan/double boiler
flan tin/pie pan
frying pan/skillet
greaseproof paper/wax paper
grill/broil
liquidize/blend
loaf tin/loaf pan
piping bag/pastry bag
stoned/pitted
Swiss roll tin/jelly roll pan

British/American
Ingredients
aubergine/eggplant
bicarbonate of soda/baking soda
biscuits/crackers, cookies
cocoa powder/unsweetened cocoa
cornflour/cornstarch
courgettes/zucchini
cream, single/cream, light
cream, double/cream, heavy
essence/extract
flour, plain/flour, all-purpose
glacé cherries/candied cherries
icing/frosting
lard/shortening
shortcrust pastry/basic pie dough
spring onion/scallion
sultanas/seedless white raisins
yeast, fresh/yeast, compressed

NOTE: **When making any of the recipes in this book, only follow one set of measures as they are not interchangeable.**

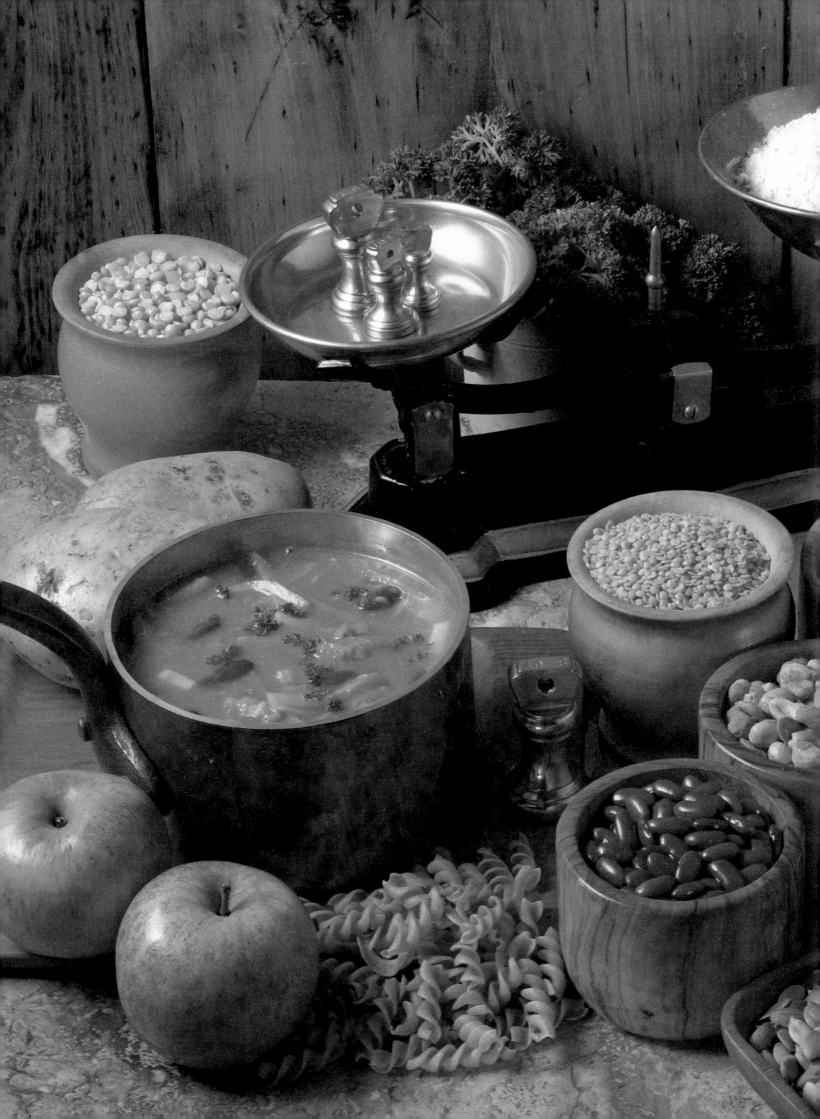

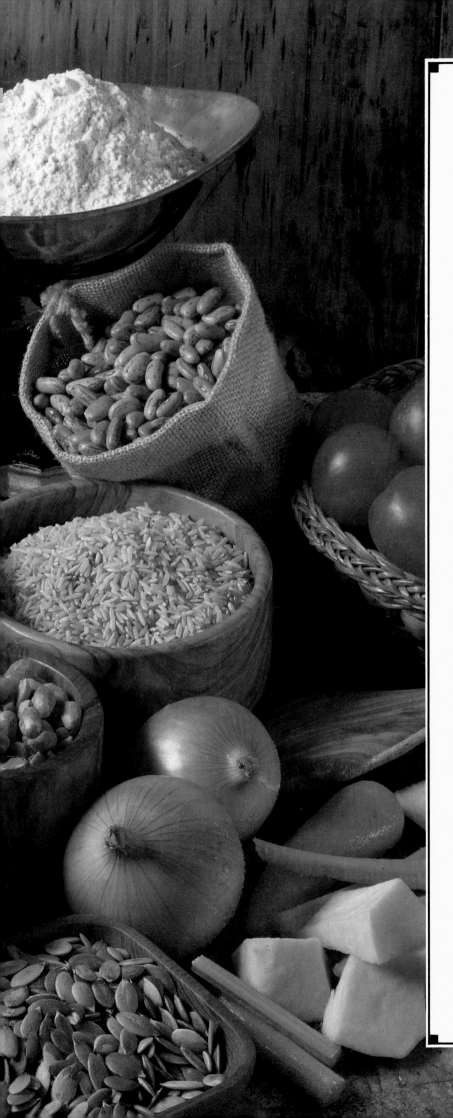

Introduction

To become healthy, and stay that way for the rest of our lives, we all need to eat sufficient dietary fibre. Yet for centuries, we've been hard at work refining our food, and removing most of the fibre from it. So we have lost much of the vital element in our daily diet which eases natural digestion and the elimination of waste products. Don't confuse it with meat fibres, which are almost completely digested and absorbed by the body.

The wonder-working substance, with which this book is concerned, is contained in all cereals, pulses, fruit, nuts and vegetables to some extent. Bran is not another name for fibre, although it does contain a very high percentage. But if you eat sensibly, you will not need to consume bran by the bowlful, especially when you choose wholewheat breads, pastas and flour for cooking. Fibre-rich breakfast cereals are also an obvious choice to begin the day well.

At first you will notice that you are consuming more bulk and perhaps fear you may put on weight. But providing you keep a watchful eye on your fat intake, there is little danger of this, since fibrous foods are naturally low in calories. In fact, high fibre foods are an integral part of the most successful slimming plans.

Highly refined foods, once regarded as delicate and desirable fare, are now blamed by the medical profession for many modern ills. Make the switch to healthier eating now. It will be easier and more fun than you think.

Hi-fi dishes need not be dreary or unappetizing. Turn the pages of this book and study the illustrations; you'll see how tempting they look. Include them in your family meal menus and discover how delicious they are.

Fibre Content of Food

Many standard items high on the average shopping list contain plenty of roughage. Others, as you will see from the list of non-fibrous foods, are entirely lacking in it. But it is worth learning the relative fibre values of different cereals, vegetables and fruit, because even these foods vary surprisingly in their fibre content.

Fibre content given per 25 g/1 oz unless otherwise stated

Breakfast cereals	Fibre grams
Jordan's Country Muesli (U.S. ⅓ cup)	0.7
Original Crunchy with bran and apple (U.S. ¼ cup)	0.7
Kellogg's All Bran (U.S. ½ cup)	8.0
Bran Buds (U.S. ½ cup)	7.0
30% Bran Flakes (U.S. scant 1 cup)	4.4
Cornflakes (U.S. 1 cup)	0.4
Rice Krispies (U.S. 1¼ cups)	0.25
Sultana Bran (U.S. ¾ cup)	3.8
Nabisco Shredded Wheat, 2	5.0
Quaker Puffed Wheat (U.S. 1¼ cups)	4.2
Weetabix, 2	4.8
Whitworth's Oatmeal (U.S. scant ¼ cup)	2.0
Rolled oats (U.S. generous ¼ cup)	2.0
Unprocessed bran (U.S. ½ cup)	12.4
Wheatgerm (U.S. ½ cup)	0.6

Fibre content given per 25 g/1 oz (U.S. ¼ cup)

Flour	Fibre grams
White, plain or self-raising (U.S. self-rising)	1.0
strong (U.S. white bread flour)	0.8
White, high fibre flour	2.4
Brown (wheatmeal)	2.1
Wholemeal (U.S. wholewheat)	2.7
Granary (U.S. fancy wholewheat)	2.0
Rye	3.3
Cornflour (U.S. cornstarch)	0.8

Fibre content given per 25 g/1 oz unless otherwise stated

Bread products	Fibre grams
White (U.S. 1 small slice)	0.75
Wheatgerm (U.S. 1 small slice)	1.3
Wholemeal (U.S. 1 small slice wholewheat)	2.4
Malt (U.S. 1 small slice)	1.4
French (U.S. about 2.5-cm/1-inch length	0.75
Brown (wheatmeal) (U.S. 1 small slice)	1.45
Soda (white)	0.65
Granary (U.S. 1 slice fancy wholewheat)	1.4
Breadcrumbs, white, fresh (U.S. ½ cup)	0.75
brown (wheatmeal) (U.S. ½ cup)	1.4
wholemeal (U.S. ½ cup wholewheat)	2.4

	Fibre grams
Bap (U.S. hamburger bun), white	1.4
Wholemeal roll (U.S. wholewheat roll)	4.2
White bread roll, crisp	1.5
soft	1.4
Brown bread roll, crisp	2.9
soft	2.7
Scone, white (U.S. biscuit)	1.2
wholemeal (U.S. wholewheat biscuit)	3.2
Doughnut, plain ring	0.8

Fibre content given per single item

Crispbreads and biscuits (U.S. cookies)	Fibre grams
Crispbreads, light	0.2
wholemeal	0.8
bran	1.2
Biscuits, digestive (U.S. Graham cracker), 1 large	0.8
Fig roll	0.7
Oatmeal or peanut cookies	0.5
Wholemeal shortbread	1.4
Cream cracker (U.S. plain cracker for cheese)	0.2
Farmhouse (U.S. savoury cracker for cheese)	0.4

Fibre content given per 150 ml/¼ pint (U.S. ⅔ cup)

Yogurt	Fibre grams
Natural or fruit flavoured	—
Hazelnut (U.S. filbert)	2.0
Muesli	0.7

Fibre content given per 100 g/4 oz (U.S. ¼ lb)

Fruit, fresh, small	Fibre grams
Apricots	2.4
Blackberries (U.S. black raspberries)	8.2
Blackcurrants	9.8
Cherries	1.7
Cranberries	4.8
Damsons (U.S. damson plums)	4.2
Figs, fresh	1.0
Gooseberries, cooking	0.3
eating	2.8
Grapes, white or green black (U.S. purple)	7.0
Greengages (U.S. greengage plums)	0.4
Loganberries	2.6
Lychees, weigh with shells	8.4
Mulberries	9.2
Plums	2.9
Raspberries	2.5
Redcurrants	9.2
Rhubarb	2.9
Strawberries	2.5

Fruit, fresh, large	Fibre grams
Apple, eating, 1 medium-sized unpeeled	2.7
1 medium-sized peeled	2.2
cooking, 1 medium-sized unpeeled	4.3
Apple purée, 100 ml/4 fl oz (U.S. ½ cup apple sauce)	2.3
Avocado, half medium-sized fruit	2.1
Banana, 1 medium-sized	3.4
Grapefruit, 1 medium-sized half	0.5
Mandarin orange, 1 medium-sized	0.9
Melon, Honeydew or Canteloupe, 1 medium-sized slice about 225 g/8 oz (U.S. ½ lb)	1.3
Melon, Charentais, Galia or Ogen, ½ small fruit about 225 g/8 oz (U.S. ½ lb)	1.65
Melon, watermelon, 1 medium-sized slice about 225 g/8 oz (U.S. ½ lb)	0.65
Nectarine, 1 medium-sized	2.5
Orange, 1 medium-sized	3.4
Passion fruit, 1 medium-sized	5.7
Peach, 1 medium-sized	1.4
Pear, 1 medium-sized unpeeled	5.2
1 medium-sized peeled	2.3
Pineapple, 1 medium-sized slice about 175 g/6 oz (weight with skin and core)	0.9
Tangerine, 1 medium-sized	0.9

Fibre content given per 100 ml/4 fl oz (U.S. ½ cup) fruit with juice or syrup

Fruit, canned	Fibre grams
Apricot, halves	1.5
Grapefruit, segments	0.6
Lychees	0.4
Mandarin, segments	0.3
Peach, slices	1.1
Pear, halves	1.9
Pineapple, rings (2)	1.0

Fibre content given per 100 g/4 oz (U.S. ¼ lb)

Fruit, dried	Fibre grams
Apricots	27.2
Currants	5.2
Dates, stoned (U.S. pitted)	9.6
Figs	20.8
Peaches	16.0
Prunes, with stones (U.S. pits)	15.2
Raisins, seedless (U.S. ⅔ cup)	5.6
Sultanas (U.S. ⅔ cup seedless white raisins)	5.6

Fibre content given per 25 g/1 oz, shelled

Nuts	Fibre grams
Almonds, whole (U.S. scant ¼ cup)	4.1
ground (U.S. ¼ cup)	4.1
Brazils, 4 nuts	1.2
Cashews (U.S. scant ¼ cup)	4.0
Chopped nuts, most kinds (U.S. ¼ cup)	4.0
Coconut, desiccated (U.S. ⅓ cup shredded)	6.6
fresh, chopped (U.S. ⅓ cup)	3.8
Peanuts, fresh or roasted (U.S. scant ¼ cup)	2.3
Pecans, halved (U.S. ¼ cup)	1.5
Walnuts, halved (U.S. ¼ cup)	1.5

Fibre content given per 100 g/4 oz (U.S. ½ cup) uncooked

Rice	Fibre grams
Brown	4.8
White, long or short grain	1.4

Note: Cooked rice retains fibre content of uncooked grain but trebles in volume, i.e. 100 g/4 oz (U.S. ½ cup) uncooked brown rice with a fibre content of 4.8 grams becomes 350 g/12 oz (U.S. 1½ cups) cooked rice with a fibre content of 4.8 grams.

Fibre content given per 100 g/4 oz (U.S. ¼ lb) uncooked

Pasta	Fibre grams
Lasagne, green or white	3.4
wholewheat	11.2
Macaroni, white	3.4
wholewheat	11.2
Pasta shapes, green or white	3.4
wholewheat	11.2
Spaghetti, green or white	3.4
wholewheat	11.2
Tagliatelle, green or white	3.4

Fibre content given per 295-g/10.4-oz can condensed

Soups	Fibre grams
Chicken and sweetcorn	1.8
Cream of celery	1.5
Cream of tomato	3.0
Pea and ham	10.8
Cream of mushroom	0.9
Lentil	6.6
French onion	2.4
Turkey and vegetable broth	3.0

Fibre content given per 25 g/1 oz dry weight unless otherwise stated

Grains	Fibre grams
Pearl barley (U.S. generous ⅛ cup)	0.6
Ground rice (U.S. scant ¼ cup)	0.7
Semolina (U.S. scant ¼ cup)	0.8
Tapioca (U.S. scant ¼ cup)	0.8
Oatmeal (U.S. scant ¼ cup)	2.0

Fibre content given per 100 g/4 oz (U.S. ¼ lb) dry weight unless otherwise stated

Pulses, dried	Fibre grams
Aduki beans	28.0
Black-eye beans	28.8
Butter beans	24.4
Chick peas	17.2
Haricot beans (U.S. navy beans)	28.8
Mung beans	24.8
Red kidney beans	28.0

Soya beans	4.8
Peas, green dried	17.0
Peas, split	13.6

Fibre content given per 225-g/8-oz can

Pulses, canned	Fibre grams
Butter beans	8.0
Cannellini beans	8.3
Red kidney beans	9.5
Broad beans (U.S. fava or lima beans)	6.0
Baked beans in tomato sauce	16.0
Soya beans in brine	7.0
Green peas, canned fresh peas	8.9
canned processed dried peas	8.0

Fibre content given per 100 g/4 oz (U.S. $\frac{1}{4}$ lb) raw weight, unless otherwise stated

Vegetables, fresh	Fibre grams
Asparagus, 6 spears	2.4
Aubergine (U.S. eggplant)	2.8
Beansprouts	1.2
French, runner or green beans (U.S. green beans)	3.3
Beetroot (U.S. beet), cooked	2.8
Broccoli	4.1
Brussels sprouts	4.8
Cabbage, red	3.8
green	3.4
white	3.0
Carrots	3.2
Cauliflower	2.4
Celeriac, cooked	5.6
Celery, 1 large stalk	1.0
cooked 100 g/4 oz (U.S. $\frac{2}{3}$ cup sliced cooked)	2.5
Chinese leaves (U.S. Chinese cabbage)	2.4
Corn, canned or cooked, kernels only (U.S. $\frac{2}{3}$ cup)	5.3
Courgettes (U.S. zucchini)	2.0
Cucumber, 10-cm/4-inch length	0.4
Leeks	3.5
Lettuce, 2 large leaves	0.4
Marrow (U.S. squash)	2.0
Mushrooms	2.8
Okra	3.6
Onion, 1 medium-sized	1.5
Parsnips	4.5
Peppers, red or green, 1 medium-sized	1.2
Potato, raw peeled	2.4
raw with skin	2.8
baked in jacket	2.8
crisps (U.S. chips), 1 small pack 25 g/1 oz	3.4
Pumpkin	0.6
Radishes	2.0
Spinach, cooked and drained (U.S. $\frac{1}{2}$ cup chopped cooked)	7.1
Swede (U.S. rutabaga)	3.0
Sweet potato	2.8

Tomatoes, fresh	1.6
canned, drained 50 g/2 oz (U.S. $\frac{1}{3}$ cup)	0.5

Note: Tomatoes are peeled before being canned and this accounts for the drop in fibre content.

Turnip	3.2
Watercress, 4 large sprigs	0.9

Fibre content given per 1 level tablespoon

Spreads	Fibre grams
Golden syrup (U.S. light corn syrup)	–
Jam	0.2
Maple syrup	–
Marmalade	0.1
Redcurrant jelly	–
Black treacle (U.S. molasses)	–
Peanut butter	1.2

Daily fibre intake To judge how much fibre you are recommended to eat each day, the normal consumption is about 20 g, but an increase of 10-15 g would be beneficial according to medical authorities.

The fibre content of these foods is either nil or negligible for an average serving

Non-fibrous foods	Fibre grams
Alcoholic drinks	–
Beef	–
Butter	–
Cheese	–
Chicken	–
Chocolate	–
Cocoa (U.S. unsweetened cocoa)	–
Coffee	–
Drinking chocolate (U.S. sweetened cocoa)	–
Dripping	–
Eggs	–
Fish	–
Fruit juices	–
Ice cream	–
Lamb	–
Lard	–
Lemonade (U.S. 7 Up)	–
Low fat spreads	–
Margarine	–
Milk – fresh, low fat, non-fat, dried, condensed or evaporated	–
Oil	–
Pork	–
Shellfish	–
Suet	–
Tea	–

Good morning start (recipe page 35)

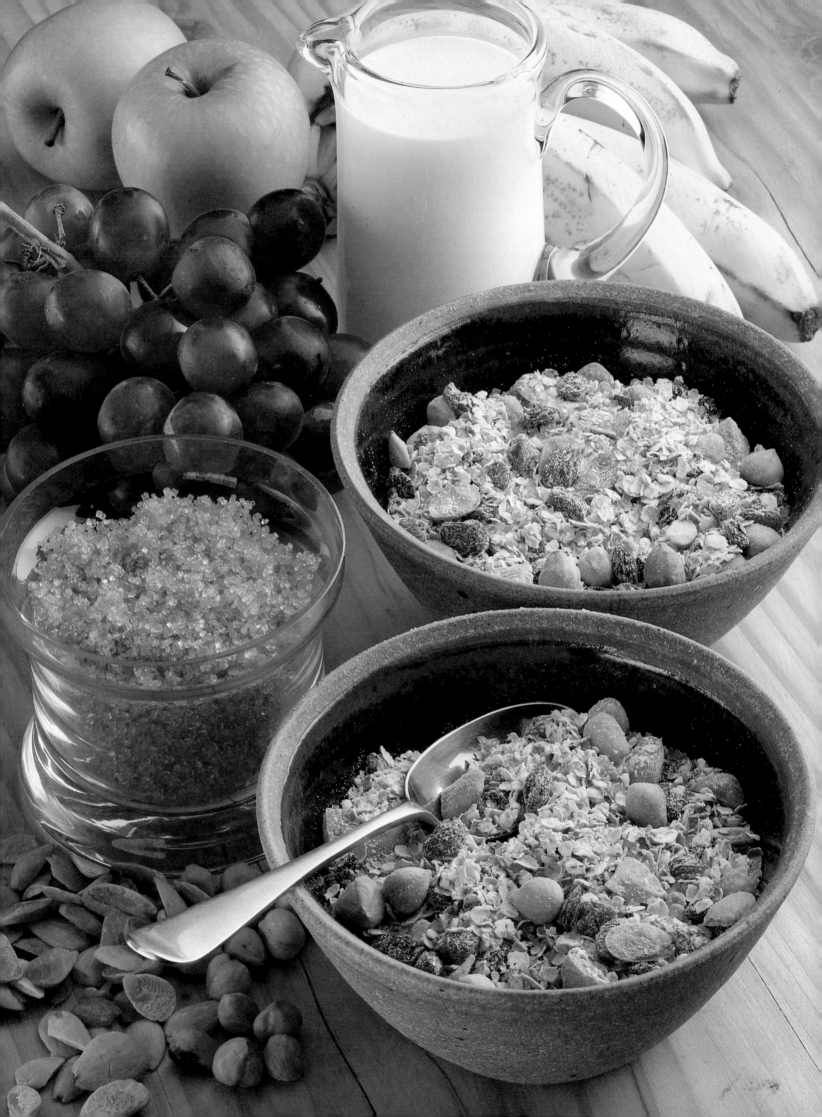

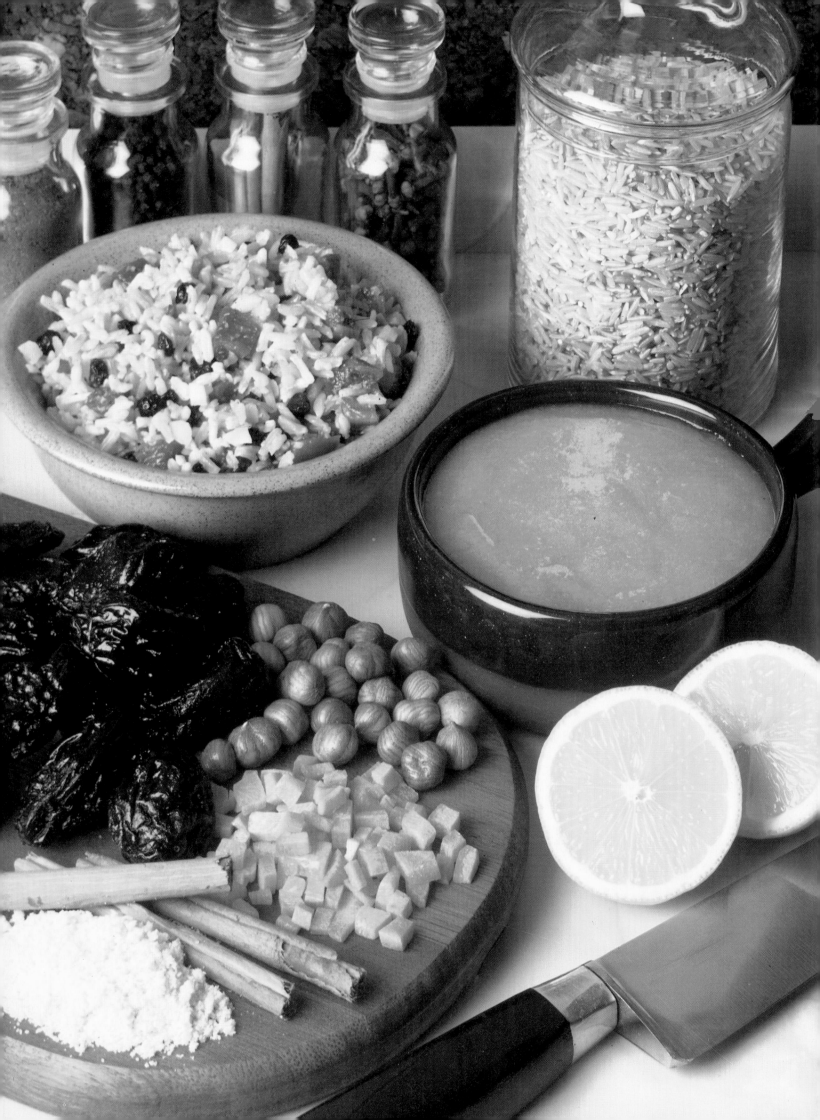

Good Slimming Sense

There is no such thing as a slimming diet that is equally good for everyone who wishes to lose weight. There are those of us who can easily give up desserts and chocolate, and those to whom this is a real deprivation. Those who can eat a hearty breakfast and miss lunch entirely; and those who prefer to eat little or nothing until at least mid-day, and then hardly stop until midnight chimes.

Here are some golden rules that apply to all sensible weight-reducing diets. Choose the diet that works for you. But don't make the mistake of giving up foods high in fibre, because you assume them to be high in calories. This is not necessarily so.

1 Adjust your food-consumption time clock as far as possible to the early segment of the waking day. If you can, eat breakfast (not just coffee and half a slice of toast); then nothing until lunchtime. Eat a good lunch, rather than a snack. Eat an early evening meal, and no naughty tit-bits between then and going to bed. It is often the chocolate bars and cookies eaten absentmindedly while watching TV, after you've finished working your food intake off with exercise, that over-top your calorie allowance. Impossible? Then set a time, say 9 o'clock, after which you eat nothing more till next morning, and stick to it.

2 Read up the subject just enough to have a good idea at the back of your mind on the calorie and fibre content of the foods you eat and enjoy often. Then a mental warning bell rings if you are indulging too many calorie-weighted favourites in one day or falling behind on your fibre intake. Don't become a diet bore, but do know the score!

3 Suppose there is a special item you crave, know you shouldn't eat, and which tends to wreck your diet. Say it's a chocolate bar or a big portion of golden-fried potatoes. Indulge yourself now and again, but make a production of it. Set the time, approach it with pleasurable anticipation, sit down and devote yourself to enjoying your treat. Don't gulp it down in a hurry, and then reproach yourself because you hardly feel as if you have eaten it, and already want another. Tell yourself, when the treat has been demolished, that you feel positively satiated, and won't need it again for quite a while. Approached in the proper spirit, this method succeeds.

4 Increase the amount of fibre you eat. Why does this help you to slim? Quite simply because you tend not to eat so much. High fibre foods are filling and satisfying, and take a great deal more chewing than does a scrambled egg or ice cream! You really do have to eat more slowly and perhaps for the first time appreciate and get full enjoyment out of the flavour of what you are eating. There's a big psychological plus in eating slowly rather than rushing one's meal.

5 The digestive process can't be hurried. Fibrous food takes quite a time to digest and while this is going on, you won't experience those unpleasant hunger pangs which so often beset the dieter.

6 Another unexpected bonus is that a small proportion of fibrous foods do not become fully digested on their way through your body. Not only does the fibre pass harmlessly straight through without building up your calorie count, it takes other food elements with it, before your system has consigned them to the body's storehouse; that's to say the layer of unnecessary fat you build up when you are overweight.

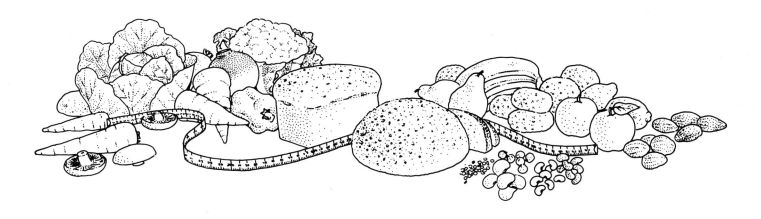

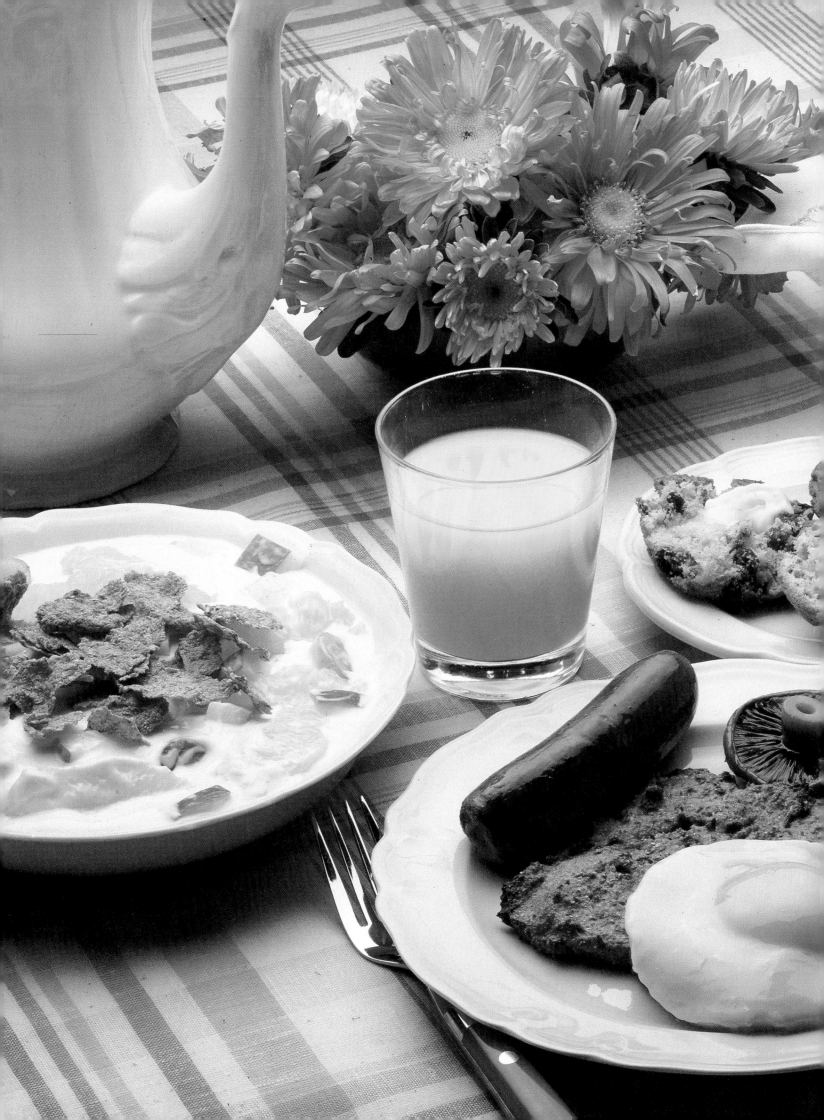

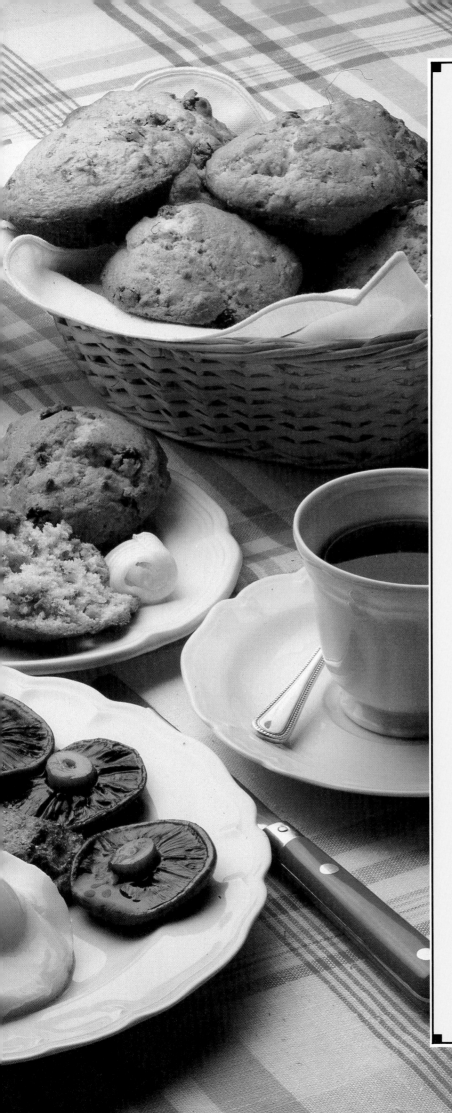

Breakfast and Snacks

The best way to start the day is with a meal that gives you sufficient energy to function at what doctors call your 'optimum efficiency'. There is a great temptation to fill the gap until lunch time with foods of the quick snack variety that do little to promote health. Resist it.

Breakfast-time gives you the best opportunity of the day to consume a sizeable proportion of your fibre intake in the form of hot or cold cereals. You may be one of the crowd who love crisp, crunch-in-the-mouth cereals with tempting additions of dried fruit and nuts, well moistened with cold milk. Splendid. Or you may feel that no day gets off to a good start without a bowl of creamy, hot oats taken either as the Scots like it with a big pinch of salt; or, as most of us prefer, with lashings of brown sugar melting into delicious toffee-like puddles. For those who do not want cereal, choose a crispbread or bread that is fibre-rich.

By all means enjoy bacon and eggs if you wish, so long as you accompany them by wholemeal bread or toast, or even muffins with extra bran, to help out the classic breakfast choice. For, sad to say, this contains no dietary fibre at all. It's a very good habit to put the fruit bowl on the table at breakfast-time. Late risers may just grab an apple or pear before they rush out of the house, and if it is eaten without being peeled, so much the better.

Snack meals do not have a very good reputation where health considerations are concerned. But they can be as fibre-full as you like. Sandwiches made with wholemeal breads, baps or buns have a respectable quota of roughage. The fillings may also be composed of foods you will see in the chart on pages 10-12. Or, if you have a meat or cheese sandwich, add a salad layer.

From the left – Citrus bran flakes (recipe page 18), Poached eggs on bran cakes (recipe page 20), Lemon breakfast muffins (recipe page 22)

Apricot yogurt crunch

(Illustrated opposite)

175 g/6 oz (U.S. 1¼ cups) no-need-to-soak
dried apricots
40 g/1½ oz chopped hazelnuts
(U.S. ⅓ cup chopped filberts)
25 g/1 oz (U.S. generous ¼ cup) rolled oats
1 tablespoon light muscovado sugar
(U.S. light brown sugar)
300 ml/½ pint (U.S. 1¼ cups) natural yogurt, chilled

Place the apricots in a pan, pour over water just to cover and cook gently for 20 minutes, until the fruit is just tender. Lift out the apricots, divide among 4 serving dishes and leave to cool.

Combine the nuts, oats and sugar. Spoon the yogurt over the fruit and sprinkle the nut mixture on top. Serve at once, or prepare the night before and chill until required. **Serves 4**

Note If preferred, serve the ingredients in heatproof dishes and place these under a hot grill (U.S. broiler) for 2 minutes, or until the topping browns.

Fruity breakfast kedgeree

(Illustrated opposite)

100 g/4 oz (U.S. generous ½ cup)
long grain brown rice
2 tablespoons (U.S. 3 tablespoons) oil
100 g/4 oz (U.S. generous ½ cup) peanuts,
toasted and skins removed
75 g/3 oz (U.S. ⅔ cup) no-need-to-soak prunes,
stoned (U.S. pitted) and chopped
1 egg, hard-boiled (U.S. hard-cooked),
shelled and chopped
salt and freshly ground black pepper
cayenne pepper
Garnish
1 egg, hard-boiled (U.S. hard-cooked),
shelled and sliced
chopped parsley

Cook the rice in a pan of boiling salted water for about 25 minutes, or until tender. Drain well.

Heat the oil in a pan and fry the nuts for 2 minutes. Put in the rice, prunes, egg and seasoning to taste. Reheat over low heat, stirring gently. When piping hot, divide among 4 warm dishes and top each with slices of egg and a sprinkling of parsley. Serve hot. **Serves 4**

Muesli medley

(Illustrated opposite)

75 g/3 oz (U.S. scant 1 cup) rolled oats
75 g/3 oz (U.S. ½ cup) chopped dried fruit salad
75 g/3 oz (U.S. ¾ cup) chopped nuts
To serve
milk or natural yogurt
toasted coconut flakes

Combine the oats, fruit and nuts and divide among 4 shallow plates. At serving time, moisten with milk or yogurt and top with a sprinkling of coconut flakes.

For greater convenience, multiply the dry ingredients and store in an airtight container. **Serves 4**

Dried fruit compôte

(Illustrated opposite)

450 g/1 lb no-need-to-soak dried fruit
(figs, apricots, prunes)
finely grated rind and juice of 1 lemon
150 ml/¼ pint (U.S. ⅔ cup) apple juice

Put the fruit in a pan, add water barely to cover, then put in the lemon rind and juice and the apple juice. Bring to the boil, cover and simmer for 20 minutes, or until the fruit is just tender.

Serve the fruit and liquid hot or cold, either plain or topped with natural yogurt and toasted flaked almonds (U.S. slivered almonds). **Serves 4**

Citrus bran flakes

(Illustrated on page 16)

450 ml/¾ pint (U.S. 2 cups) natural yogurt
1 teaspoon ground cinnamon
finely grated rind of 1 lemon
1 orange, peeled and divided into segments
1 grapefruit, peeled and divided into segments
1 red-skinned apple, cored and chopped
few grapes, halved and seeds removed (U.S. pitted)
bran flakes

Beat the yogurt with the cinnamon and lemon rind. Fold in the fruit. Divide the mixture among serving bowls and sprinkle with bran flakes. **Serves 4–6**

Clockwise from top left – Apricot yogurt crunch, Fruity breakfast kedgeree, Muesli medley, Dried fruit compôte

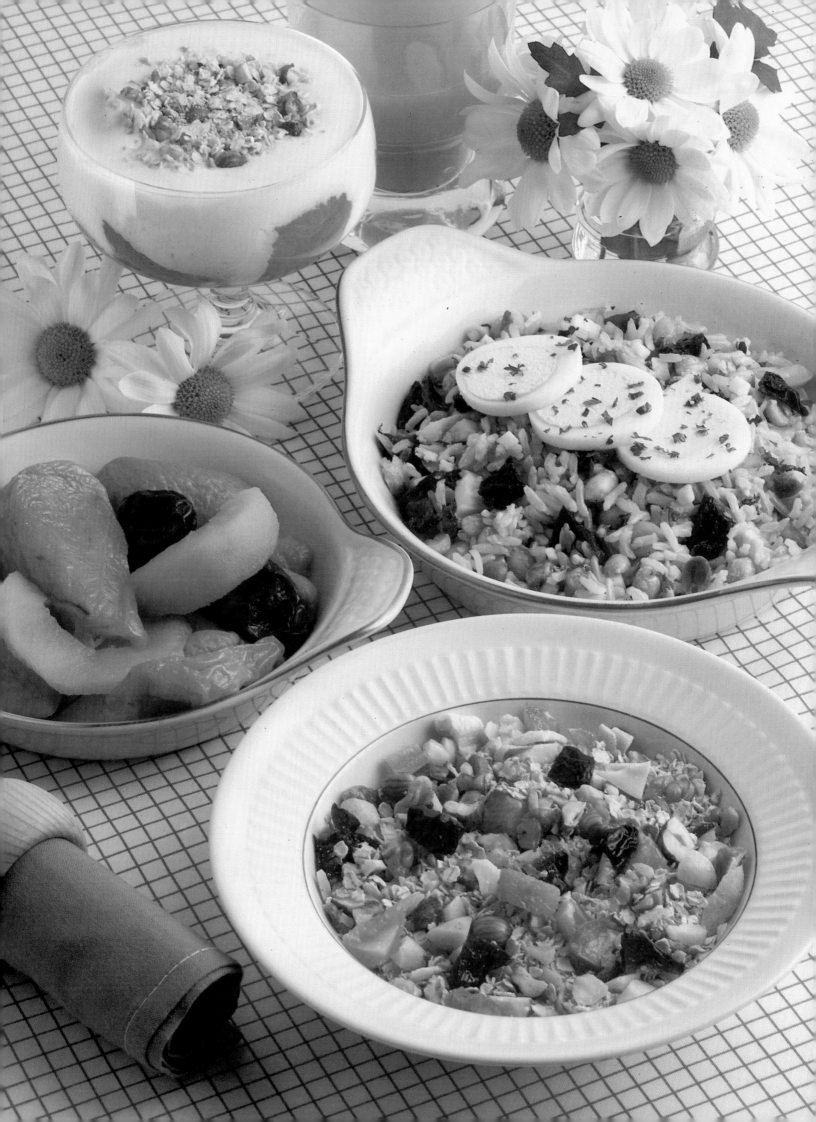

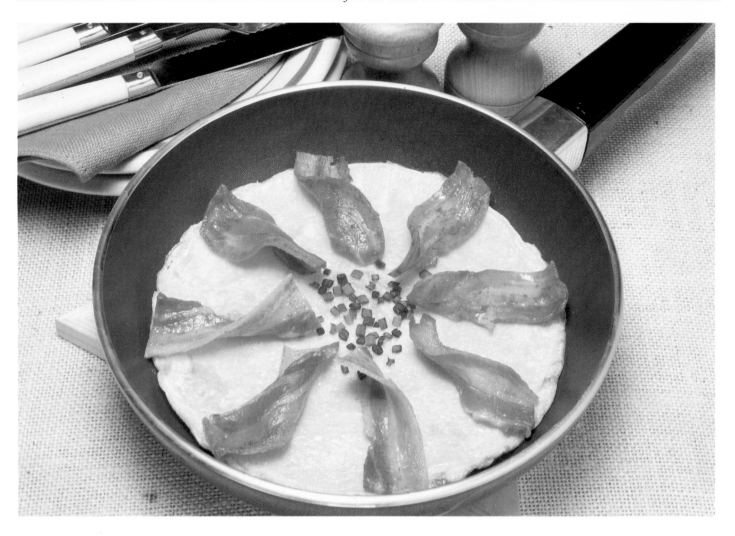

Bacon and egg cake

(Illustrated above)

100 g/4 oz streaky bacon rashers
(U.S. $\frac{1}{4}$ lb bacon slices), rind removed
1 teaspoon wholemeal flour (U.S. wholewheat flour)
3 tablespoons (U.S. 4 tablespoons) milk
2 eggs
salt and pepper
15 g/$\frac{1}{2}$ oz (U.S. 1 tablespoon) butter
1 tablespoon chopped chives to garnish

Place the bacon rashers on a rack in a grill pan (U.S. broiler pan) and cook under high heat, turning occasionally, until crisp.

Meanwhile, whisk the flour into the milk and eggs. Season lightly. Melt the butter in a frying pan (U.S. skillet), pour in the egg mixture and cook over moderately high heat, lifting the edges of the omelette to allow uncooked mixture to run underneath and set. When the centre is cooked but still creamy, slide the 'cake' on to a warm plate or serve from the pan with the bacon arranged on top like the spokes of a wheel. Sprinkle with chives and serve immediately. **Serves 2**

Poached eggs on bran cakes

(Illustrated on page 16)

5 eggs
150 ml/$\frac{1}{4}$ pint (U.S. $\frac{2}{3}$ cup) milk
75 g/3 oz (U.S. 1$\frac{1}{2}$ cups) All Bran
25 g/1 oz plain flour (U.S. $\frac{1}{4}$ cup all-purpose flour)
$\frac{1}{2}$ teaspoon salt
butter or margarine for frying and spreading
4 pork sausages, grilled (U.S. 4 pork links, broiled)
12 medium-sized mushrooms, sautéed

Mix together one egg, the milk and All Bran. Leave to stand for about 10 minutes, or until all the liquid has been absorbed. Meanwhile, heat the oven to 220°C/425°F, Gas Mark 7 and grease a baking sheet.

Stir the flour and salt into the All Bran mixture and divide into 4 equal portions. Spread each into a 10-cm/4-inch square on the prepared sheet. Bake for about 20 minutes, or until crisp. At the same time, poach the remaining eggs.

Spread each cake with butter and top with an egg. Serve with sausages and mushrooms. **Serves 4**

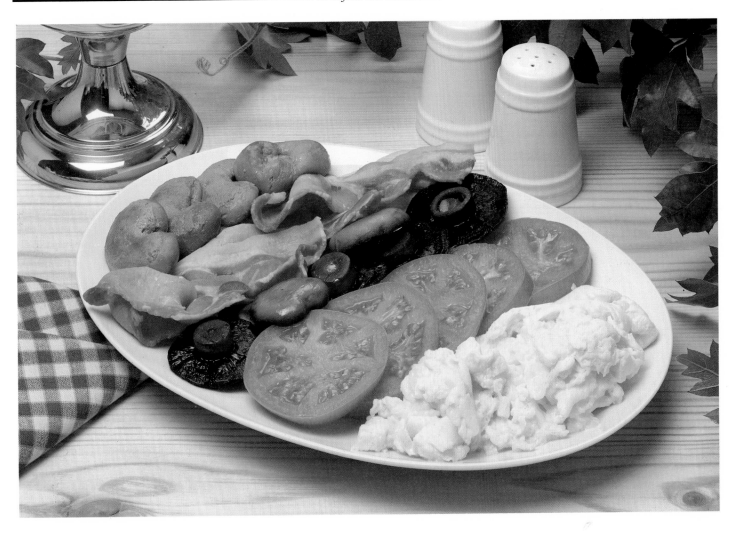

Family breakfast platter

(Illustrated above)

4 lambs' kidneys
butter for cooking
4 middlecut bacon rashers (U.S. 8 Canadian bacon
slices), rind removed
8 mushrooms
2 large tomatoes, cut into thick slices
4 eggs
4 tablespoons milk or single cream
(U.S. 6 tablespoons milk or light cream)
salt and pepper

Remove the skin from the kidneys, rinse and dry them. Heat about 25 g/1 oz (U.S. 2 tablespoons) butter in a frying pan (U.S. skillet) and gently fry the kidneys for 4-5 minutes, turning them occasionally, until cooked through. Remove from the pan and arrange on a serving dish. Keep warm in the oven.

Cut the bacon rashers in half (U.S. leave slices whole) and grill (U.S. broil) or fry for about 2 minutes on each side, until cooked. Arrange next to the kidneys on the serving dish and keep warm. Fry the mushrooms gently and add to the serving dish. Arrange the tomato slices alongside or, if preferred, fry them lightly first on both sides. Return the dish to the oven.

Beat the eggs and milk together lightly and season to taste. Melt a little butter in a small pan, add the egg mixture and stir constantly over low heat until soft and creamy. Remove from the heat and spoon on to the serving dish with the rest of the breakfast. Serve immediately with wholemeal toast (U.S. whole-wheat toast). **Serves 4**

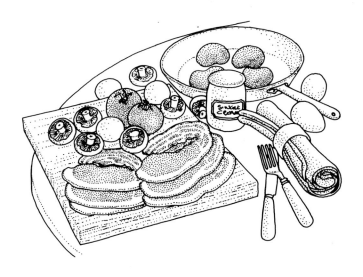

Spanish bacon omelette

(Illustrated opposite)

6 middle cut bacon rashers (U.S. 12 small Canadian
bacon slices), rind removed
25 g/1 oz (U.S. 2 tablespoons) butter
450 g/1 lb potatoes, peeled and diced
1 medium-sized onion, peeled and finely chopped
1 small red pepper, seeds removed and finely chopped
100 g/4 oz (U.S. $\frac{3}{4}$ cup) frozen peas
salt and freshly ground black pepper
6 eggs, beaten
sprigs of parsley to garnish

Cut the streaky end off the bacon and chop finely
(U.S. finely chop half the bacon slices). Cook the
chopped bacon in a greased frying pan (U.S. skillet)
until crisp. Add the butter to the pan and when
melted put in the potato and onion. Cook gently,
stirring now and then, for about 10 minutes, or until
the potato is tender. Add the pepper and peas to the
pan and season to taste. Stir in the egg and cook very
gently, stirring occasionally, until the egg has set.

While the omelette is cooking, grill (U.S. broil) the
remaining bacon. Remove from the heat and slip the
omelette, still in the pan, under the hot grill (U.S.
broiler) until the top just turns golden. Serve topped
with the bacon and garnish with parsley sprigs.
Serves 4

Devilled gammon brunch

(Illustrated opposite)

oil for frying
750 g/1$\frac{1}{2}$ lb potatoes, peeled and coarsely grated
4 smoked gammon steaks (U.S. ham steaks)
175 g/6 oz (U.S. 1$\frac{1}{2}$ cups) button mushrooms
2 tomatoes, cut into wedges
sprigs of parsley to garnish
Sauce
3 tablespoons (U.S. generous 4 tablespoons) mango
chutney
2 tablespoons (U.S. generous 3 tablespoons)
soy sauce
3 tablespoons (U.S. 4 tablespoons) tomato ketchup
1 teaspoon ground ginger
1 teaspoon ground coriander
1 teaspoon ground cumin
1 clove garlic, crushed

First make the sauce. Put all the ingredients together

in a pan and stir until boiling. Keep hot while cooking
the remainder of the meal.

Heat 4 tablespoons (U.S. 6 tablespoons) oil in a
large frying pan (U.S. skillet) and add tablespoonfuls
of potato, keeping them slightly apart. Fry until
golden brown underneath, then turn and cook until
the second side is golden. Drain on absorbent kitchen
towel and keep hot while frying the rest of the potato.

Snip the rind of the gammon steaks at 1.25-cm/
$\frac{1}{2}$-inch intervals. Add a little extra oil to the pan if
necessary, and fry the steaks, two at a time, for about
4 minutes on each side. Drain well and keep warm.
Lightly fry the mushrooms in the pan.

Arrange the gammon steaks, potato crunchies,
mushrooms and tomato wedges on a warm serving
platter and garnish with parsley. Pour a little of the
sauce over the steaks and hand the rest separately in a
sauce boat. **Serves 4**

Lemon breakfast muffins

(Illustrated on pages 16-17)

50 g/2 oz (U.S. 1 cup) All Bran or Bran Buds
150 ml/$\frac{1}{4}$ pint (U.S. $\frac{2}{3}$ cup) milk
50 g/2 oz (U.S. $\frac{1}{4}$ cup) butter or margarine, softened
50 g/2 oz light muscovado sugar (U.S. $\frac{1}{4}$ cup light
brown sugar)
1 egg, beaten
finely grated rind of $\frac{1}{2}$ lemon
1 tablespoon lemon curd
25 g/1 oz sultanas (U.S. scant $\frac{1}{4}$ cup seedless white
raisins)
100 g/4 oz plain flour (U.S. 1 cup all-purpose flour)
4 teaspoons (U.S. 2 tablespoons) baking powder

Heat the oven to 200°C/400°F, Gas Mark 6 and
grease 15 deep bun tins (U.S. muffin pans).

Put the All Bran in a large bowl and pour the milk
over. Leave to stand for about 5 minutes, or until the
cereal is soft. Add the butter, sugar, egg, lemon rind,
lemon curd and sultanas, and beat until blended. Sift
the flour with the baking powder and fold into the
mixture. Divide among the prepared tins.

Bake for about 20 minutes, or until golden brown
and springy to the touch. Serve warm with butter or
margarine. **Makes about 15**

Variation
Orange walnut muffins Omit the lemon rind and
sultanas and substitute the finely grated rind of $\frac{1}{2}$
orange and 25 g/1 oz (U.S. $\frac{1}{4}$ cup) chopped walnuts.

*Above: Spanish bacon omelette. Below: Devilled gammon
brunch*

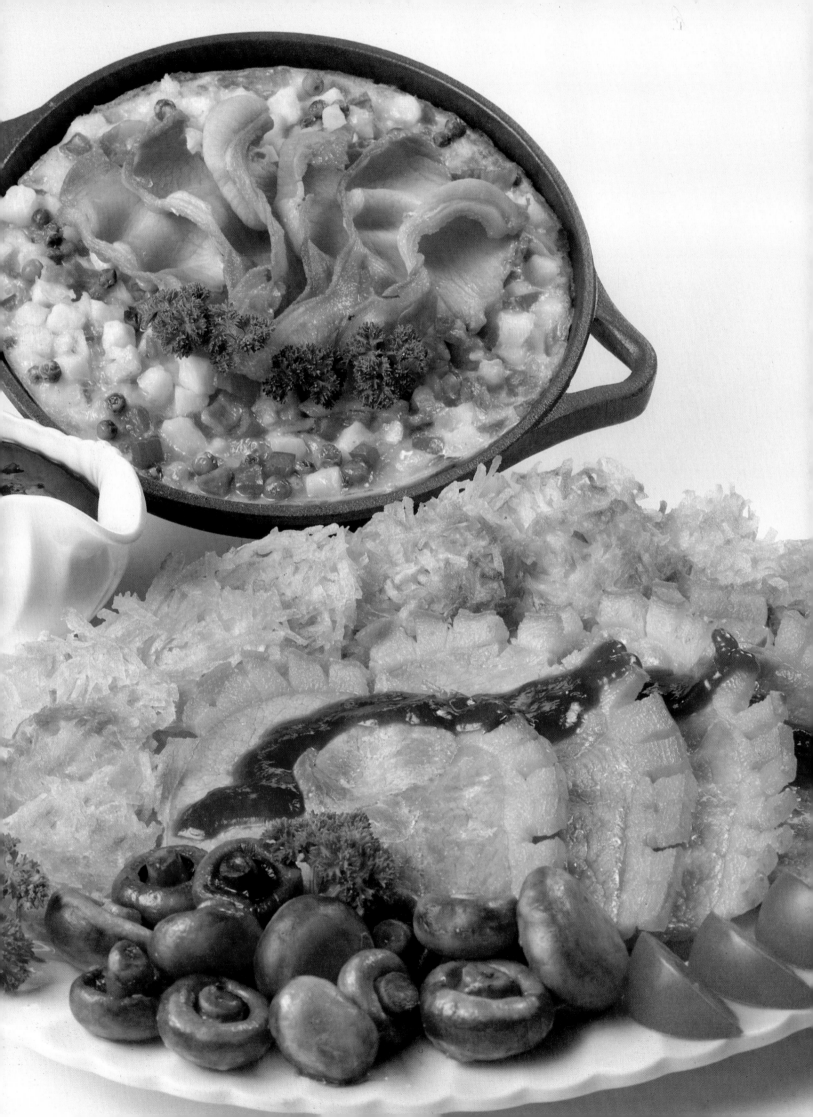

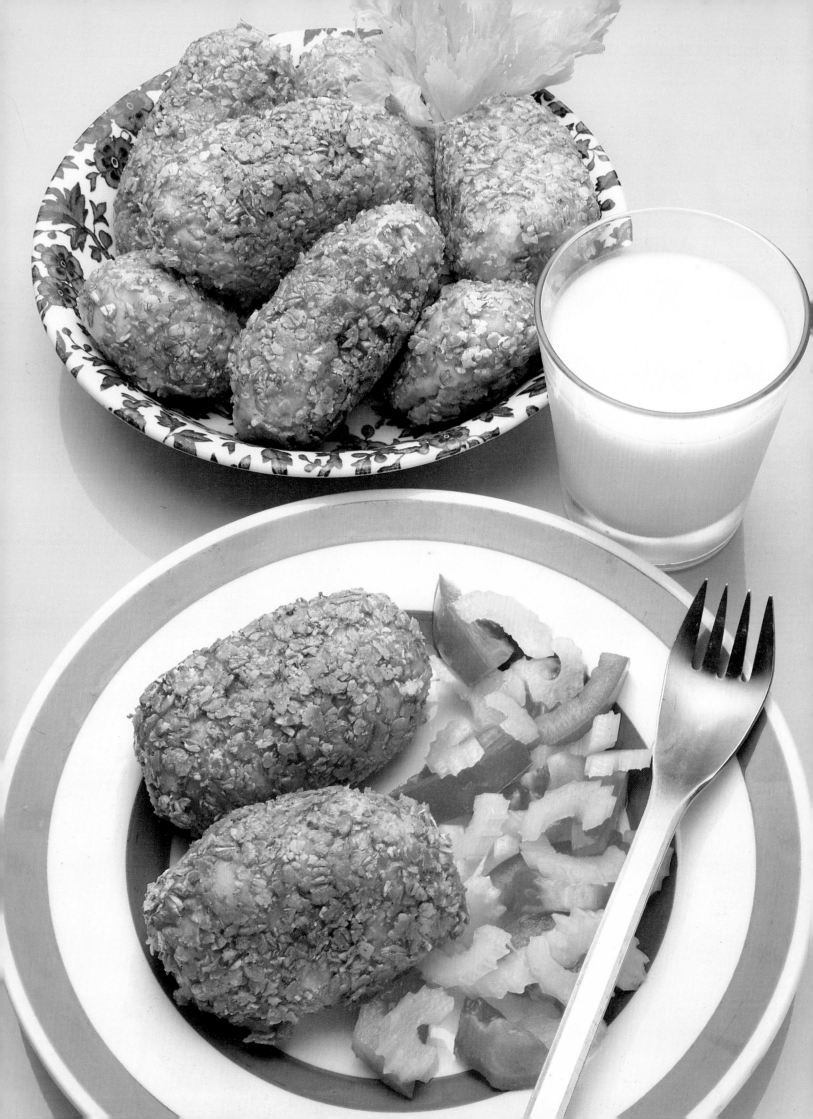

Barbecued bean tostadas

(Illustrated on page 29)

6 ready-made tostada shells
2 (450-g/16-oz) cans barbecue beans
275 g/10 oz (U.S. 2½ cups) chopped cooked chicken
salt and freshly ground black pepper (optional)
12.5-cm/5-inch length cucumber
½ small red pepper, seeds removed and finely chopped
sprigs of parsley to garnish

Heat the oven to 190°C/375°F, Gas Mark 5. Put the tostada shells on a baking sheet (U.S. cookie sheet) and place in the oven for 5 minutes.

Meanwhile, put the beans and chicken in a pan and heat through thoroughly over low heat, stirring frequently. Season, if wished.

Thinly slice enough cucumber to make an overlapping border round each tostada. Finely dice the remaining cucumber. Spoon the bean mixture on to the tostadas and sprinkle with cucumber and chopped pepper. Garnish with parsley and serve at once.
Serves 6

Oaty crunch parcels

(Illustrated opposite)

1 egg, separated
550 g/1¼ lb (U.S. 2½ cups) mashed potato
salt and pepper
1 (225-g/8-oz) can curried beans with sultanas
50 g/2 oz (U.S. ½ cup) chopped roasted peanuts
50 g/2 oz (U.S. ½ cup) grated Cheddar cheese
rolled oats or lightly crushed bran flakes for coating
oil for deep frying

Mix the egg yolk into the potato and season to taste. Divide into 8 equal portions. Using floured hands, shape each portion into a round flat cake. Combine the beans, peanuts and cheese, and divide among the potato cakes. Carefully work the potato mixture around the bean filling to completely encase it.

Lightly whisk the egg white and place in a shallow bowl. Put some oats or bran flakes on a plate. Dip each potato parcel in egg white and then roll in the cereal until completely covered. Add more cereal as necessary. Chill for 10 minutes.

Heat oil to a temperature of 180°C/350°F or until a cube of day-old bread turns golden brown in 60 seconds. Fry the parcels, a few at a time, for about 5

Oaty crunch parcels

minutes, or until golden brown and crisp on the outside. Drain on absorbent kitchen towel and keep hot. Serve as soon as all the parcels are cooked.
Makes 8

Scotch muffins

1 egg
3 tablespoons (U.S. 4 tablespoons) oil
225 ml/8 fl oz (U.S. 1 cup) milk
100 g/4 oz wholemeal flour (U.S. 1 cup wholewheat flour)
½ teaspoon salt
1 tablespoon (U.S. 4 teaspoons) baking powder
90 g/3½ oz (U.S. 1 cup) rolled oats

Heat the oven to 220°C/425°F, Gas Mark 7 and grease 12 deep bun tins (U.S. muffin pans).

Whisk the egg and oil into the milk. Mix the flour with the salt and baking powder in a bowl. Add the oats and mix again. Make a well in the centre, pour in the milk liquid and mix with a fork until the dry ingredients are just moistened. Do not beat the mixture, which may be slightly lumpy. Divide among the tins, filling them about two-thirds full.

Bake for 20 minutes, or until well risen, and firm to the touch. Serve warm with butter or margarine.
Makes 12

American peanut rolls

225 g/8 oz wholemeal flour (U.S. 2 cups wholewheat flour
2½ teaspoons (U.S. 1 tablespoon) baking powder
½ teaspoon salt
50 g/2 oz (U.S. ¼ cup) peanut butter
25 g/1 oz (U.S. 2 tablespoons) margarine
about 150 ml/¼ pint (U.S. ⅔ cup) buttermilk
25 g/1 oz (U.S. ¼ cup) roasted peanuts, chopped

Heat the oven to 220°C/425°F, Gas Mark 7 and grease a 17.5-cm/7-inch square shallow tin.

Put the flour, baking powder and salt in a bowl and rub or cut in the peanut butter and margarine until the mixture resembles breadcrumbs. Mix in enough buttermilk to make a fairly soft dough.

Turn out on a floured surface and pat out to a square to fit the prepared tin. Put the dough in the tin and, using a sharp knife, mark into 9 squares, cutting about half-way through the dough. Brush the top with a little buttermilk and sprinkle with the nuts.

Bake for about 20 minutes, or until well risen and the centre roll is golden. Separate the squares and serve warm with butter. **Makes 9 rolls**

Bean busters

(Illustrated opposite)

225 g/8 oz wholemeal flour
(U.S. 2 cups wholewheat flour)
75 g/3 oz (U.S. $\frac{1}{3}$ cup) solid vegetable fat,
frozen for 30 minutes
75 g/3 oz (U.S. $\frac{1}{3}$ cup) butter or block margarine,
frozen for 30 minutes
175 ml/6 fl oz (U.S. $\frac{3}{4}$ cup) ice cold water
beaten egg for brushing
Filling
6 spring onions (U.S. scallions), chopped
1 (450-g/16-oz) can baked beans in tomato sauce
$\frac{1}{4}$ teaspoon freshly ground black pepper
175 g/6 oz (U.S. 1 cup) diced Cheddar cheese

Place the flour in a bowl and grate the fats directly
into it. Add the water and mix to a dough. Cover and
chill for 30 minutes.

Sprinkle the dough and a working surface with
flour. Roll out the dough to a rectangle measuring
about 45 cm/18 inches × 15 cm/6 inches, having a short
side towards you. Fold up the bottom third of the
pastry strip then fold down the top third, seal the
edges by pressing with the rolling pin and give the
dough a one quarter turn. Repeat the rolling, folding
and sealing process twice. Cover and chill for 30
minutes.

Divide the pastry into 6 equal portions and roll
each out to a 17.5-cm/7-inch circle. Mix together the
ingredients for the filling and divide among the pastry
rounds. Brush the pastry edges with egg, bring up
opposite sides over the filling and seal firmly together.
Flute decoratively and make a small steam vent in
each pasty. Arrange on a lightly greased baking sheet
(U.S. cookie sheet) and chill for 30 minutes. Heat the
oven to 220°C/425°F, Gas Mark 7.

Bake for about 25 minutes, or until golden brown.
Serve hot or cold with a crunchy salad. **Makes 6**

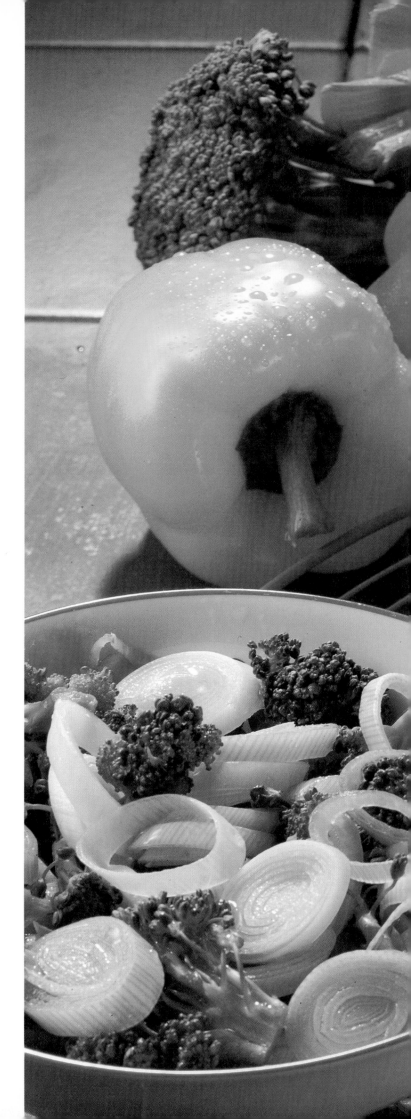

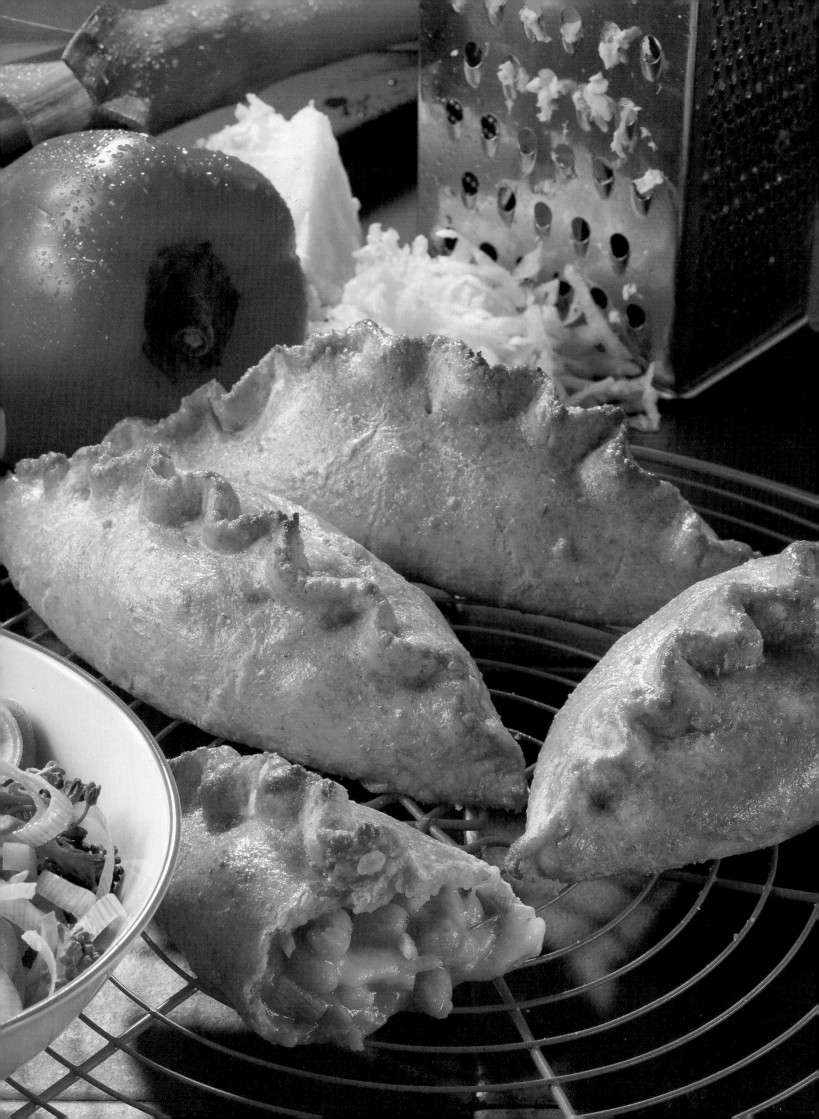

Wheatgerm drop pancakes

75 g/3 oz wholemeal flour (U.S. $\frac{3}{4}$ cup wholewheat flour)
$\frac{1}{2}$ teaspoon bicarbonate of soda (U.S. baking soda)
pinch of salt
1 teaspoon cream of tartar
25 g/1 oz (U.S. $\frac{1}{2}$ cup) wheatgerm
1 egg
150 ml/$\frac{1}{4}$ pint (U.S. $\frac{2}{3}$ cup) milk
2 tablespoons (U.S. 3 tablespoons) oil
little oil for cooking

Put the flour, bicarbonate of soda, salt, cream of tartar and wheatgerm in a bowl and mix thoroughly. Make a well in the centre, drop in the egg, milk and oil and whisk the mixture until smooth.

Heat a heavy frying pan (U.S. skillet) and brush the surface with oil. Make pancakes, using 2 table-spoons of mixture for each one, and cook until bubbles burst on the surface. Turn and cook until the other side is brown.

Place the pancakes on a plate, cover with a clean cloth to prevent them from drying out, and keep warm while cooking the remainder of the batter. Serve warm with sausages and maple syrup, or cold spread with butter and marmalade. **Makes about 12**

Chilli bean toasts

1 tablespoon oil
1 large onion, peeled and chopped
350 g/12 oz minced beef (U.S. $\frac{3}{4}$ lb ground beef)
1 teaspoon mild chilli powder
$\frac{1}{2}$ teaspoon ground coriander
300 ml/$\frac{1}{2}$ pint beef stock (U.S. 1$\frac{1}{4}$ cups beef bouillon)
1 (298-g/10$\frac{1}{2}$-oz) can condensed tomato soup
1 (425-g/15-oz) can red kidney beans, drained
4 large slices wholemeal bread
(U.S. wholewheat bread)
butter or margarine for spreading
25 g/1 oz (U.S. $\frac{1}{4}$ cup) grated Cheddar cheese

Heat the oil in a pan and fry the onion gently until soft. Add the beef and fry, stirring, until brown and crumbly. Mix in the chilli powder and coriander and cook for a further 2 minutes. Add the stock and soup and bring to the boil, stirring. Cover and simmer for 20 minutes, stirring occasionally. Mix in the beans and reheat.

Meanwhile, toast the bread slices and spread them with butter or margarine. Arrange on warm plates and spoon the chilli beef over them. Top each portion with a little grated cheese and serve at once. **Serves 4**

Yogurt topped peaches

150 ml/$\frac{1}{4}$ pint (U.S. $\frac{2}{3}$ cup) natural yogurt
2 tablespoons (U.S. 3 tablespoons) clear honey
2 tablespoons (U.S. 3 tablespoons) muesli
300 ml/$\frac{1}{2}$ pint (U.S. 1$\frac{1}{4}$ cups) water
juice of $\frac{1}{2}$ lemon
2 tablespoons (U.S. 3 tablespoons) sugar
4 medium-sized ripe peaches

Mix together the yogurt, honey and muesli and leave to stand while preparing the fruit. Heat the water, lemon juice and sugar in a pan, stirring until the sugar has dissolved. Halve the peaches, stone (U.S. pit) and place the fruit in the syrup. Cook gently for 5 minutes, turning the peach halves occasionally.

Lift out the peach halves and place in 4 breakfast dishes. Boil the syrup until reduced to about a quarter of the original quantity. Spoon over the peaches and leave to cool. Top with the yogurt mixture at breakfast time. **Serves 4**

Tacos with beef and beans

(Illustrated opposite)

2 tablespoons (U.S. 3 tablespoons) oil
1 small onion, peeled and finely chopped
350 g/12 oz minced beef (U.S. $\frac{3}{4}$ lb ground beef)
2 green peppers, seeds removed and finely chopped
2 tablespoons (U.S. 3 tablespoons) taco sauce
4 tablespoons (U.S. 6 tablespoons) red wine
salt and freshly ground black pepper
6 ready-made taco shells
1 (450-g/16-oz) can baked beans in tomato sauce
6 black olives, stoned (U.S. 6 ripe olives, pitted)

Heat the oil in a pan and fry the onion gently until soft. Add the beef and fry, stirring, until brown and crumbly. Stir in three-quarters of the green pepper, the taco sauce, wine and a little seasoning. Simmer for about 15 minutes, or until the beef is tender. Meanwhile, heat the oven to 190°C/375°F, Gas Mark 5.

Arrange the taco shells on a baking sheet (U.S. cookie sheet) with the curved edges upwards. Heat through in the oven for 5 minutes. At the same time, stir the beans into the beef mixture, adjust the seasoning and reheat.

Fill the tacos with the beef and bean mixture and top each with a little of the remaining chopped pepper and an olive. Serve immediately. **Serves 6**

Above: Barbecued bean tostadas (recipe page 25). Below: Tacos with beef and beans

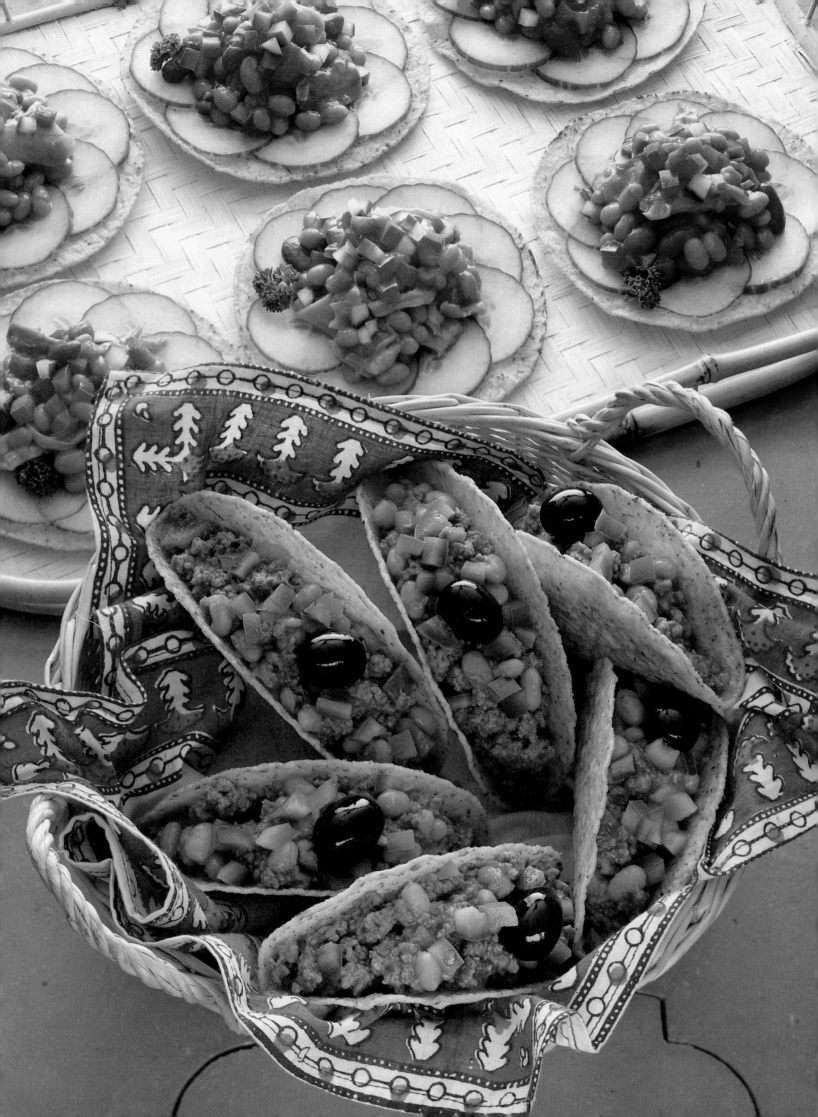

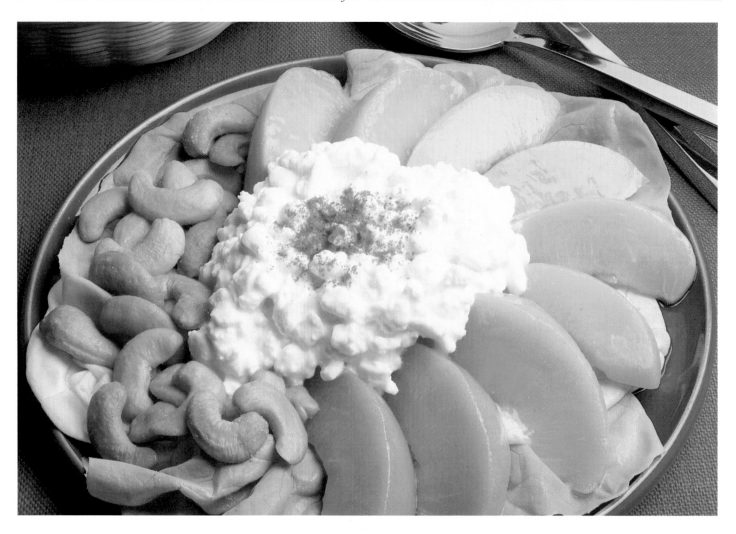

Chewy banana squares

100 g/4 oz (U.S. $\frac{1}{4}$ lb) dried bananas
100 g/4 oz (U.S. $\frac{1}{4}$ lb) dried dates
100 g/4 oz sultanas (U.S. $\frac{2}{3}$ cup seedless white raisins)
juice of $\frac{1}{2}$ lemon
6 tablespoons (U.S. 9 tablespoons) water
350 g/12 oz (U.S. $\frac{3}{4}$ lb) cooking apples,
peeled, cored and chopped
2 tablespoons light muscovado sugar
(U.S. 3 tablespoons light brown sugar)
225 g/8 oz (U.S. 1 cup) margarine
6 tablespoons golden syrup (U.S. 9 tablespoons
light corn syrup)
350 g/12 oz (U.S. $3\frac{1}{2}$ cups) rolled oats

Heat the oven to 190°C/375°F, Gas Mark 5 and grease a shallow tin measuring 17.5 cm/7 inches by 27.5 cm/11 inches and about 2.5 cm/1 inch deep.

Roughly chop the bananas and dates and place in a pan with the sultanas, lemon juice and water. Stir then simmer for 5 minutes. Mix in the apple and cool.

Place the sugar, margarine and syrup in a pan and heat gently, stirring, until the fat melts. Remove from the heat and stir in the oats. Spread half this mixture in the prepared tin and press down evenly with the back of a spoon. Cover with the fruit filling then sprinkle the remaining oat mixture evenly on top and press down quite firmly all over.

Bake for about 35 minutes, or until golden brown. Allow to stand for 30 minutes, then mark into 15 squares with a sharp knife. Leave until cold before removing from the tin. These squares make a delicious snack served with a yogurt.

Makes 15 squares

Peach sunrise

(Illustrated above)

lettuce leaves
1 (411-g/14$\frac{1}{2}$-oz) can sliced peaches, drained
225 g/8 oz (U.S. 1 cup) cottage cheese
cayenne pepper
50 g/2 oz (U.S. $\frac{1}{3}$ cup) roasted cashew nuts

Make a bed of the lettuce leaves on a serving plate. Arrange the peach slices decoratively in a semi-circle to one side and spoon the cottage cheese into the centre. Sprinkle it with cayenne pepper. Scatter the cashews around the cheese and serve with wholemeal rolls (U.S. wholewheat rolls). **Serves 2-3**

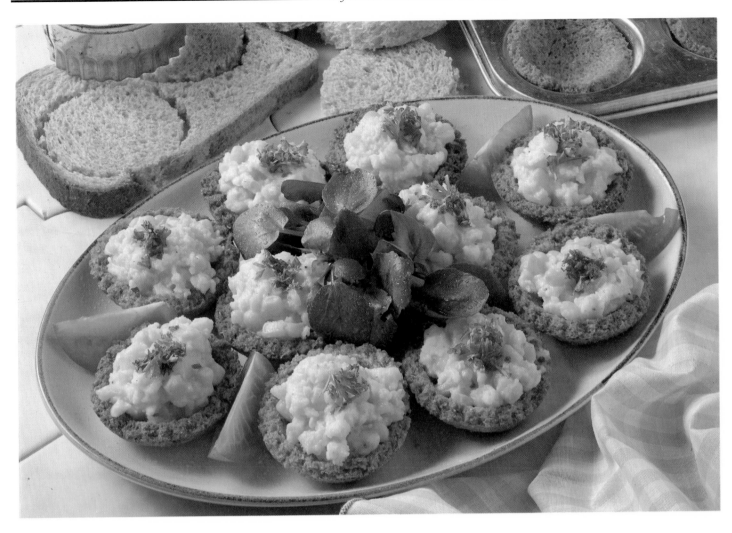

Sunshine tartlets

(Illustrated above)

6 large slices wholewheat bread
100 g/4 oz (U.S. ½ cup) butter or margarine
3 eggs, beaten
50 ml/2 fl oz single cream (U.S. ¼ cup light cream)
50 g/2 oz (U.S. ½ cup) cooked or canned corn kernels
salt and pepper
1 teaspoon chopped parsley
sprig of watercress to garnish

Heat the oven to 180°C/350°F, Gas Mark 4 and have ready 12 deep bun tins (U.S. muffin pans).

Cut 2 (6.25-cm/2½-inch) circles from each bread slice. Melt 75 g/3 oz (U.S. ⅓ cup) of the butter and dip the bread circles into this. Press them into the bun tins. Bake for about 15 minutes, or until the bread has formed crisp golden cases.

Meanwhile, melt the remaining butter in a pan and add the egg and cream. Stir over low heat until the egg starts to scramble but is still creamy. Add the sweetcorn and season to taste.

Ease the bread cases out of the tin and fill with the egg mixture. Sprinkle with parsley and serve the tartlets on a warm dish garnished with a sprig of watercress. Alternatively, allow the egg mixture to cool before filling the cases and then serve cold.
Makes 12

Variations

Mushroom and egg tartlets Omit the corn and substitute 50 g/2 oz (U.S. ½ cup) sliced button mushrooms. Sauté very lightly in the butter before pouring in the egg and cream. Add a pinch of ground nutmeg with the seasoning.

Chicken and pepper tartlets Omit the eggs and corn and substitute 175 g/6 oz (U.S. 1½ cups) chopped cooked chicken and 1 tablespoon very finely chopped red pepper. Sauté the pepper in the butter until soft, stir in the chicken and cream and reheat thoroughly. Season with a pinch of curry powder and salt to taste.

Hot baps with savoury filling

4 large wholemeal baps (U.S. 4 wholewheat hamburger buns)
2 tablespoons (U.S. 3 tablespoons) peanut butter
50 g/2 oz soft liver sausage (U.S. ⅓ cup soft
liverwurst)
100 g/4 oz (U.S. 1 cup) chopped cooked chicken
2 tablespoons (U.S. 3 tablespoons) chopped parsley
2 tablespoons (U.S. 3 tablespoons) tomato ketchup
salt and freshly ground black pepper (optional)

Heat the oven to 200°C/400°F, Gas Mark 6.

Cut the baps in half and take out a little of the soft
crumb inside. Mix about 1 tablespoon of the crumbs
with the peanut butter, liver sausage, chicken, parsley
and ketchup. Add seasoning only if desired. Divide
the filling among the halved baps, then sandwich
them together in pairs and place on a greased baking
sheet (U.S. cookie sheet).

Bake for 10 minutes, or until crisp on the outside
and lightly browned. Serve hot with carrot and
cucumber sticks. **Serves 4**

Variation

Hot baps with sardine filling Omit the chicken,
liver sausage and peanut butter and substitute
1 (100-g/4-oz) can sardines in tomato sauce, mashed
with 50 g/2 oz (U.S. ¼ cup) curd cheese, all the
breadcrumbs, the ketchup and parsley. Season well
before filling the rolls.

Potato, carrot and sweetcorn omelette

450 g/1 lb potatoes, peeled and diced
1 large carrot, peeled and finely chopped
7 size 5/medium-sized eggs (U.S. large eggs)
½ teaspoon garlic salt
freshly ground black pepper
2 tablespoons chopped sweet brown pickle
(U.S. 3 tablespoons relish)
2 tablespoons (U.S. 3 tablespoons) oil
1 medium-sized onion, peeled and finely chopped
1 (198-g/7-oz) can corn kernels
1 tablespoon chopped parsley to garnish

Put the potatoes and carrot in a large pan, pour over
salted water to cover and bring to the boil. Cook for
5 minutes, or until the vegetables are just tender but
not breaking up. Drain well. Beat together the eggs,
garlic salt, pepper to taste and the pickle.

Heat the oil in a large pan and cook the onion
gently until soft. Remove from the heat. Pour half the
egg mixture into the pan. Spoon the potato, carrot
and sweetcorn evenly over this, then pour in the
remaining egg mixture. Return to the heat and cook
very gently for about 10 minutes, or until the
omelette is cooked but still creamy on the top.
Meanwhile, heat the grill (U.S. broiler).

Slip the pan under the heat and cook the omelette
for about 3 minutes, or until the top is just turning
golden. Use spatulas to help slide the omelette on to a
warm serving dish, sprinkle with the parsley and cut
into wedges. **Serves 4**

Note: This omelette makes a filling meal served with
hot garlic bread and a salad.

Avocado deluxe

(Illustrated opposite)

1 (539-g/19-oz) can grapefruit segments
2 ripe avocado pears, halved and stoned (U.S. pitted)
10 walnut halves
4 tablespoons (U.S. 6 tablespoons) oil
1 teaspoon mild continental mustard
salt and freshly ground black pepper
shredded lettuce
4 sprigs of mint to garnish

Drain the syrup from the grapefruit segments and
reserve. Brush the avocado flesh with a little of the
syrup. Break each walnut half into 2-3 pieces.

Put the oil, mustard and 6 tablespoons (U.S. 9
tablespoons) of the grapefruit syrup in a bowl. Add
seasoning to taste and whisk until blended. Transfer
to a serving container.

Arrange a bed of lettuce on 4 serving plates and top
each with an avocado half. Fill with the grapefruit
segments and nuts. Garnish each with a sprig of mint.
Hand the dressing separately and serve with brown
bread and butter or margarine. **Serves 4**

Avocado deluxe

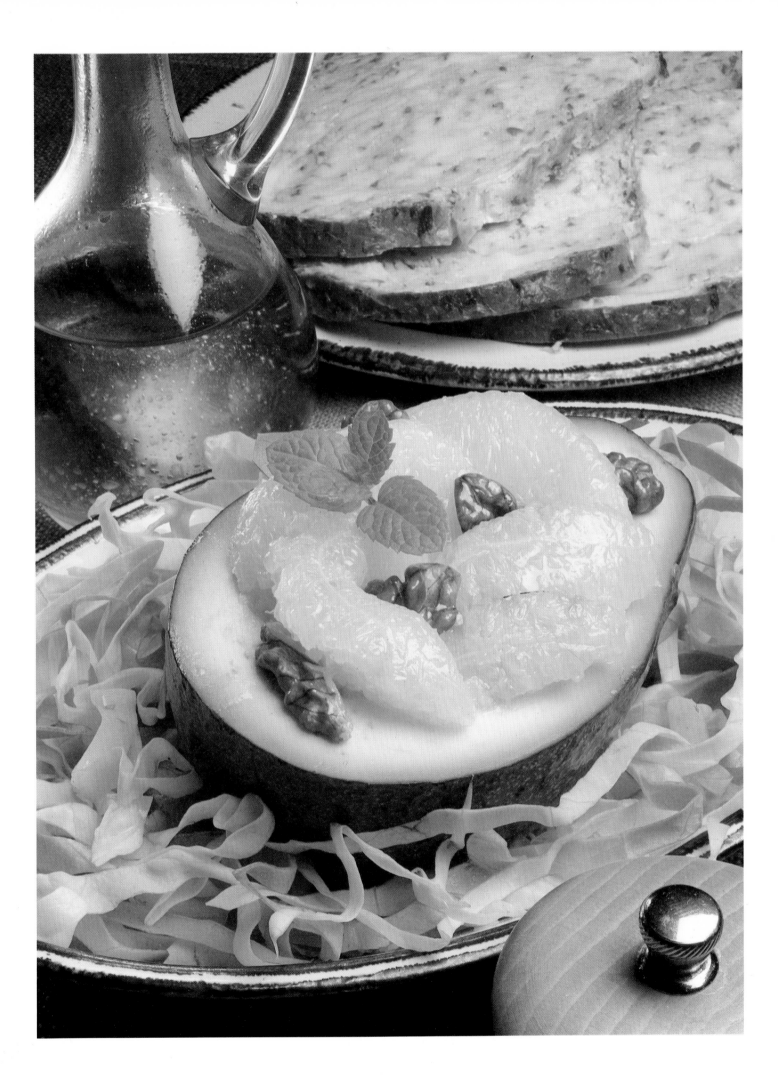

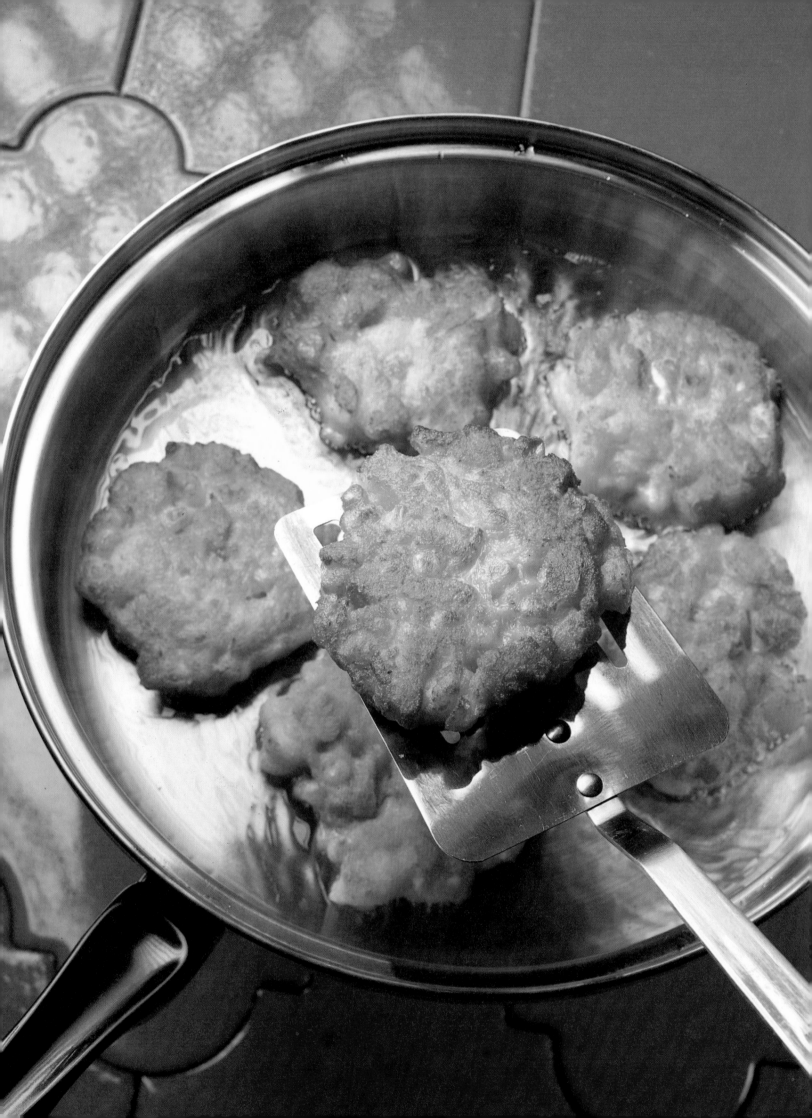

Fish fritters

(Illustrated opposite)

150 g/5 oz wholemeal flour
(U.S. 1¼ cups wholewheat flour)
pinch of salt
¼ teaspoon freshly ground black pepper
1 egg, beaten
150 ml/¼ pint (U.S. ⅔ cup) milk
225 g/8 oz (U.S. ½ lb) smoked cod or haddock fillets, skinned
350 g/12 oz (U.S. ¾ lb) white fish fillets, skinned
100 g/4 oz (U.S. ¾ cup) canned or cooked corn kernels
oil for shallow frying

Mix together the flour, salt and pepper in a bowl. Add the egg and half the milk, and whisk until smooth. Gradually whisk in the remaining milk. Cut the fish into small pieces, add to the batter with the corn and mix lightly.

Heat a little oil in a frying pan (U.S. skillet) and fry tablespoons of the mixture over moderately high heat for about 3 minutes on each side, or until golden brown. Drain well on absorbent kitchen towel and keep hot. Serve as soon as all the fritters are cooked. **Serves 4-6**

Good morning start

(Illustrated on page 13)

225 g/8 oz (U.S. 2¼ cups) rolled oats
75 g/3 oz demerara sugar
(U.S. ⅓ cup light brown sugar)
50 g/2 oz chopped hazelnuts or almonds
(U.S. ½ cup chopped filberts or almonds)
50 g/2 oz seedless raisins or sultanas
(U.S. ⅓ cup seedless dark or white raisins)
4 whole dried apricots, chopped

Mix together the oats, sugar and nuts and spread on a baking sheet (U.S. cookie sheet). Place under a moderately hot grill (U.S. broiler) for about 5 minutes, stirring the ingredients frequently and levelling them out again, until evenly toasted. Leave to cool then mix in the fruit. Store in an airtight container.

Serve for breakfast with milk and fresh fruit such as chopped apple or pear, sliced banana, or halved and seeded (U.S. pitted) grapes. **Serves 6**

Note The proportions of fruit and nuts in the recipe can be increased if wished.

Fish fritters

Crumbed chicken-liver mushrooms

2 medium-sized leeks, trimmed
4 tablespoons (U.S. 6 tablespoons) oil
1 large carrot, grated
salt and freshly ground black pepper
8 large 'flat' mushrooms
25 g/1 oz (U.S. 2 tablespoons) margarine
225 g/8 oz (U.S. ½ lb) chicken livers, chopped
½ teaspoon dried marjoram
75 g/3 oz fresh wholemeal breadcrumbs (U.S. 1½ cups fresh wholewheat bread crumbs)

Heat the oven to 190°C/375°F, Gas Mark 5 and grease a shallow ovenproof dish.

Thinly slice the white and pale green parts of the leeks, place the slices in a colander and wash thoroughly. Drain well. Heat half the oil in a pan, add the carrot and leek and stir well. Cover and cook over moderate heat for 5 minutes, shaking the pan frequently, or until the vegetables begin to soften. Season, transfer to the prepared dish and spread flat.

Carefully ease out the stalks from the mushrooms and chop the stalks. Melt the margarine in the pan used to cook the leeks and carrot. Put in the chicken livers and mushroom stalks and cook briskly for 4 minutes, stirring. Add the marjoram and season to taste. Arrange the mushrooms caps, rounded side downwards, on the vegetables in the dish and mound up the chicken liver filling on these. Heat the remaining oil in a clean pan and cook the bread-crumbs over high heat for 1 minute, stirring all the time. Spoon the crumbs over the ingredients in the dish.

Bake for 20 minutes, or until the topping is golden brown. Serve hot. **Serves 4**

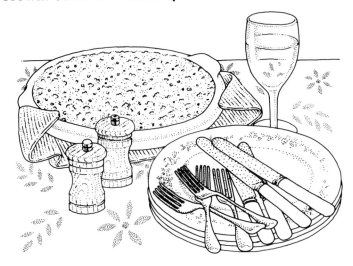

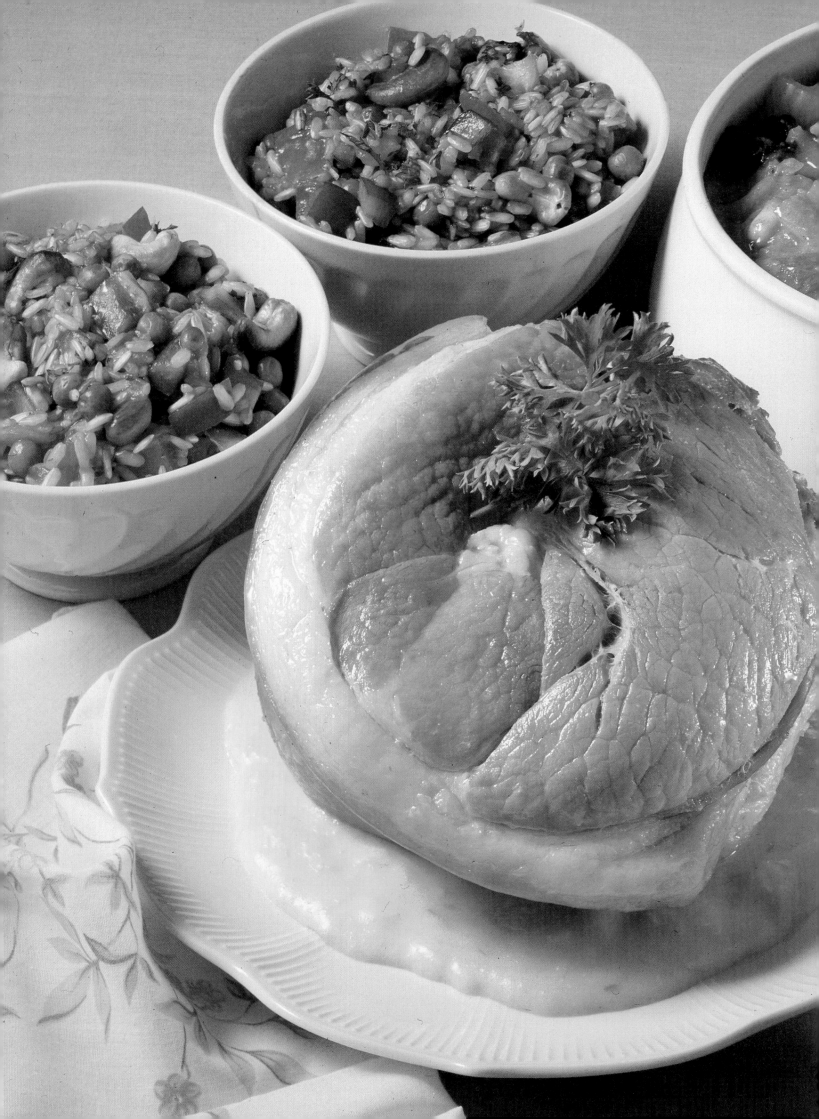

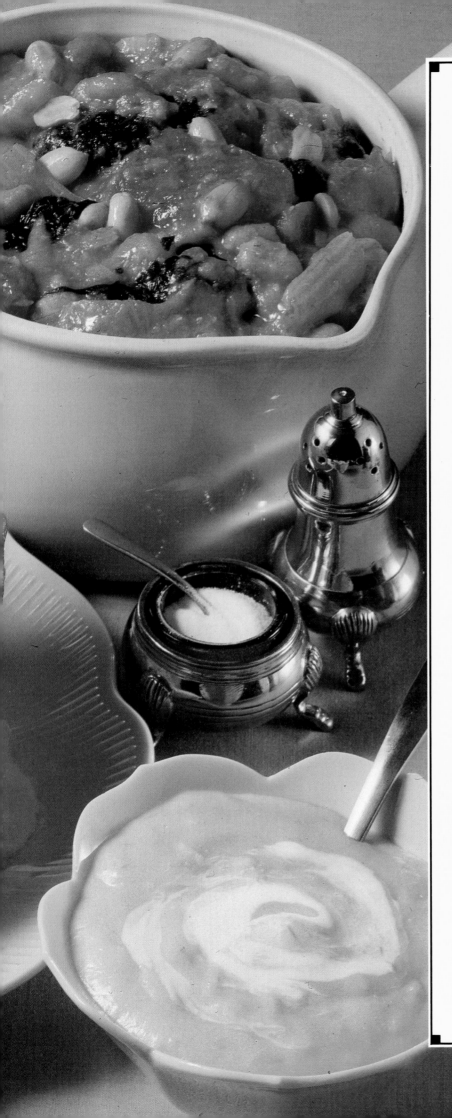

Soups, Sauces and Light Meals

The addition of fibre-full ingredients has added a new dimension to soups as simple meal starters or hearty complete meals. It is wonderfully easy to base them on vegetables or pulses that are high in roughage; to thicken them with a little wholemeal flour, or add wholewheat pasta or brown rice. Easiest of all, if you like the idea, sprinkle a little bran over the cooked soup. Certainly, croûtons as a garnish for soups should always be made with wholemeal bread which makes them look and taste particularly good.

Brown melba toast is elegant enough to serve with clear soups for guests and miniature fancy brown rolls (see page 129) would grace a dinner party table.

Sauces are not often, in themselves, high in fibre, but a creamy, velvety sauce turns a healthy vegetable into a delicious meal. This is rather a new concept for those who cannot see themselves enjoying strictly vegetarian food. Providing you choose a concentrated soup with a pulse or grain in it (beans, sweetcorn, peas or lentils for example), you can soon concoct the right kind of sauce. Pour it over a lightly cooked but well flavoured vegetable such as broccoli, Brussels sprouts or parsnips.

Attractive recipes for fibre-rich light meals are legion. Dried beans you soak and cook yourself are the basis of many of them, but canned beans which are ready cooked, make very light work of quite elaborate recipes, and canning robs them of none of the precious roughage. Nuts of all kinds add lots of crunchy texture and interesting flavour to quickly cooked dishes, and a sizeable contribution to your daily fibre intake.

Above left: Cashew nut risotto (recipe page 38). Above right: Mild curried vegetables (recipe page 38). Below: Boiled ham with Spiced apricot sauce (recipe page 38)

Mild curried vegetables

(Illustrated on page 37)

3 stalks celery, sliced
2 onions, peeled and sliced
150 ml/¼ pint (U.S. ⅔ cup) water
1 teaspoon concentrated curry sauce
1 (225-g/8-oz) can tomatoes
1 (300-g/10.6-oz) can condensed lentil soup
150 ml/¼ pint (U.S. ⅔ cup) natural yogurt
50 g/2 oz (U.S. ⅓ cup) roasted peanuts
450 g/1 lb frozen spinach, thawed and strained

Place the celery, onion and water in a large pan. Bring to the boil and simmer for 5 minutes. Add the curry sauce, tomatoes and liquid from the can and the soup. Stir well and bring to the boil. Remove from the heat if crunchy vegetables are required or, if softer vegetables are preferred, simmer for a further 10-15 minutes. Stir in the yogurt and peanuts.

Heat the spinach and transfer to a warm serving dish. Pour the curried vegetables over and lift the spinach here and there, so that some of the sauce runs underneath, but do not stir the two together. Serve at once. **Serves 4**

Cashew nut risotto

(Illustrated on page 36)

225 g/8 oz (U.S. generous 1 cup) long grain brown rice
1 (295-g/10.4-oz) can condensed French onion soup
150 ml/¼ pint (U.S. ⅔ cup) water
1 teaspoon sesame seeds
1 teaspoon cumin seeds
50 g/2 oz (U.S. scant ⅓ cup) roasted cashew nuts
1 red or green pepper, seeds removed and chopped
2 tomatoes, chopped
225 g/8 oz (U.S. ½ lb) shelled fresh or frozen peas
2 tablespoons (U.S. 3 tablespoons) chopped parsley

Place the rice, soup and water in a pan and bring to the boil. Stir once, cover and simmer for 20 minutes, or until the rice is tender.

Meanwhile, put the sesame seeds, cumin seeds and cashew nuts in a greased frying pan (U.S. skillet) and heat gently, shaking the pan frequently, until the seeds and nuts are brown. Do not allow them to burn.

Add the pepper, tomato, peas, seeds and nuts to the risotto. Stir well, bring back to simmering point, cover and continue cooking for a further 5-10 minutes, or until the peas are cooked and the liquid absorbed. Fork in the parsley and serve hot. **Serves 4**

Spiced apricot sauce

(Illustrated on pages 36-37)

100 g/4 oz (U.S. ¼ lb) dried apricots
½ teaspoon ground fenugreek
1 (295-g/10.4-oz) can condensed cream of chicken soup
1 teaspoon Continental mustard
4 tablespoons single cream or natural yogurt
(U.S. 6 tablespoons light cream or natural yogurt)

Put the apricots in a pan and just cover with water. Leave to soak for 3 hours. Bring to the boil then drain off the liquid and reserve 75 ml/3 fl oz (U.S. scant ½ cup).

Liquidize the apricots with the reserved liquid, the fenugreek, soup and mustard. Transfer to a pan and heat gently to simmering point. Blend in the cream or yogurt. Serve hot with boiled ham or bacon. **Serves 4-6**

Cheese cream sauce

(Illustrated opposite)

1 (170-g/6-oz) can cream
75 g/3 oz (U.S. ¾ cup) grated Cheddar cheese
4 tablespoons (U.S. 6 tablespoons) milk
salt and pepper

Turn the cream into a small pan and heat gently to boiling point. Put in the cheese and stir until the sauce is smooth. Blend in the milk and add seasoning to taste.

Serve immediately with freshly cooked broccoli or cauliflower. **Makes about 300 ml/½ pint (U.S. 1¼ cups)**

Note On cooling, the sauce becomes firm and makes a delicious cheese spread.

Broccoli with Cheese cream sauce

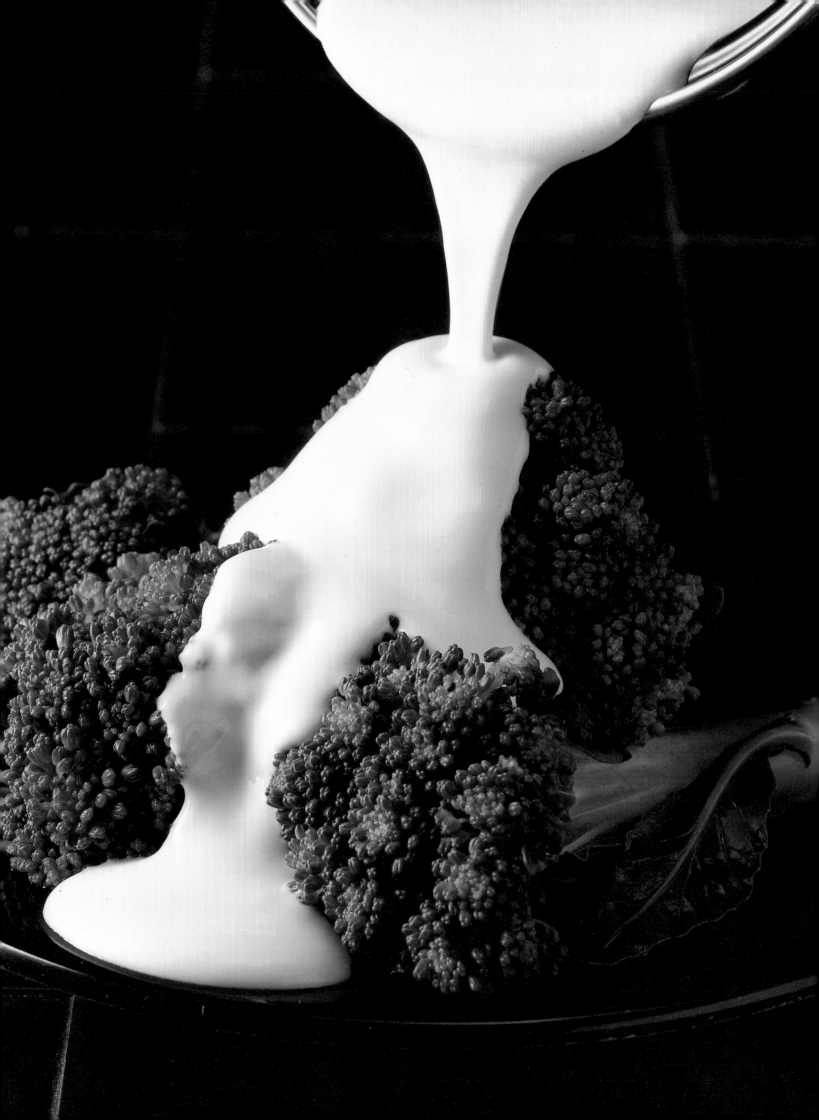

Brussels sprout soup with sesame toasts

50 g/2 oz (U.S. ¼ cup) margarine
1 large onion, peeled and chopped
1 kg/2¼ lb Brussels sprouts, trimmed and roughly
chopped
25 g/1 oz wholemeal flour (U.S. ¼ cup wholewheat
flour)
600 ml/1 pint (U.S. 2½ cups) milk
½ teaspoon ground nutmeg
salt and freshly ground black pepper
150 ml/¼ pint single cream (U.S. ⅔ cup light cream)
4 slices wholemeal bread (U.S. wholewheat bread)
butter or margarine for spreading
about 2 tablespoons (U.S. 3 tablespoons) sesame
seeds

Melt the margarine in a large pan, add the onion and sprouts and stir well. Cover the pan and place over low heat, stirring occasionally, for 5 minutes. Sprinkle on the flour, stir and cook for 1 minute.

Gradually add the milk and bring to the boil, stirring constantly. Add the nutmeg and season lightly, cover and simmer for 25 minutes. Liquidize the soup and return to the rinsed pan. Blend in the cream and adjust the seasoning if necessary.

Meanwhile, toast the bread on one side, turn the slices, spread with butter or margarine and sprinkle with sesame seeds. Toast until the seeds are golden brown. Cut the toast into fingers and serve with the hot soup. **Serves 4**

Barn-dance turkey supper

4 stalks celery, sliced
1 chicken stock cube (U.S. chicken bouillon cube),
crumbled
300 ml/½ pint (U.S. 1¼ cups) water
1 (425-g/15-oz) can butter beans (U.S. lima beans),
drained
350 g/12 oz (U.S. 3 cups) chopped cooked turkey
1 tablespoon soy sauce
2 teaspoons cornflour (U.S. 3 teaspoons cornstarch)
salt and pepper
2 thick slices wholemeal bread (U.S. wholewheat
bread)
2 tablespoons (U.S. 3 tablespoons) oil
15 g/½ oz (U.S. 1 tablespoon) margarine

Put the celery, stock cube and water in a pan. Bring to the boil, stirring, cover and simmer for about 15 minutes, or until the celery is tender. Put in the beans, turkey and soy sauce. Stir gently until piping hot.

Moisten the cornflour with a little cold water, add to the pan and bring to the boil, stirring constantly. Simmer for 3 minutes and add seasoning if necessary. Keep hot.

Cut the slices of bread into triangles. Heat the oil and margarine and fry the bread triangles over moderately high heat, turning them frequently, until golden brown. Drain on absorbent kitchen towel and serve hot with the turkey mixture. **Serves 4**

Fish and bacon chowder

(Illustrated opposite)

50 g/2 oz (U.S. ¼ cup) butter or margarine
1 large onion, peeled and thinly sliced
100 g/4 oz (U.S. ¼ lb) bacon, rind removed and
chopped
4 stalks celery, chopped
1 small green pepper, seeds removed and diced
1 large potato, peeled and diced
300 ml/½ pint chicken stock (U.S. 1¼ cups chicken
bouillon)
225 g/8 oz (U.S. ½ lb) smoked cod or haddock fillets,
skinned
225 g/8 oz (U.S. ½ lb) white fish fillets, skinned
300 ml/½ pint (U.S. 1¼ cups) milk
1 tablespoon cornflour (U.S. cornstarch)
salt and freshly ground black pepper
100 g/4 oz (U.S. ¼ lb) cooked or canned shelled
mussels, drained
3 tomatoes, chopped
4 tablespoons single cream (U.S. 6 tablespoons
light cream)
1 tablespoon chopped parsley to garnish

Melt the butter in a large pan and gently fry the onion, bacon, celery, pepper and potato for 5 minutes. Add the stock, bring to the boil and simmer for about 10 minutes, or until the potato is just tender. Cut the fish into cubes and add to the pan. Gradually blend the milk into the cornflour until smooth. Pour into the chowder and bring to the boil, stirring frequently. Add a little seasoning and simmer for 5 minutes.

Put in the mussels, tomato and cream, stir well and reheat thoroughly over low heat. Adjust the seasoning and serve hot, sprinkled with parsley and accompanied by crusty bread. **Serves 4-5**

Fish and bacon chowder

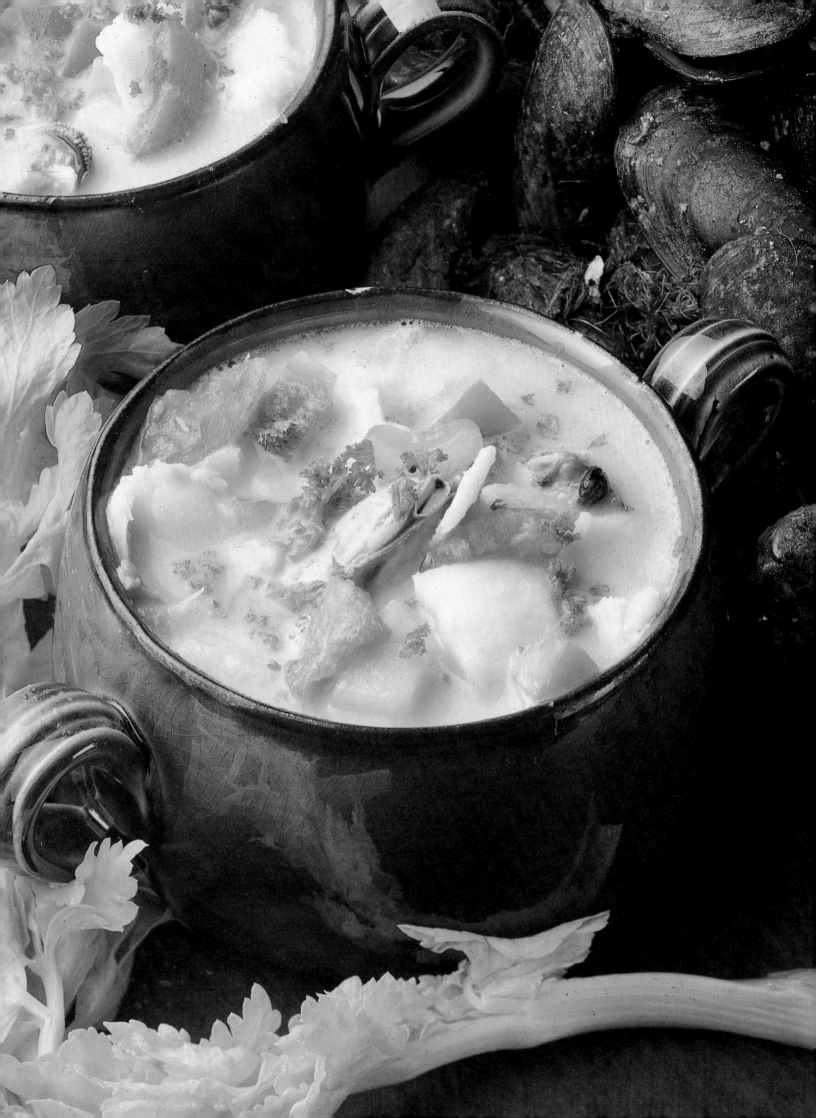

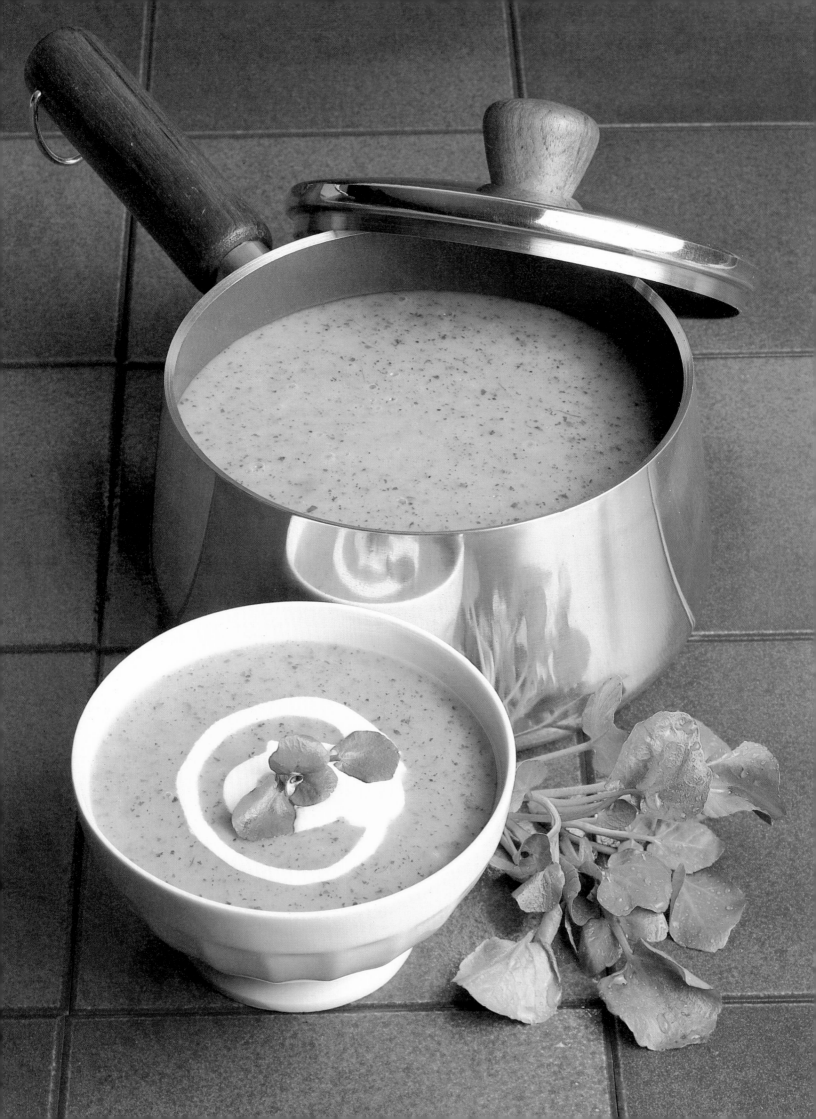

Watercress
and potato soup

(Illustrated opposite)

2 bunches of watercress
25 g/1 oz (U.S. 2 tablespoons) butter or margarine
1 medium-sized onion, peeled and chopped
450 g/1 lb potatoes, peeled and chopped
300 ml/½ pint (U.S. 1¼ cups) milk
600 ml/1 pint chicken stock (U.S. 2½ cups chicken bouillon)
salt and freshly ground black pepper
4 tablespoons single cream
(U.S. 6 tablespoons light cream)

Reserved a few watercress leaves for the garnish and shred the remainder, along with any tender stalks.

Melt the butter in a non-stick pan and gently cook the onion and watercress until the onion is soft. Add the potato, milk and chicken stock and bring to the boil, stirring all the time. Season lightly and simmer for 20 minutes.

Liquidize the soup and return it to the rinsed pan. Adjust the seasoning and reheat. Swirl in the cream and serve hot or cold, garnished with the reserved watercress leaves. **Serves 4-6**

Pasta cheese custard

(Illustrated on page 45)

100 g/4 oz (U.S. 1⅓ cups) wholewheat short-cut macaroni
25 g/1 oz (U.S. 2 tablespoons) margarine
1 tablespoon oil
125 g/5 oz grated mature Cheddar cheese
(U.S. 1¼ cups grated sharp Cheddar cheese)
1 teaspoon dry mustard powder
2 eggs
salt and pepper
600 ml/1 pint (U.S. 2½ cups) milk
1 tablespoon finely grated Parmesan cheese
1 tablespoon sunflower seeds

Heat the oven to 180°C/350°F, Gas Mark 4.

Cook the pasta in a pan of boiling salted water as directed but for only 5 minutes. Spread the margarine over the base and sides of a shallow ovenproof dish. Drain the pasta well and return to the hot pan with the oil. Toss lightly. Layer up the pasta and Cheddar cheese in the prepared dish. Whisk the mustard, eggs and a little seasoning into the milk and pour over the pasta mixture. Sprinkle with the Parmesan cheese combined with the sunflower seeds.

Watercress and potato soup

Bake for 40 minutes, or until set and golden brown on top. Serve hot from the dish with Tasty green salad. **Serves 4**

Tasty green salad Combine 4 tablespoons (U.S. 6 tablespoons) cooked or canned chickpeas with the finely sliced flesh of a small green pepper and 1 green-skinned eating apple, cored and sliced. Quarter the heart of a round green lettuce and serve each quarter in a small bowl with part of the chickpea mixture. Fold 4 tablespoons (U.S. 6 tablespoons) very finely chopped parsley into 4 tablespoons French dressing (U.S. 6 tablespoons Italian dressing) and spoon over the salads at serving times. **Serves 4**

Parsnip, carrot
and orange soup

(Illustrated on the cover)

50 g/2 oz (U.S. ¼ cup) margarine
450 g/1 lb carrots, peeled and chopped
450 g/1 lb parsnips, peeled and chopped
1 tablespoon wholemeal flour (U.S. wholewheat flour)
1 litre/1¾ pints chicken or vegetable stock
(U.S. 4¼ cups chicken or vegetable bouillon)
½ teaspoon ground bay leaves
salt and freshly ground black pepper
finely grated rind of 1 orange
juice of 2 oranges
1 tablespoon snipped chives
Croûtons
3 slices wholemeal bread (U.S. wholewheat bread), crusts removed
25 g/1 oz (U.S. 2 tablespoons) margarine
1 tablespoon oil

Melt the margarine in a large pan and add the carrot and parsnip. Stir well, cover and cook gently for 10 minutes without allowing the vegetables to brown, shaking the pan occasionally. Stir in the flour and cook for 1 minute. Gradually add the stock and bring to the boil, stirring constantly. Put in the ground bay leaves and a little seasoning, cover and simmer for 15 minutes, or until the vegetables are really soft.

Liquidize the soup and return it to the rinsed pan. Add the orange rind and juice. Bring to boiling point, adjust the seasoning if necessary and simmer, uncovered, for 5 minutes. Sprinkle with chives.

Meanwhile, cut the bread into neat dice. Heat the margarine and oil in a pan and toss the bread dice over high heat until golden brown. Drain on absorbent kitchen towel and hand separately with the hot soup. **Serves 6**

43

Chicken Indienne

(Illustrated opposite)

25 g / 1 oz (U.S. 2 tablespoons) margarine
2 tablespoons (U.S. 3 tablespoons) oil
4 chicken pieces
2 medium-sized onions, peeled and sliced
1 clove garlic, crushed
1 tablespoon curry powder
$\frac{3}{4}$ teaspoon ground cinnamon
$\frac{1}{2}$ teaspoon ground ginger
25 g / 1 oz wholemeal flour (U.S. $\frac{1}{4}$ cup wholewheat
flour)
300 ml / $\frac{1}{2}$ pint chicken stock (U.S. 1$\frac{1}{4}$ cups chicken
bouillon)
2 tablespoons (U.S. 3 tablespoons) mango chutney,
chopped
salt
350 g / 12 oz (U.S. $\frac{3}{4}$ lb) wholewheat spaghetti
1 tablespoon lemon juice
4 canned peach halves, drained
1 tablespoon French dressing (U.S. Italian dressing)
Garnish
lemon wedges
sprig of parsley

Heat the margarine and oil in a heavy pan and fry the
chicken pieces over moderately high heat, until
golden brown on both sides. Remove the chicken.
Add the onion and garlic to the fat remaining in the
pan and fry gently until soft. Sprinkle over the curry
powder, cinnamon, ginger and flour, stir well and
cook for 1 minute. Gradually blend in the stock and
bring to the boil, stirring all the time. Add the mango
chutney and a little salt. Return the chicken to the
pan, cover and simmer for 25 minutes.

Meanwhile, cook the pasta in boiling salted water
as directed. Add the lemon juice to the curry and stir
well, then carefully add the peach halves. Cook for a
further 5 minutes.

Drain the pasta, toss with the French dressing and
transfer to a warm serving dish. Arrange the chicken
pieces and peaches on top and spoon the sauce around
them. Garnish the dish with lemon wedges and
parsley sprig. Serve at once. **Serves 4**

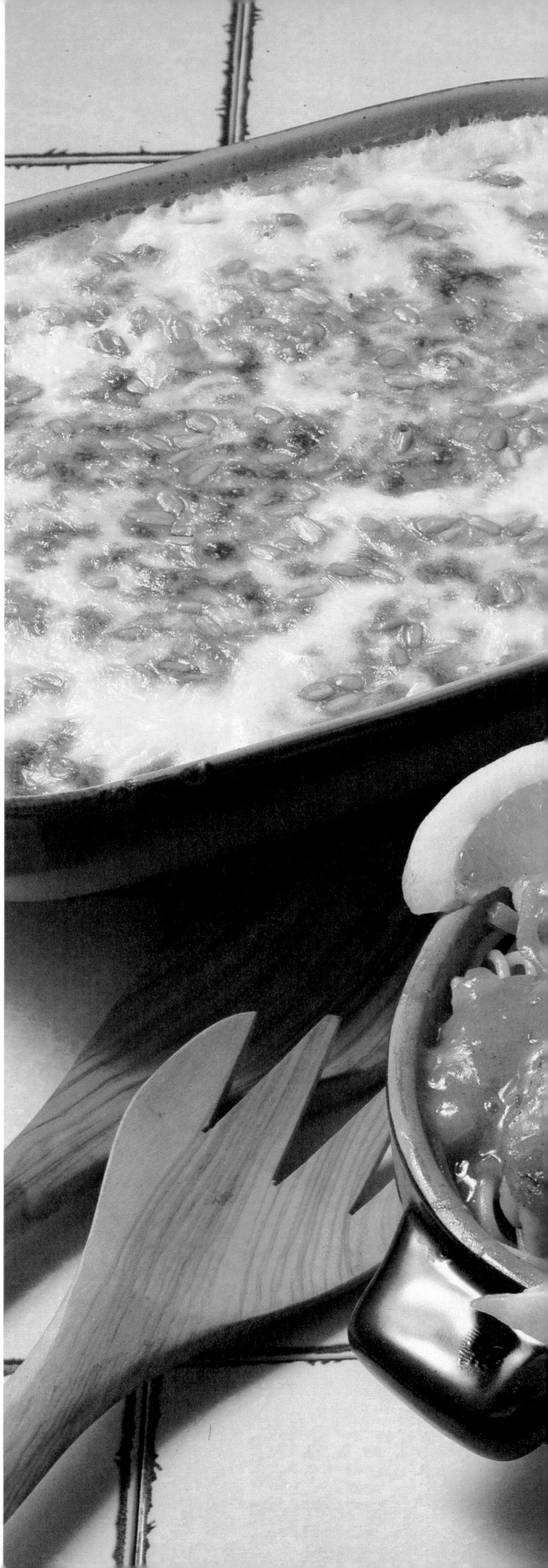

*Above: Pasta cheese custard (recipe page 43). Below: Chicken
Indienne*

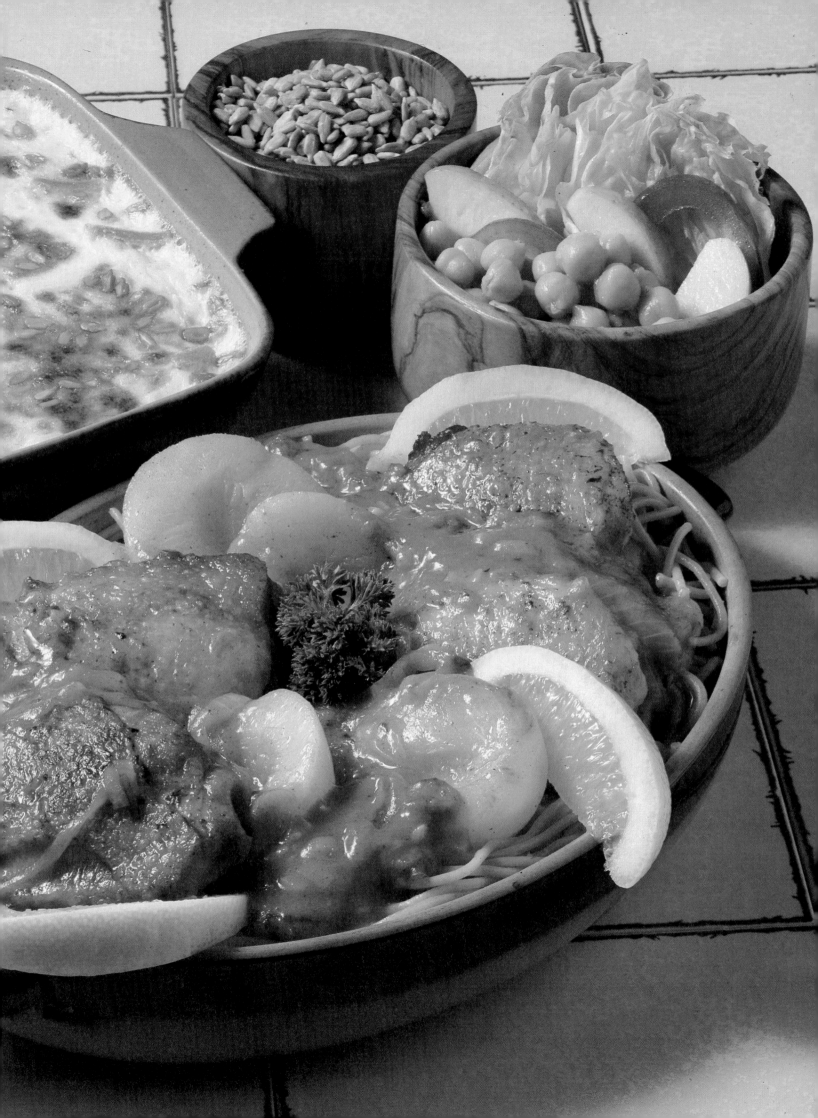

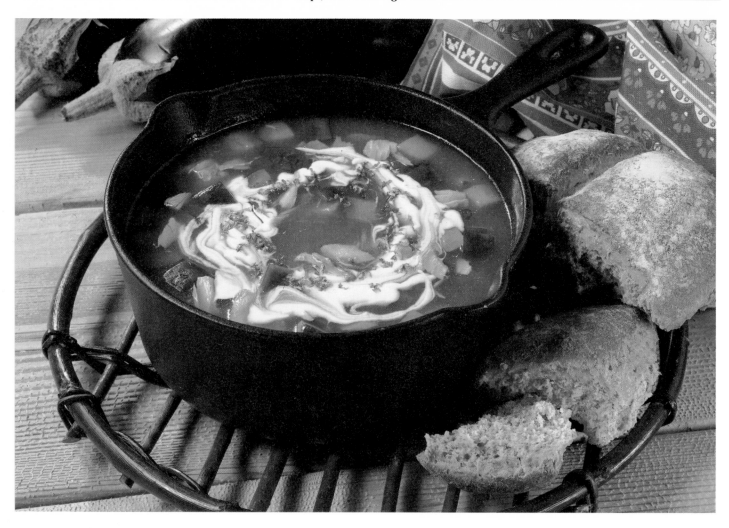

Aubergine supper soup

(Illustrated above)

2 tablespoons (U.S. 3 tablespoons) oil
225 g/8 oz aubergine (U.S. $\frac{1}{2}$ lb eggplant), cubed
1 clove garlic, crushed
900 ml/1$\frac{1}{2}$ pints vegetable stock (U.S. 3$\frac{3}{4}$ cups
vegetable bouillon)
2 tablespoons tomato purée (U.S. 3 tablespoons
tomato paste)
salt and freshly ground black pepper
1 teaspoon sugar
1 (99-g/3$\frac{1}{2}$-oz) can tuna
150 ml/$\frac{1}{4}$ pint (U.S. $\frac{2}{3}$ cup) natural yogurt
1 tablespoon chopped parsley

Heat the oil in a large pan and toss the aubergine cubes over moderately high heat until golden. Add the garlic, stock, tomato purée, a little seasoning and the sugar. Bring to the boil, cover and simmer for 15 minutes, or until the aubergine is tender.

Flake the tuna and stir into the soup with the liquid from the can. Simmer for a further 5 minutes and adjust the seasoning if necessary. Swirl the yogurt into the soup and sprinkle with parsley. Serve with wholemeal (U.S. wholewheat) bread. **Serves 4**

Sausage and apple patties

1 eating apple, peeled and coarsely grated
2 teaspoons lemon juice
450 g/1 lb pork sausagemeat (U.S. 1 lb bulk pork
sausage)
100 g/4 oz (U.S. 1 cup) chopped roasted peanuts
2 tablespoons fresh wholemeal breadcrumbs
(U.S. 3 tablespoons fresh wholewheat bread crumbs)
oil for brushing

Combine the apple, lemon juice, pork, peanuts and breadcrumbs. Divide into 8 equal portions and shape each into a round flat cake with floured hands.

Arrange the patties in an oiled grill pan (U.S. broiler pan), brush with oil and cook under high heat for about 5 minutes, on each side, until cooked through and golden brown. Serve hot with Waldorf cabbage salad (see page 110). **Serves 4**

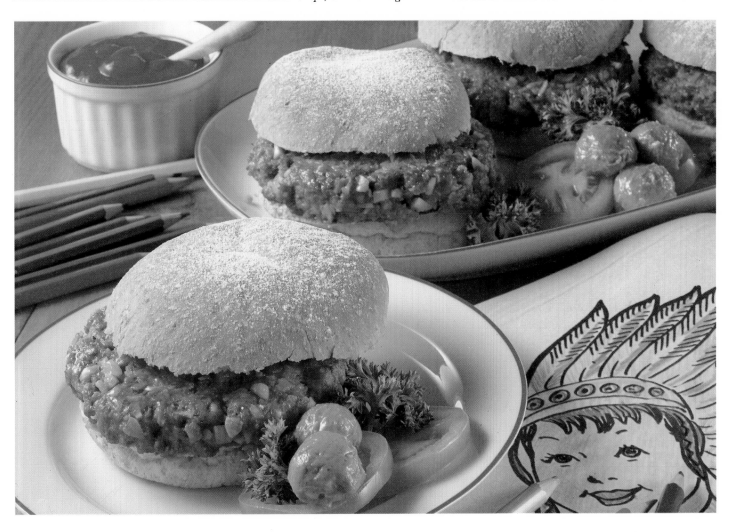

Lamb and peanut burgers

(Illustrated above)

8 teaspoons (U.S. 8 slightly rounded teaspoons)
peanut butter, chilled
450 g/1 lb minced (U.S. ground) lean lamb
1 medium-sized onion, peeled and finely chopped
40 g/1½ oz (U.S. ⅓ cup) finely chopped roasted
peanuts
½ teaspoon dried mixed herbs
salt and freshly ground black pepper
oil for shallow frying
4 wholemeal hamburger rolls (U.S. wholewheat
hamburger buns), toasted
Garnish
2 tomatoes, sliced
sprigs of parsley

Form the peanut butter into 8 balls, put them on a plate and keep chilled.

Mix together the lamb, onion, peanuts, herbs and a little seasoning in a bowl. Divide into 4 equal portions and shape each into a flat round burger with floured hands.

Heat a little oil in a frying pan (U.S. skillet) and fry the burgers over moderate heat for 6–8 minutes on each side, or until cooked through. Drain and serve in the toasted rolls, garnished with the peanut butter balls, tomato slices and parsley sprigs. **Serves 4**

Variations

Lamb and olive burgers Omit the peanut butter and peanuts. Mix the lamb, onion, herbs and seasoning with 6 chopped stuffed green olives. Serve each burger in a roll and garnish with extra olives.

Surprise lamb burgers Omit the peanut butter and peanuts. Make up the lamb mixture and shape into 8 thin burgers. Sandwich these together in pairs with a little mild mustard and a thin slice of Cheddar cheese. Press the burgers firmly together before cooking.

Curried lamb balls Omit the peanut butter and peanuts. Mix 1 teaspoon curry powder into the lamb mixture, divide it into 16 equal portions and shape each into a ball with floured hands. Fry the balls in 1 tablespoon oil, turning frequently, until brown and cooked through. Serve with cucumber slices in natural yogurt.

Barbecued lamb with apricots

(Illustrated opposite)

100 g/4 oz (U.S. $\frac{1}{4}$ lb) dried apricots, halved
3 tablespoons (U.S. 4 tablespoons) oil
1 large onion, peeled and thinly sliced
$\frac{1}{4}$ teaspoon ground ginger
8 small lamb cutlets (U.S. 8 small rib lamb chops)
1 (450-g/16-oz) can barbecue beans
$\frac{1}{2}$ cucumber, cut in thin strips and seeds removed
salt and freshly ground black pepper

Soak the apricots in cold water to cover overnight. Drain.

Heat the oil in a large frying pan (U.S. skillet) and fry the onion and apricots gently until the onion is soft. Stir in the ginger, then add the lamb cutlets and fry over low heat for about 10 minutes, turning them once, or until evenly brown on all sides but still slightly pink in the centre. Stir in the beans and cook gently for 5 minutes. Put in the cucumber strips and reheat thoroughly. Season if wished.

Arrange the cutlets on a warm serving platter and top with the bean mixture. Serve hot with potatoes baked in their jackets. **Serves 4**

Crispy stuffed pancakes

225 g/8 oz minced beef (U.S. $\frac{1}{2}$ lb ground beef)
50 g/2 oz (U.S. $\frac{1}{2}$ cup) chopped mushrooms
2 (225-g/8-oz) cans curried beans with sultanas
salt
Pancakes
100 g/4 oz wholemeal flour (U.S. 1 cup wholewheat flour)
pinch of salt
1 egg
grated rind of 1 lemon
300 ml/$\frac{1}{2}$ pint (U.S. $1\frac{1}{4}$ cups) milk
oil for frying
little lemon juice
lemon wedges to garnish

Place the beef and mushrooms in a pan over medium heat and cook, stirring occasionally, until the meat looks brown and crumbly. Remove from the heat, add the beans and salt to taste.

To make the pancakes, put the flour, salt, egg and lemon rind in a bowl. Pour in half the milk and whisk until smooth. Gradually whisk in the remaining milk. Heat a small frying pan (U.S. skillet) and brush with oil. Reserve 1 tablespoon batter. Using about 2 tablespoons (U.S. 3 tablespoons) batter each time, make 8-10 pancakes. Cook until bubbles burst on the surface then turn to cook the other side. Lay the pancakes out on a clean working surface and leave to cool.

Divide the beef mixture among the pancakes, placing it in the centre. Fold in two opposite sides to slightly overlap in the centre. Fold in one of the remaining sides and put a little uncooked batter on top. Bring in the last side to cover the batter and press lightly. Put the stuffed pancakes on a board, seam side downwards, and chill for at least 15 minutes.

Heat oil to a temperature of 190°C/375°F, or until a cube of day-old bread turns golden brown in about 40 seconds. Fry the pancakes, in batches, for about 3 minutes, or until crisp and golden. Drain on absorbent kitchen towel and keep hot until all the pancakes are cooked. Serve piled up on a warm serving dish, sprinkle with lemon juice and garnish with lemon wedges. **Serves 4**

Prawn and bean pilaff

(Illustrated opposite)

3 tablespoons (U.S. 4 tablespoons) oil
1 medium-sized onion, peeled and finely chopped
175 g/6 oz (U.S. scant 1 cup) long grain brown rice
300 ml/$\frac{1}{2}$ pint (U.S. $1\frac{1}{4}$ cups) dry white wine
450 ml/$\frac{3}{4}$ pint chicken stock (U.S. 2 cups chicken bouillon)
175 g/6 oz peeled prawns (U.S. 1 cup shelled cooked shrimp)
2 (225-g/8-oz) cans curried beans with sultanas
salt and freshly ground black pepper
1 tablespoon chopped parsley to garnish

Heat the oil in a strong pan and fry the onion gently until soft. Add the rice and stir over the heat until coated with oil. Stir in the wine and bring to the boil. Simmer, uncovered, for about 10 minutes, until the wine has almost evaporated. Stir in the stock, bring back to the boil and simmer for about 15 minutes, or until the rice is tender and has almost absorbed the liquid. Fork in the shellfish and beans and add seasoning to taste. Cover and heat through thoroughly.

Serve on a warm dish, sprinkled with parsley, and accompanied by a simple cucumber and yogurt salad. **Serves 4**

Above: Barbecued lamb with apricots. Below: Prawn and bean pilaff

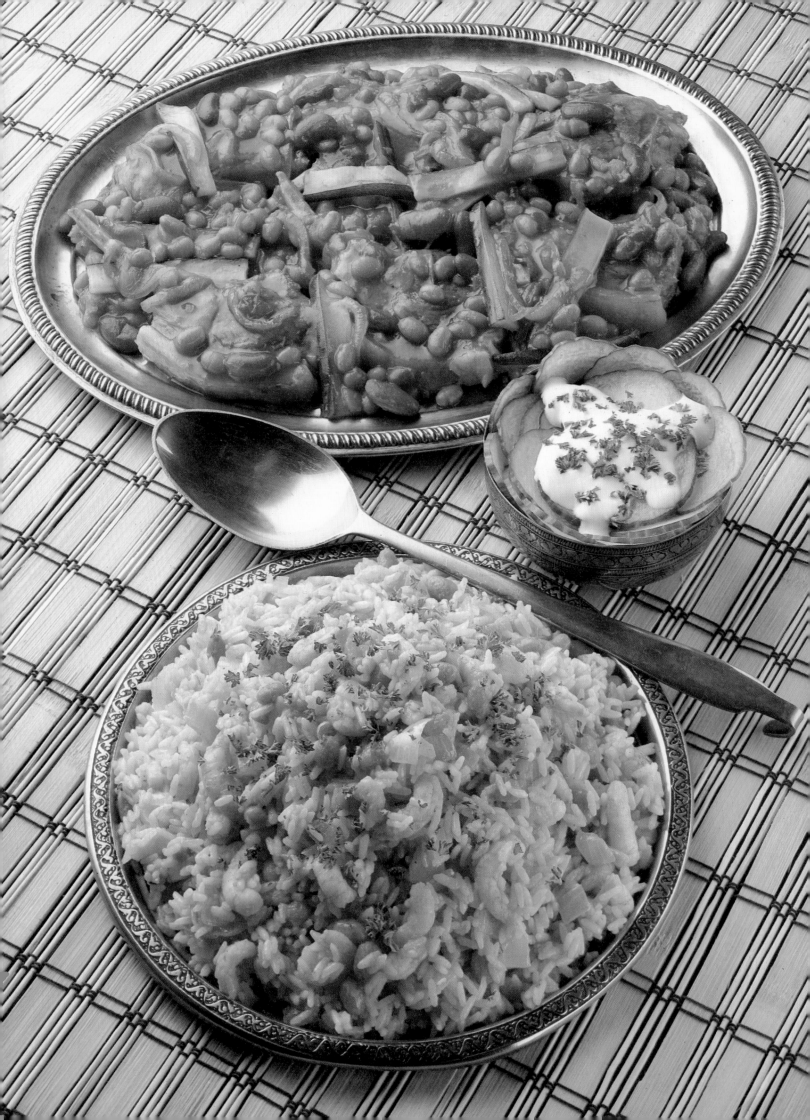

Chicken risotto

(Illustrated opposite)

2 tablespoons (U.S. 3 tablespoons) oil
100 g/4 oz (U.S. generous $\frac{1}{2}$ cup) long grain brown
rice
1 large onion, peeled and sliced
1 large carrot, peeled and diced
1 green pepper, seeds removed and chopped
450 g/1 lb raw boneless chicken flesh, cubed
1 tablespoon sweet paprika pepper
3 tablespoons tomato purée (U.S. 4 tablespoons
tomato paste)
1 (425-g/15-oz) can tomatoes
50 g/2 oz (U.S. $\frac{1}{3}$ cup) seedless raisins
50 g/2 oz (U.S. $\frac{1}{2}$ cup) blanched almonds
100 g/4 fl oz (U.S. $\frac{1}{2}$ cup) water
salt
1 tablespoon flaked almonds (U.S. slivered almonds),
toasted

Heat the oil in a pan and fry the rice gently for 3 minutes, stirring frequently. Put in the onion and carrot and cook until the onion softens. Stir in the pepper and chicken and cook, stirring occasionally, until the chicken pieces begin to turn golden.

Add the paprika, tomato purée, tomatoes and liquid from the can, the raisins, whole almonds and water. Season with a little salt, stir well and bring to the boil. Cover and simmer for about 25 minutes, or until the rice is tender and the liquid almost absorbed.

Add more salt to taste, transfer the risotto to a warm serving dish and fluff up with a fork. Serve sprinkled with the toasted almonds. **Serves 4**

Saucy pork

(Illustrated opposite)

4 pork chops, trimmed
about 40 g/1$\frac{1}{2}$ oz (U.S. $\frac{1}{3}$ cup) ground almonds
25 g/1 oz (U.S. 2 tablespoons) butter or margarine
1 medium-sized onion, peeled and chopped
$\frac{1}{2}$ green pepper, seeds removed and cut into strips
1 red pepper, seeds removed and sliced
100 g/4 oz (U.S. $\frac{1}{4}$ lb) ready-to-eat figs, halved
300 ml/$\frac{1}{2}$ pint chicken stock (U.S. 1$\frac{1}{4}$ cups chicken
bouillon)
salt and freshly ground black pepper

Heat the oven to 180°C/350°F, Gas Mark 4.

Coat the chops with ground almonds, pressing them on well. Heat the butter in a frying pan (U.S. skillet) and fry the chops for about 5 minutes on each side, until browned. Transfer to a shallow ovenproof casserole.

Add the onion and peppers to the fat remaining in the pan and fry gently, stirring occasionally, until the onion is soft. Stir in the figs and stock, and bring to the boil. Season to taste and pour over the chops. Cover and cook for 1$\frac{1}{4}$ hours.

Strain the cooking liquid into a pan and boil rapidly until reduced by one third. Pour back over the ingredients in the dish and serve hot with freshly boiled brown rice. **Serves 4**

Variation

Pruned pork Omit the figs and substitute no-need-to-soak prunes.

Chicken patties

(Illustrated opposite)

150 g/5 oz (U.S. $\frac{3}{4}$ cup) long grain brown rice,
cooked and cooled
225 g/8 oz minced (U.S. 2 cups ground)
cooked chicken
1 small onion, peeled and finely chopped
100 g/4 oz (U.S. $\frac{1}{2}$ cup) cottage cheese, sieved
1 tablespoon finely chopped parsley
2 teaspoons (U.S. 1 tablespoon) lemon juice
salt and freshly ground black pepper
1 small egg, beaten
about 50 g/2 oz (U.S. $\frac{1}{3}$ cup) seedless raisins
about 75 g/3 oz (U.S. $\frac{3}{4}$ cup) ground almonds
oil for shallow frying
Garnish
lemon slices
sprigs of parsley

Combine the rice, chicken, onion, cheese, parsley, lemon juice and seasoning to taste. Add enough egg to bind the mixture together. Cover and chill for 2 hours.

Divide into 10 equal portions and shape each into a round flat cake with floured hands, enclosing a few raisins in the centre of each. Coat the patties in almonds, pressing them on well.

Heat a little oil in a frying pan (U.S. skillet) and fry the patties over moderate heat for about 4 minutes on each side, or until crisp and golden brown. Drain well on absorbent kitchen towel and serve in a warm dish, garnished with lemon slices and parsley sprigs. **Serves 4-5**

From the top – Chicken risotto, Saucy pork, Chicken patties

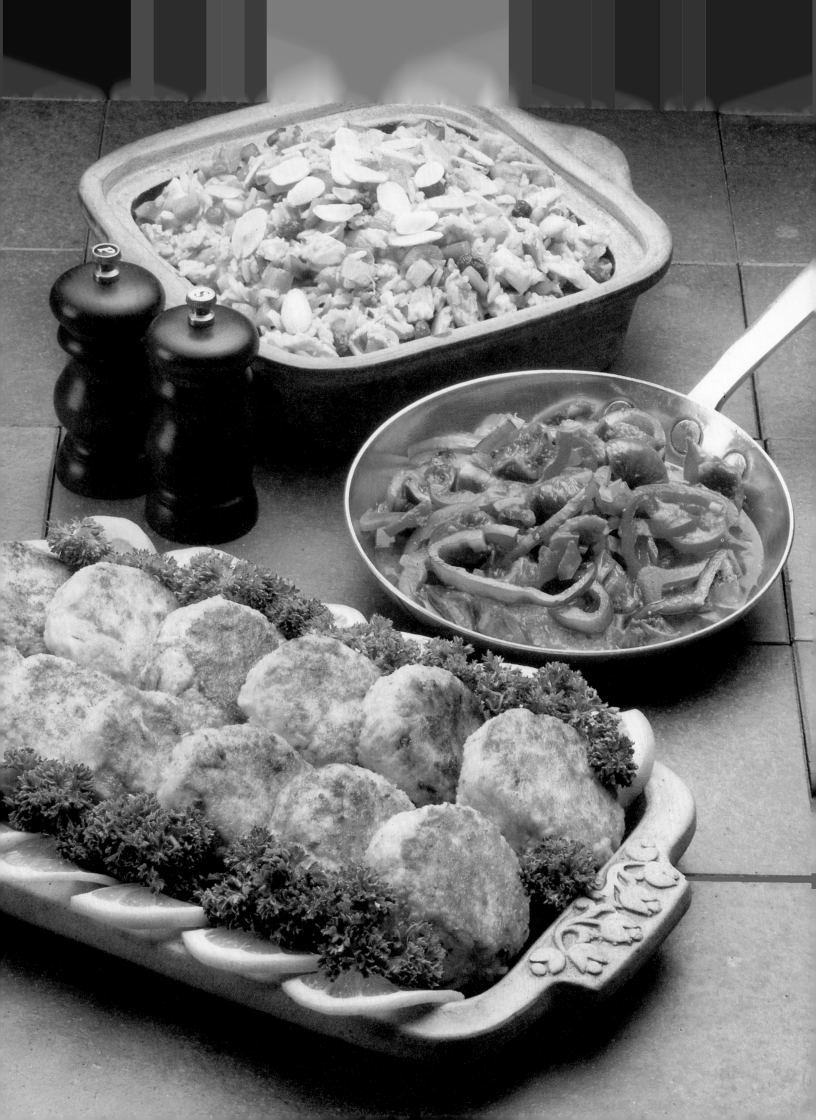

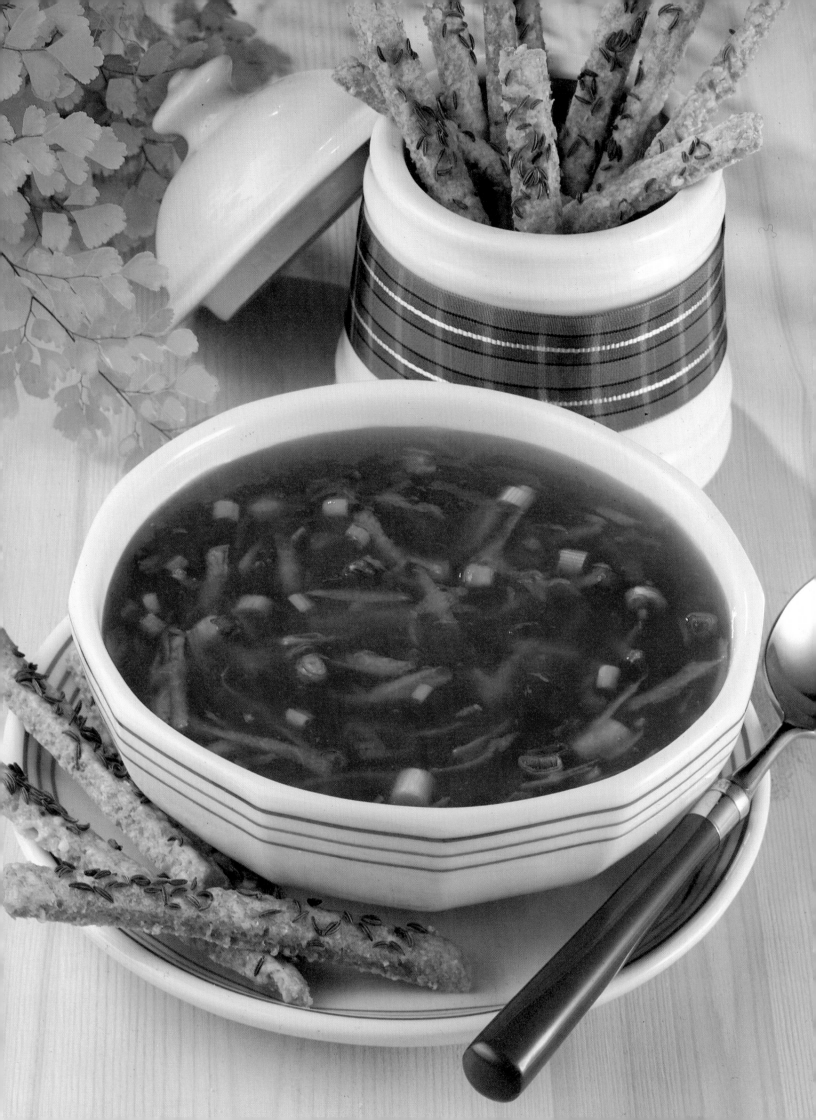

Jellied consommé with cheese straws

(Illustrated opposite)

600 ml/1 pint light stock (U.S. 2½ cups light bouillon)
1 tablespoon powdered gelatine (U.S. 1 envelope unflavored gelatin)
1 (425-g/15-oz) can game consommé
2 medium-sized carrots, peeled and grated
2 large spring onions (U.S. scallions), trimmed and chopped
Cheese straws
100 g/4 oz wholemeal flour (U.S. 1 cup wholewheat flour)
½ teaspoon salt
large pinch of cayenne pepper
50 g/2 oz (U.S. ¼ cup) butter or margarine
50 g/2 oz (U.S. ½ cup) grated Cheddar cheese
1 tablespoon rolled oats
little milk
caraway seeds

Put about 3 tablespoons (U.S. 4 tablespoons) of the stock into a medium-sized bowl and sprinkle on the gelatine. Leave to stand for 5 minutes, then place the bowl over a pan of simmering water until the gelatine has completely dissolved. Stir in the remaining stock and the consommé. Mix well then chill for several hours.

Meanwhile, make the cheese straws. Heat the oven to 200°C/400°F, Gas Mark 6 and grease 2 baking sheets (U.S. cookie sheets). Put the flour in a bowl and add the seasoning. Rub or cut in the butter until the mixture resembles breadcrumbs, then stir in the cheese and oats. Add enough water to make a stiff dough. Roll out half the dough thinly on a floured surface and trim to a rectangle measuring 17.5 cm/ 7 inches by 10 cm/4 inches. Repeat with the remaining dough. Transfer to the prepared sheets, brush with milk and sprinkle with caraway seeds. Cut each piece of dough into 5-mm/¼-inch wide strips.

Bake for about 10 minutes, or until pale golden. Cool on a wire rack.

Ladle the consommé into soup bowls and stir carrot and onion into each portion. Serve with the cheese straws. **Serves 6**

Jellied consommé with cheese straws

Creamy lamb and lentil soup

25 g/1 oz (U.S. 2 tablespoons) margarine
1 large onion, peeled and chopped
2 medium-sized carrots, peeled and sliced
150 g/5 oz (U.S. ⅔ cup) dried red lentils
1 litre/1¾ pints chicken or lamb stock (U.S. 4¼ cups chicken or lamb bouillon)
½ teaspoon ground rosemary
225 g/8 oz (U.S. ½ lb) boneless lean lamb, diced
salt and freshly ground black pepper
75 ml/3 fl oz single cream (U.S. ⅓ cup light cream)

Melt the margarine in a large pan and fry the onion and carrot, stirring, for 1 minute. Cover and leave over low heat for 4 minutes, shaking the pan occasionally. Put in the lentils and stir for 1 minute. Add the stock and rosemary and bring to the boil, stirring. Cover and simmer for 45 minutes, or until the lentils are really soft.

Liquidize the soup and return to the rinsed pan. Add the lamb and bring to boiling point. Cover and simmer for a further 20 minutes, stirring occasionally.

Taste and add seasoning if necessary, stir in the cream and reheat but do not allow the soup to boil. Serve very hot with crusty brown rolls. **Serves 4**

Fresh green pea soup

450 g/1 lb shelled or frozen peas (U.S. green peas)
1 medium-sized potato, peeled and sliced
1 medium-sized onion, peeled and sliced
1 lettuce heart, quartered
900 ml/1½ pints strong chicken stock (U.S. 3¾ cups strong chicken bouillon)
juice of ½ lemon
1 teaspoon cornflour (U.S. cornstarch)
150 ml/¼ pint (U.S. ⅔ cup) milk
salt and freshly ground black pepper
100 g/4 oz (U.S. ¼ lb) cooked ham, diced

Place the peas, potato, onion and lettuce in a large pan with half the stock and the lemon juice. Bring to the boil, cover and simmer for 15 minutes.

Liquidize the soup and return to the rinsed pan. Add the remaining stock. Blend the cornflour with the milk, pour into the soup and stir until boiling. Cook for 3 minutes and add seasoning if necessary. Serve hot with a scattering of ham dice in each portion. **Serves 4-6**

Whisked vegetable sauces

Basic sauce
50 g/2 oz (U.S. $\frac{1}{4}$ cup) butter or margarine
50 g/2 oz wholemeal flour (U.S. $\frac{1}{2}$ cup wholewheat flour)
600 ml/1 pint (U.S. $2\frac{1}{2}$ cups) milk
1 chicken or vegetable stock cube (U.S. chicken or vegetable bouillon cube), crumbled

Place all the ingredients in a heavy pan and whisk over moderate heat until the sauce boils and thickens. Simmer for 3 minutes then fold in the chosen vegetable purée (below) and spice. **Makes about 750 ml/1$\frac{1}{4}$ pints (U.S. 3 cups) basic sauce**

Vegetable choices

Onion sauce Peel and finely chop 1 large onion. Place in a pan with 25 g/1 oz (U.S. 2 tablespoons) butter or margarine and 2 tablespoons (U.S. 3 tablespoons) water. Cover and cook gently until the onion is soft. Stir into the hot sauce, add a pinch of ground cloves and seasoning if wished.

Carrot and swede sauce (U.S. Carrot and rutabaga sauce) Purée 175 g/6 oz cooked carrot and swede (U.S. 1 cup puréed carrot and rutabaga). Fold into the hot sauce, add a pinch of ground nutmeg and extra seasoning if needed. Reheat.

Mushroom sauce Chop 100 g/4 oz (U.S. $\frac{1}{4}$ lb) button mushrooms. Place in a pan with 25 g/1 oz (U.S. 2 tablespoons) butter or margarine and 1 tablespoon water. Stir, cover and cook gently for 5 minutes, or until soft. Blend into the hot sauce, add a pinch of ground allspice and seasoning to taste.

Spinach and watercress sauce Strip the leaves from 100 g/4 oz (U.S. $\frac{1}{4}$ lb) spinach, wash and drain. Place in a pan with just the water clinging to the leaves. Cover and cook briskly, shaking the pan frequently, until the spinach is limp. Purée in a blender or food processor with the leaves from 4 large sprigs of watercress. Stir into the hot sauce, add $\frac{1}{4}$ teaspoon ground mace and extra seasoning if desired.

Leek sauce Finely slice the white and pale green parts of 2 medium-sized leeks. Rinse thoroughly in a colander, drain and place in a pan with 25 g/1 oz (U.S. 2 tablespoons) butter or margarine and 2 tablespoons (U.S. 3 tablespoons) water. Cover and cook until the leek is soft. Stir into the hot sauce, add a large pinch of ground coriander and seasoning if necessary.

Herring and oatmeal fries

900 g/2 lb fresh whole herring or mackerel
salt and freshly ground black pepper
2 eggs, beaten
100 g/4 oz (U.S. 1$\frac{1}{3}$ cups) rolled oats
$\frac{1}{2}$ teaspoon dry mustard powder
wholemeal flour (U.S. wholewheat flour) for coating
oil for deep frying
2 oranges, sliced
sprig of parsley to garnish

To clean the fish, remove the heads, split along the undersides, remove the entrails then open the fish and place, skin side upwards, on a board. Press firmly along the back, turn over and remove the bones. Wash and dry on absorbent kitchen towel.

Season the egg and place in a shallow dish. Mix the oats with the mustard and put in a plastic bag. Cut the fish into 5-cm/2-inch strips and coat with flour. Dip the strips in egg then add them, a few at a time, to the bag of oats and shake until completely covered.

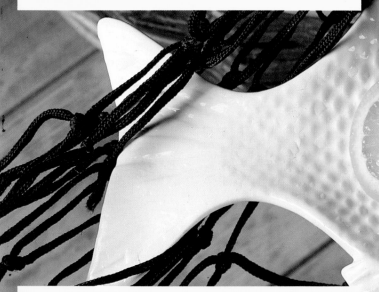

Remove the coated strips and repeat until all the fish strips are prepared.

Heat the oil to a temperature of 180°C/350°F or until a cube of day-old bread turns golden brown in about 1 minute. Deep fry the strips in batches for about 5 minutes, or until golden brown. Drain well on absorbent kitchen towel. Keep hot until all the strips are cooked.

Use the orange slices to line a warm serving dish, pile the hot fries on top and serve garnished with a sprig of parsley. **Serves 4-5**

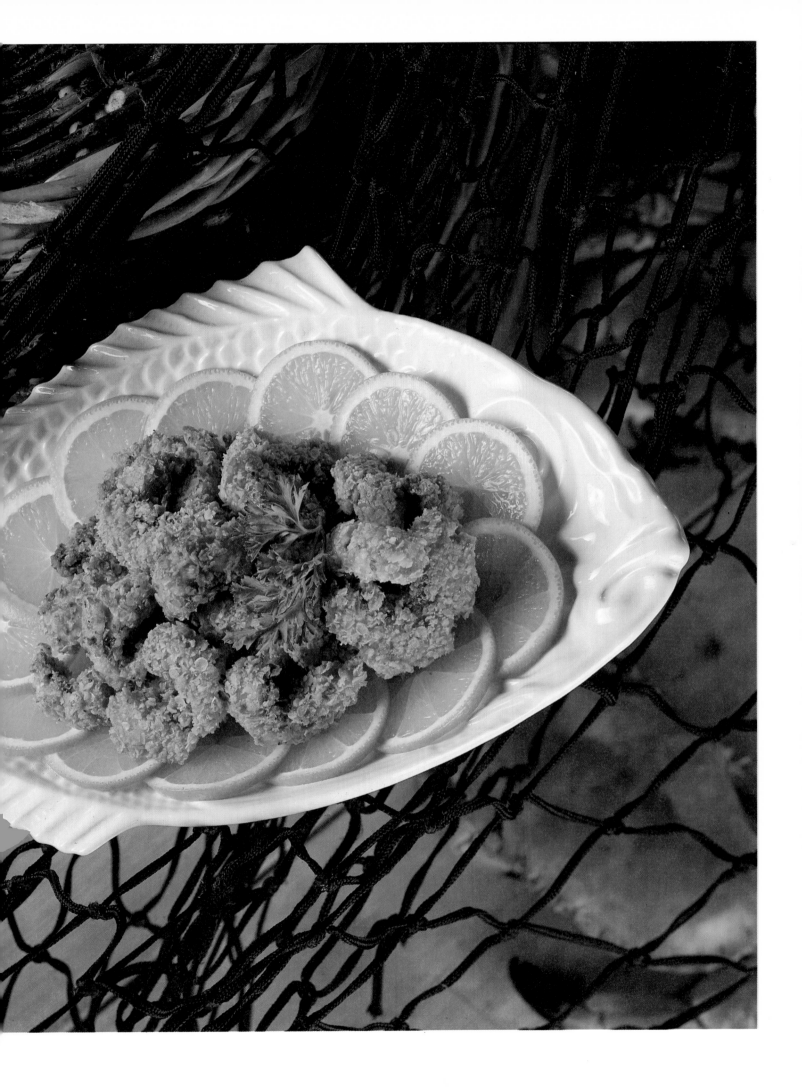

Noodles with bean sauce

(Illustrated opposite)

350 g/12 oz (U.S. ¾ lb) fresh or dried green noodles
4 tablespoons (U.S. 6 tablespoons) olive oil
4 rashers back bacon (U.S. 4 Canadian bacon slices),
rind removed and cut into strips
1 clove garlic, crushed
4 spring onions (U.S. scallions), trimmed
and chopped
salt and freshly ground black pepper
1 (425-g/15-oz) can baked beans in tomato sauce
grated Parmesan cheese

Cook the noodles in a pan of boiling salted water as directed, adding 1 tablespoon (U.S. about 1½ tablespoons) of the olive oil to the water.

Meanwhile, heat the remaining oil in a pan and add the strips of bacon, the garlic and just the white parts of the onions. Season lightly and fry for 3 minutes, stirring. Mix in the beans and heat through thoroughly.

Drain the noodles well and transfer to a warm serving dish. Top with the hot bean sauce and sprinkle with the green bits of onion. Serve with Parmesan cheese handed separately. **Serves 4**

Bean and ham supper

4 thick slices of cooked ham (about 225 g/8 oz
(U.S. ½ lb) total weight)
25 g/1 oz (U.S. 2 tablespoons) margarine
20 g/¾ oz wholemeal flour (U.S. scant ¼ cup
wholewheat flour)
450 ml/¾ pint (U.S. 2 cups) milk
2 teaspoons mild Continental mustard
1 (198-g/7-oz) can corn kernels
1 (425-g/15-oz) can butter beans (U.S. lima beans)
salt and pepper
2 tablespoons double cream (U.S. 3 tablespoons
heavy cream)
50 g/2 oz grated mature Cheddar cheese (U.S. ½ cup
grated sharp Cheddar cheese)
Garnish
tomato slices
sprig of parsley

Heat the oven to 190°C/375°F, Gas Mark 5 and grease an ovenproof casserole dish.

Place 2 slices ham in the base of the prepared casserole. Melt the margarine in a pan and stir in the flour. Cook for ½ minute, then gradually blend in the milk and bring to the boil, stirring all the time. Cook for 2 minutes then add the mustard, corn and liquid

from the can and the beans. Season to taste and pour half this mixture over the ham in the dish. Top with the remaining ham and then the rest of the sauce mixture. Spoon the cream over the surface and sprinkle with the cheese.

Bake for 25 minutes. Serve hot from the dish, garnished with the tomato slices and parsley sprig. **Serves 4**

Spicy pasta with prawns

(Illustrated opposite)

225 g/8 oz (U.S. ½ lb) pasta shells
2 tablespoons (U.S. 3 tablespoons) olive oil
100 g/4 oz peeled prawns (U.S. ¼ lb shelled cooked
shrimp)
2 (225-g/8-oz) cans curried beans with sultanas
150 ml/¼ pint single cream (U.S. ⅔ cup light cream)
100 g/4 oz (U.S. ¼ lb) button mushrooms, thinly
sliced
2 tablespoons (U.S. 3 tablespoons) chopped parsley
to garnish

Cook the pasta shells in a pan of boiling salted water as directed, adding half the oil to the water.

Meanwhile, heat the remaining oil in a pan and cook the shellfish for 3 minutes over moderate heat, shaking the pan frequently. Stir in the beans, cream and mushrooms and place over low heat, stirring occasionally, until piping hot.

Drain the pasta shells thoroughly, transfer to a warm serving dish and spoon the spicy bean mixture over the top. Sprinkle with the parsley and serve immediately. **Serves 4**

Above: Noodles with bean sauce. Below: Spicy pasta with prawns

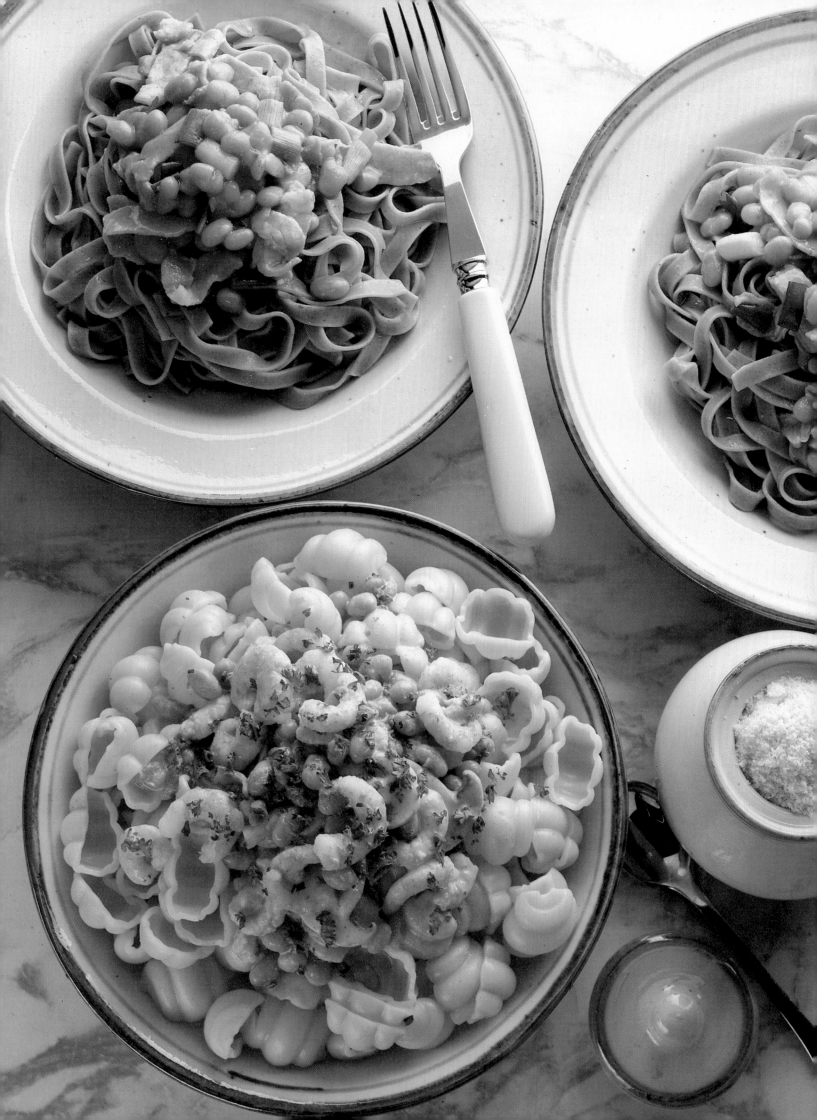

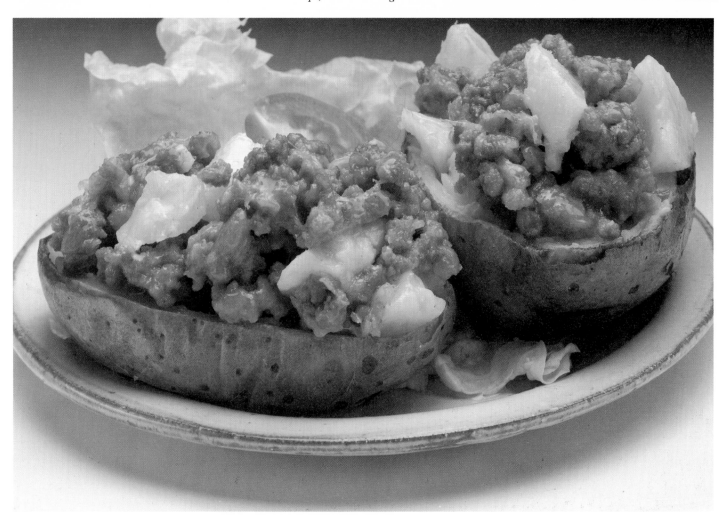

Curry baked potatoes

(Illustrated above)

4 large potatoes, scrubbed
25 g/1 oz (U.S. 2 tablespoons) butter
225 g/8 oz lean minced beef (U.S. $\frac{1}{2}$ lb lean ground beef)
2 teaspoons (U.S. 1 tablespoon) curry powder
100 g/4 oz (U.S. 1 cup) finely grated Gouda cheese
salt
Garnish
lettuce leaves
tomato wedges

Heat the oven to 180°C/350°F, Gas Mark 4. Bake the potatoes for about 1$\frac{1}{2}$ hours, or until just tender.

Meanwhile, melt the butter in a frying pan (U.S. skillet) and gently cook the beef, stirring, until it changes colour. Add the curry powder and mix well. Continue cooking gently, stirring occasionally, for 15 minutes.

Cut the hot potatoes in half and scoop out the insides leaving a thin shell. Stir the cheese into the beef mixture and add salt to taste. Fold in the potato and spoon back into the potato shells. Serve hot and garnish with lettuce and tomato. **Serves 4**

Moroccan lamb with rice

450 g/1 lb boneless lean lamb, finely diced
1 clove garlic, crushed
1 medium-sized onion, peeled and chopped
300 ml/$\frac{1}{2}$ pint (U.S. 1$\frac{1}{4}$ cups) water
1 chicken stock cube (U.S. chicken bouillon cube)
2 carrots, peeled and roughly chopped
100 g/4 oz (U.S. $\frac{2}{3}$ cup) long grain brown rice
2 (225-g/8-oz) cans curried beans with sultanas
4 tablespoons (U.S. 6 tablespoons) chopped parsley
salt

Place the meat in a pan with the garlic and onion. Cook over moderate heat, stirring all the time, until the meat changes colour. Add the water and stock cube, cover and simmer for 20 minutes.

Put in the carrots and rice. Stir well, bring back to the boil, cover and simmer for a further 15 minutes, stirring occasionally. Add the beans and parsley and a very little extra water if necessary. Heat through for 5 more minutes. Check seasoning, adding salt to taste. When the rice is tender and has absorbed the liquid, transfer to a warm platter. **Serves 4**

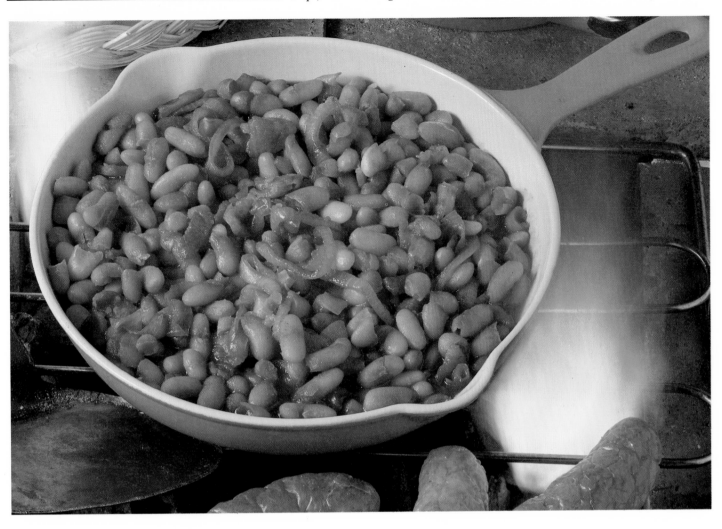

Boston baked beans

(Illustrated above)

15 g/$\frac{1}{2}$ oz (U.S. 1 tablespoon) lard or butter
1 small onion, peeled and sliced
4 rashers streaky bacon (U.S. 4 bacon slices), rind
removed and cut in strips
40 g/1$\frac{1}{2}$ oz muscovado sugar (U.S. $\frac{1}{4}$ cup brown sugar)
1 tablespoon black treacle (U.S. molasses)
1 tablespoon dry mustard powder
$\frac{1}{4}$ teaspoon freshly ground black pepper
1 teaspoon salt
150 ml/$\frac{1}{4}$ pint (U.S. $\frac{2}{3}$ cup) boiling water
1 (425-g/15-oz) can cannellini beans, drained

Heat the oven to 180°C/350°F, Gas Mark 4 and have
ready an ovenproof casserole dish.

Melt the lard in a pan and fry the onion until soft.
Add the bacon and fry, stirring frequently, until
golden. Mix in the sugar, treacle, mustard, pepper,
salt and water. Bring to the boil, then simmer for 10
minutes. Stir in the beans and transfer to the dish.

Cover and cook in the oven for 35 minutes. If
necessary, this dish can be reheated on top of the
cooker, or barbecue in summer. Serve with pork
sausages (U.S. pork links). **Serves 4**

Kipper and bean soufflés

1 (425-g/15-oz) can butter beans (U.S. lima beans)
1 tablespoon lemon juice
350 g/12 oz (U.S. $\frac{3}{4}$ lb) kipper fillets, cooked and
skinned
3 tablespoons single cream (U.S. 4 tablespoons light
cream)
3 eggs, separated
salt and freshly ground black pepper

Heat the oven to 190°C/375°F, Gas Mark 5 and
grease 4 individual ovenproof dishes. Stand them on a
baking sheet (U.S. cookie sheet).

Liquidize the beans with the liquid from the can,
the lemon juice and fish until really smooth. (Alternatively, pound the beans and fish until smooth and
gradually add the liquid.) Beat in the cream and egg
yolks, and season to taste. Whisk the egg whites in a
clean bowl until really stiff and fold into the fish
mixture. Transfer to the prepared dishes.

Bake for about 45 minutes, or until well risen and
golden on the top. Serve hot from the oven. **Serves 4**

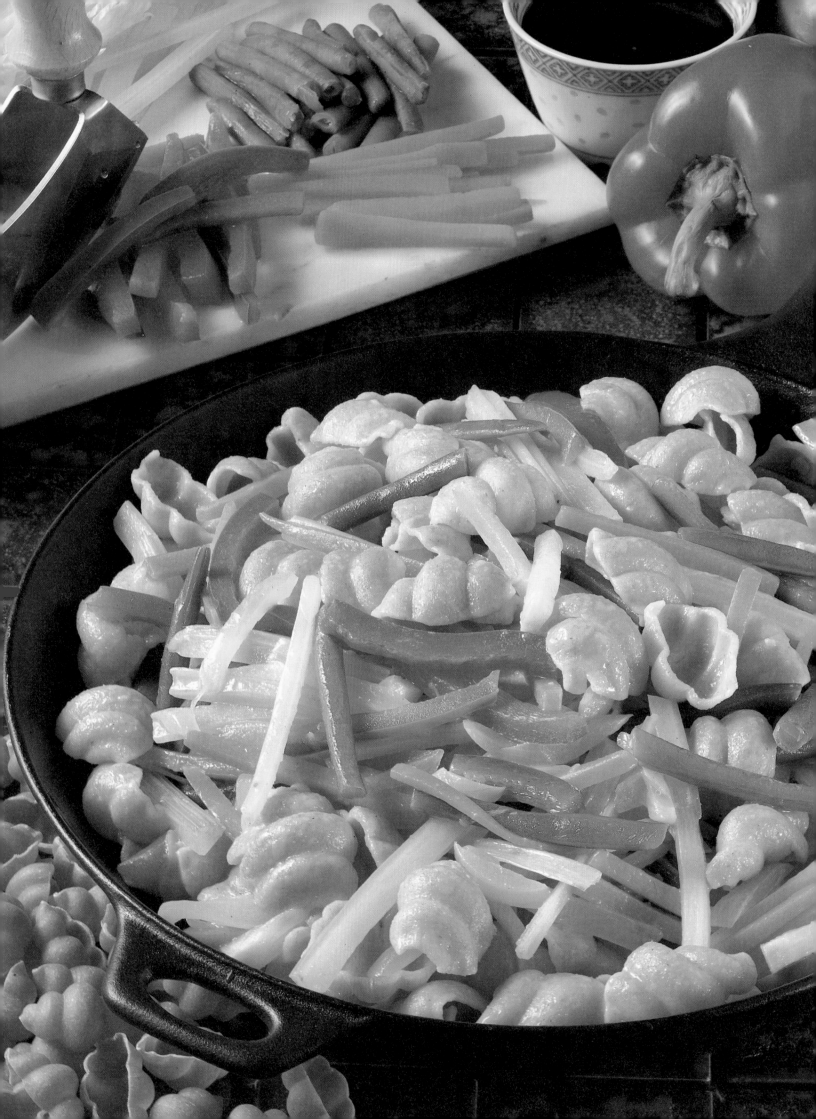

Pasta and vegetable stir fry

(Illustrated opposite)

450 g/1 lb wholewheat pasta shells
75 g/3 oz (U.S. ⅓ cup) butter or margarine
1 large onion, peeled and sliced
3 stalks celery, cut into strips
2 large carrots, peeled and cut into strips
100 g/4 oz French beans (U.S. ¼ lb green beans),
topped and tailed
½ red pepper, seeds removed and sliced
½ green pepper, seeds removed and sliced
2 tablespoons (U.S. 3 tablespoons) soy sauce
salt and freshly ground black pepper

Cook the pasta in a pan of boiling salted water as directed.

Meanwhile, melt the butter in a heavy frying pan (skillet) or wok and add all the prepared vegetables. Fry gently for 10 minutes, stirring frequently, until the vegetables soften. While they are cooking, drain the pasta and rinse with hot water. Drain, add to the pan with the soy sauce and mix all the ingredients together. Cook for further 2 minutes. Season to taste and serve at once. If wished, hand grated cheese separately. **Serves 4**

Brown rice with pimentoes

3 rashers streaky bacon (U.S. 3 bacon slices), rind removed and chopped
1 tablespoon oil
1 medium-sized onion, peeled and chopped
200 g/7 oz (U.S. 1 cup) long grain brown rice
600 ml/1 pint chicken or vegetable stock (U.S. 2½
cups chicken or vegetable bouillon)
½ teaspoon curry powder
10-cm/4-inch length cucumber, diced
2 canned red pimentoes, cut into strips
2 tablespoons (U.S. 3 tablespoons) liquid from can of
pimentoes
salt and freshly ground black pepper

Heat the bacon gently in a large pan until the fat runs. Raise the heat and fry until the bacon bits are golden. Remove them from the pan with a slotted spoon and reserve. Add the oil and onion to the pan and cook

gently until the onion is soft. Stir in the rice and continue cooking, stirring frequently, until the rice looks almost opaque. Add the stock and curry powder, bring to the boil, stir once then cover and simmer for 30 minutes.

Put in the cucumber, pimento strips and liquid from the can, season lightly and stir once. Bring back to the boil, cover and simmer for a further 5 minutes, or until the rice is tender and has absorbed the liquid. Adjust the seasoning if necessary, fork in the bacon bits and transfer to a warm dish. **Serves 4**

Baked vegetarian pasta

(Illustrated on page 115)

100 g/4 oz green pasta twists (U.S. 1⅓ cups green
pasta shapes)
25 g/1 oz plain flour (U.S. ¼ cup all-purpose flour)
25 g/1 oz (U.S. 2 tablespoons) butter
300 ml/½ pint (U.S. 1¼ cups) milk
100 g/4 oz (U.S. 1 cup) grated Edam cheese
1 tablespoon mild Continental mustard
1 tablespoon horseradish sauce
1 teaspoon tarragon vinegar
salt and freshly ground black pepper
1 red pepper, seeds removed and sliced
1 green pepper, seeds removed and sliced
225 g/8 oz (U.S. ½ lb) carrots, peeled, sliced and
cooked
1 (212-g/7½-oz) can corn kernels, drained
1 (225-g/8-oz) can red kidney beans, drained
Topping
25 g/1 oz (U.S. 2 tablespoons) butter, melted
25 g/1 oz (U.S. ¼ cup) chopped nuts
25 g/1 oz fresh wholemeal breadcrumbs (U.S. ½ cup
fresh wholewheat bread crumbs)
50 g/2 oz (U.S. ½ cup) grated Edam cheese

Heat the oven to 180°C/350°F, Gas Mark 4 and grease a shallow ovenproof dish.

Cook the pasta in plenty of boiling salted water as directed on the pack. Drain well. Meanwhile, put the flour, butter and milk in a large pan and whisk over moderate heat until the sauce boils and thickens. Simmer for 2 minutes. Remove from the heat and stir in the cheese, mustard, horseradish, vinegar, seasoning to taste and finally the pasta. Fold the pepper slices, carrot, corn and beans into the sauce and transfer to the prepared dish. Mix together all the ingredients for the topping and sprinkle evenly over the surface.

Bake for 30 minutes, or until golden brown.
Serves 4-6

Pasta and vegetable stir fry

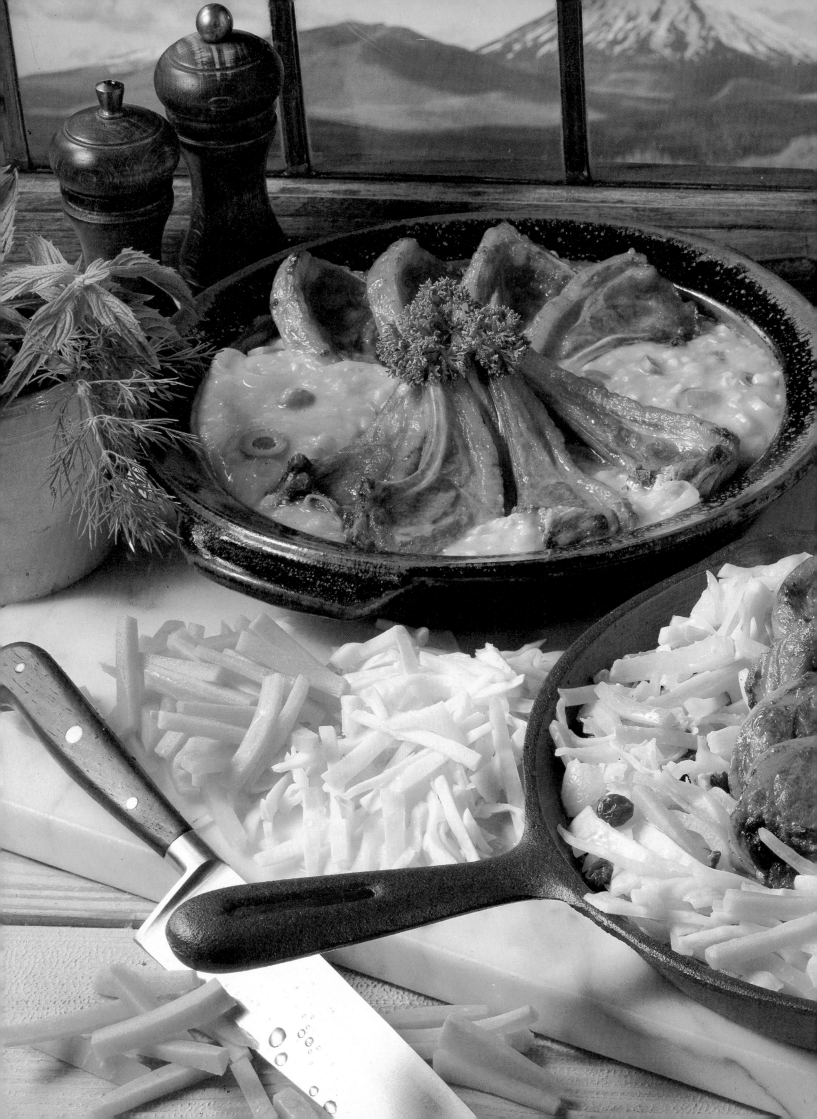

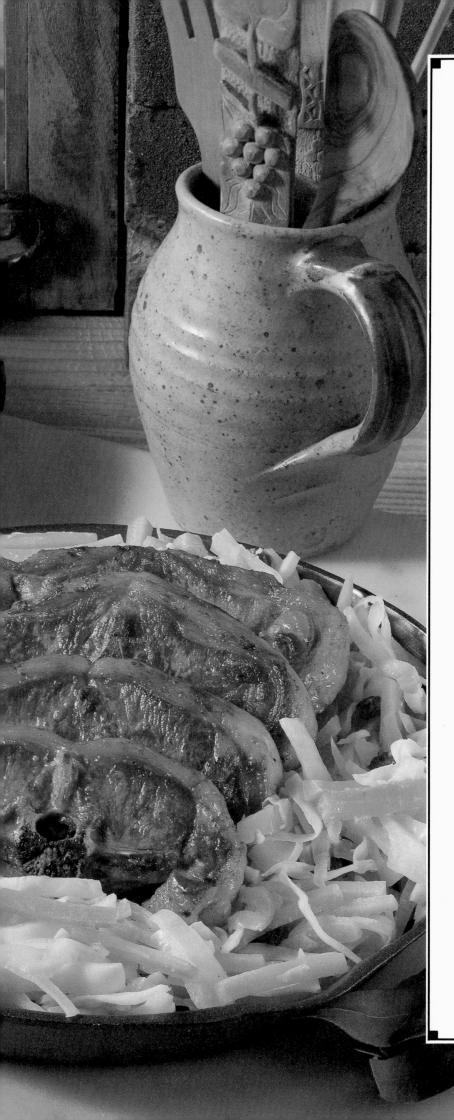

Main Meals

How pleasant it is when a whole family gathers round the dining table to enjoy the main meal of the day, piping hot and satisfying. In our busy lives, this seems to occur most often in the evening, for few housewives have time to cook an elaborate lunch and a high tea or dinner. But no matter when it is, make it an important social event.

New ideas for healthy, substantial dishes are always welcome. Back them up with accompaniments which also provide a proportion of the daily fibre intake, so necessary to everyone's well-being. Never miss an opportunity to include a high-fibre ingredient, whether it's the flour to thicken a sauce, or brown breadcrumbs for coating food instead of white. Every little helps.

Stock up with wholewheat pasta or high-fibre white pasta. Invest in packs of nutty brown rice, and bags of dried pulses. The variety available is greater than you think, and all have subtle differences in flavour – orange and green lentils, golden and yellow split peas, dark red kidney beans, creamy butter beans, snowy white cannellini. These are just a few of the store-cupboard stand-bys at your disposal. Some of them come in cans, too, to save time in soaking and cooking.

You may not be a fan of all products from the health food shop, including bulgur wheat and buckwheat flour; but fresh green peas are good for you too, and everyone seems to enjoy them. Golden sweetcorn kernels are the grains from the corn cob and it is no penance to add them to a plate of meat and potatoes. Incidentally, most root vegetables are fibre-full, so the more you add to a high-protein centrepiece of fish, meat or poultry, the more healthy is your diet.

Above: Corned lamb cutlets (recipe page 66). Below: Lamb chops with a bite (recipe page 64)

Lamb chops with a bite

(Illustrated on pages 62-63)

4 double loin or 'butterfly' lamb chops
salt and freshly ground black pepper
2 tablespoons (U.S. 3 tablespoons) oil
1 large onion, peeled and thinly sliced
2 cloves garlic, crushed
6 medium-sized carrots, peeled and cut into thin sticks
450 g/1 lb white cabbage, shredded
150 ml/¼ pint (U.S. ⅔ cup) milk
40 g/1½ oz (U.S. ¼ cup) seedless raisins

Trim any excess fat from the chops, then season well. Heat the oil in a frying pan (U.S. skillet) and fry the chops until browned on both sides. Pour off most of the fat from the pan. Add the onion and garlic and continue frying gently until the onion is soft, turning the chops occasionally. Remove the chops. Stir the carrots, cabbage and milk into the onion mixture and top with the chops, pressing them down slightly. Bring to the boil and simmer for about 5 minutes, until the chops are cooked through, the cabbage tender but still crisp and most of the liquid absorbed.

Add the raisins and adjust the seasoning. Serve the chops on top of the cabbage mixture. **Serves 4**

Turkey roast with walnut macaroni

(Illustrated on title page)

25 g/1 oz (U.S. 2 tablespoons) butter or margarine, softened
1 (1-1.2-kg/2-2½-lb) boneless turkey roast
salt and freshly ground black pepper
275 g/10 oz (U.S. 3⅓ cups) wholewheat short-cut macaroni
350 g/12 oz (U.S. ¾ lb) carrots, peeled and diced
2 tablespoons (U.S. 3 tablespoons) oil
2 medium-sized onions, peeled and sliced
1 teaspoon dried basil
75 g/3 oz (U.S. ¾ cup) chopped walnuts
1 tablespoon wholemeal flour
(U.S. wholewheat flour)
4 tablespoons (U.S. 6 tablespoons) white wine
300 ml/½ pint chicken stock (U.S. 1¼ cups chicken bouillon)
sprigs of parsley to garnish

Heat the oven to 180°C/350°F, Gas Mark 4 and grease a small roasting tin.

Spread the butter over the turkey roast and sprinkle lightly with seasoning. Place in the prepared tin and cook for 30-35 minutes per 450 g/1 lb plus 30 minutes over, basting several times with the pan juices.

Cook the macaroni and carrots together in boiling salted water for about 10 minutes, or until just tender. Drain, rinse with boiling water and drain again thoroughly.

At the same time, heat the oil in a pan and gently fry the onions until soft and turning golden. Add the basil, 50 g/2 oz (U.S. ½ cup) of the walnuts and seasoning to taste, toss well together. Combine with the macaroni and carrots, transfer to a warm serving dish and top with the cooked turkey. Keep hot.

Drain off all but 1 tablespoon fat from the juices in the roasting tin and stir in the flour. Cook for 1 minute, stirring, then gradually add the wine and stock. Bring to the boil, stirring constantly, and simmer for 2 minutes. Add the remaining walnuts, adjust the seasoning and pour into a gravy boat. Garnish the turkey with parsley and serve with the sauce. **Serves 6**

Chilli con carne

(Illustrated opposite)

1 tablespoon oil
1 large onion, peeled and chopped
1 green pepper, seeds removed and chopped
2 cloves garlic, crushed
675 g/1½ lb minced beef (U.S. ground beef)
1 (425-g/15-oz) can tomatoes, chopped
1 tablespoon chilli powder
salt
1 (425-g/15-oz) can red kidney beans, drained and rinsed

Heat the oil in a large heavy pan and gently cook the onion and pepper, stirring frequently, until the onion begins to soften. Add the garlic and beef, and stir over moderate heat until the meat looks brown and crumbly. Add the tomatoes and liquid from the can, the chilli powder and 1 teaspoon salt. Bring to the boil, stirring, cover and simmer for 45 minutes, stirring occasionally.

Mix in the beans, add more salt if necessary, bring back to the boil and simmer for a further 15 minutes. Serve hot with corn chips. **Serves 4-6**

Note To give the dish an authentic touch, substitute 1 fresh red or green chilli pepper for the green pepper. Remove the seeds and finely chop the flesh before adding.

Chilli con carne

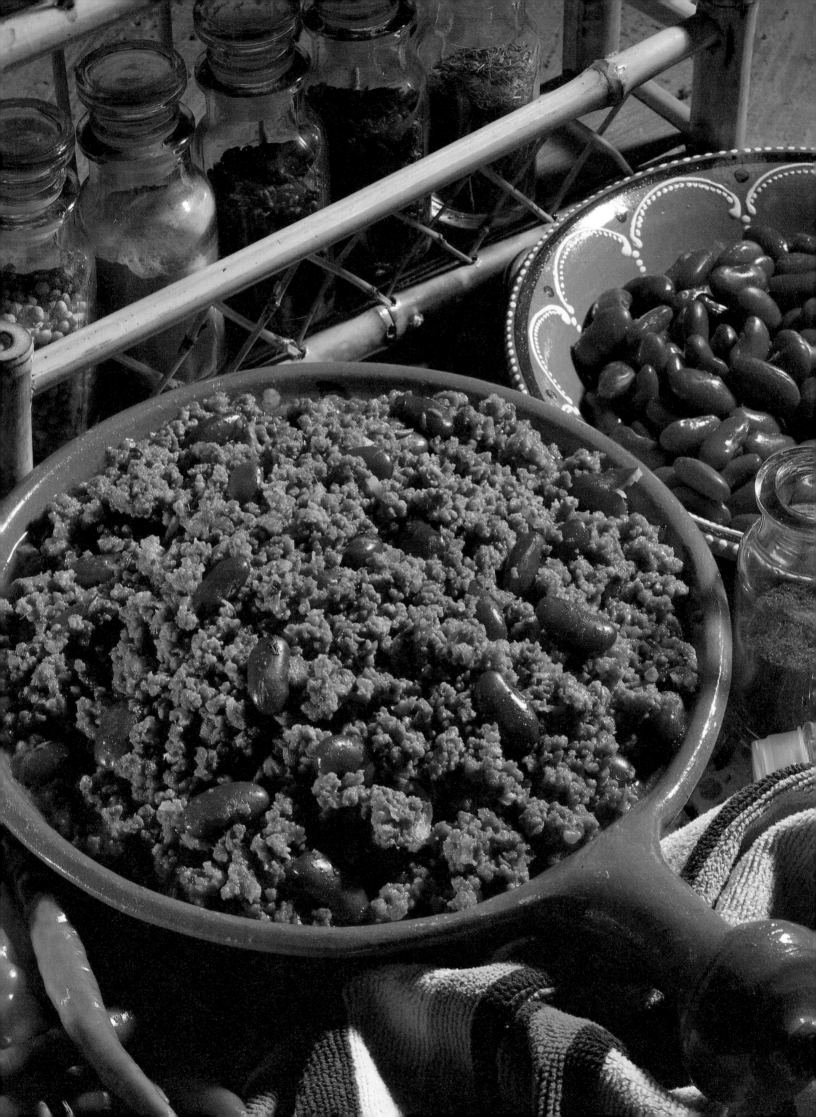

Onion cassoulet

(Illustrated opposite)

75 g/3 oz (U.S. scant ½ cup) dried black-eye beans
75 g/3 oz dried haricot beans (U.S. scant ½ cup
dried navy or lima beans)
225 g/8 oz (U.S. ½ lb) boneless lean pork, diced
150 g/5 oz Garbanzo or salami sausage, skin removed
and chopped
1 (295-g/10.4-oz) can condensed French onion soup

Put the beans in a pan and cover with boiling water.
Leave to stand for 2 hours. Drain the beans, cover
with fresh cold water, place over high heat and allow
to boil rapidly for 10 minutes. Meanwhile, heat the
oven to 180°C/350°F, Gas Mark 4 and grease an
ovenproof dish.
　Drain the beans well, transfer to the prepared dish
with the pork and sausage. Pour the soup over and
mix well.
　Cover and cook for 2 hours, stirring occasionally,
or until the beans are really tender but not broken.
Serve hot with crusty wholemeal bread (U.S. wholewheat bread) and Brussels sprouts. **Serves 4**

Corned lamb cutlets

(Illustrated on pages 62-63)

8 lamb cutlets (U.S. rib lamb chops)
salt and freshly ground black pepper
2 tablespoons (U.S. 3 tablespoons) oil
2 large onions, peeled and sliced
1 (284-g/10-oz) can cream-style corn
2 tablespoons white wine or cider (U.S. 3 tablespoons
white wine or hard cider)
8 stuffed green olives, sliced
large sprig of parsley to garnish

Trim any excess fat from the cutlets and season
lightly. Heat the oil in a frying pan (U.S. skillet) and
fry the cutlets until well browned on both sides.
Remove from the pan and keep hot.
　Add the onion to the fat remaining in the pan and
fry until soft, then drain off excess fat. Add the corn,
wine and a little seasoning to the onion and bring to
the boil, stirring. Replace the cutlets, cover the pan
and simmer for about 10 minutes. Remove the
cutlets. Stir the olives into the sauce and adjust the
seasoning if necessary.
　Pour the sauce into a warm serving dish, top with
the cutlets and garnish with the parsley sprig. Serve
with boiled potatoes and a salad or green vegetable.
Serves 4

Onion cassoulet

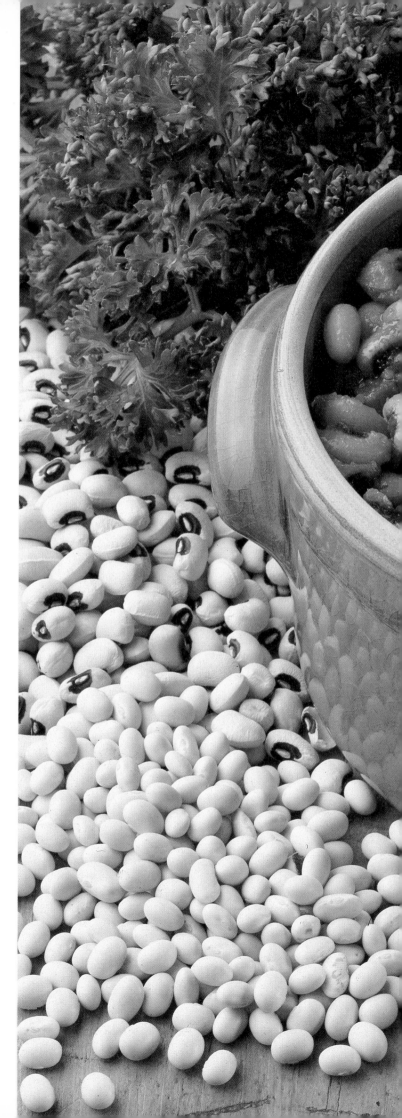

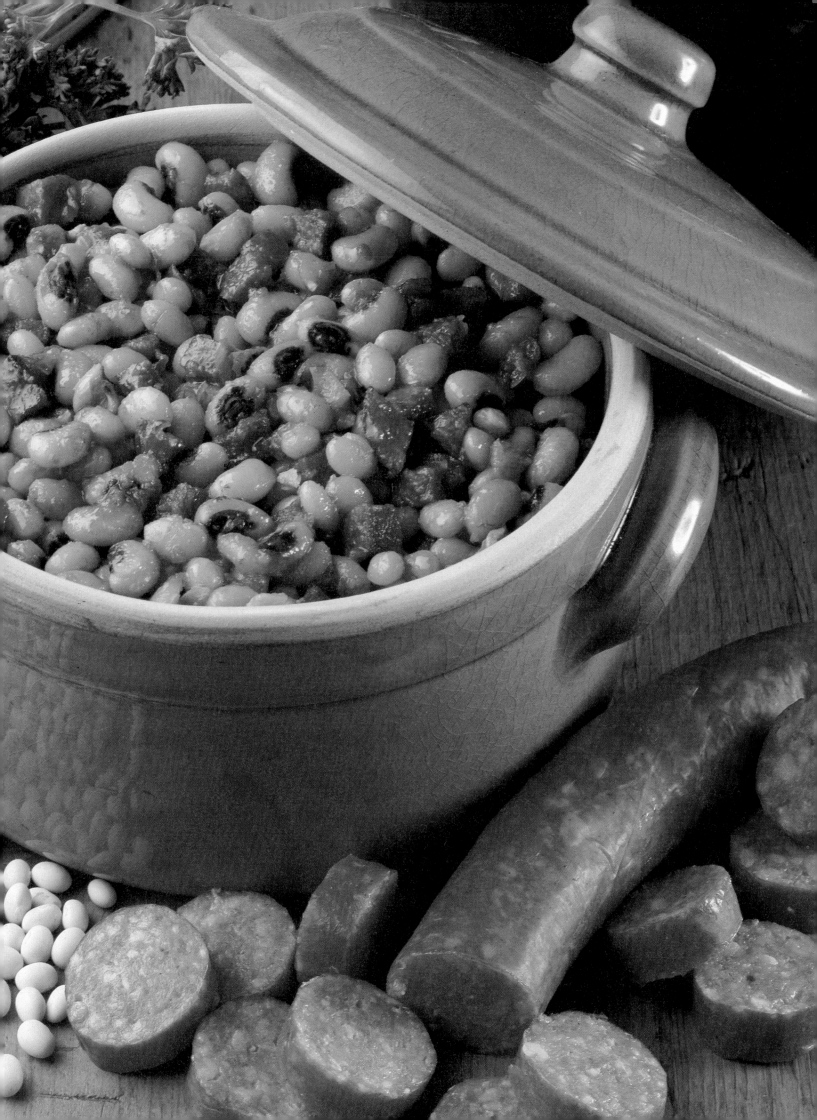

Party beanpot

(Illustrated opposite)

450 g/1 lb dried cannellini beans
900 ml/1½ pints (U.S. 3¾ cups) water
2 medium-sized onions, peeled and chopped
2 teaspoons dried mixed herbs
1 teaspoon dried rosemary
salt and freshly ground black pepper
2 (300-g/10.6-oz) cans condensed cream of tomato
soup
225 g/8 oz rashers streaky bacon (U.S. ½ lb bacon
slices), rind removed and chopped
225 g/8 oz pork sausages (U.S. ½ lb pork links),
halved
450 g/1 lb (U.S. 4 cups) diced cooked chicken
100 g/4 oz (U.S. ¼ lb) garlic sausage, thickly sliced
then chopped
4 stalks celery, sliced
450 g/1 lb frozen French beans (U.S. whole green
beans)
Topping
75 g/3 oz (U.S. ⅓ cup) butter or margarine
100 g/4 oz fresh wholemeal breadcrumbs (U.S. 2
cups fresh wholewheat bread crumbs)
50 g/2 oz (U.S. ½ cup) grated Cheddar cheese
1 teaspoon dry mustard powder

Put the beans in a large bowl and pour over boiling water to cover them well. Leave to soak overnight.

Heat the oven to 190°C/375°F, Gas Mark 5 and grease a large ovenproof casserole.

Drain the beans and place in the prepared dish with the water, onion, herbs and a little seasoning. Mix in the soup, cover and cook for 1 hour. Remove the dish from the oven and stir in the bacon, sausages, chicken, garlic sausage, celery and green beans. Return to the oven for 15 minutes.

Meanwhile, make the topping. Melt the butter in a pan and fry the breadcrumbs over moderate heat, stirring, for 3 minutes. Mix in the cheese and mustard powder and spoon over the ingredients in the casserole. Return to the oven, uncovered, for 30 minutes, or until the topping is crisp and golden. Serve hot with salad. **Serves 8**

Haricot lamb

(Illustrated opposite)

225 g/8 oz dried haricot beans (U.S. ½ lb dried navy
beans)
1 tablespoon oil
4 large chump chops (U.S. 4 sirloin lamb chops)
2 medium-sized onions, sliced
1 clove garlic, crushed
1 teaspoon dried rosemary
1 (300-g/10.6-oz) can condensed cream of tomato
soup
300 ml/½ pint (U.S. 1¼ cups) water
salt and freshly ground black pepper
finely grated rind and chopped flesh of 2 oranges
large sprig of parsley to garnish

Put the beans in a bowl and pour over warm water to cover them well. Leave to soak for at least 2 hours. Drain.

Heat the oil in a large heavy pan and fry the chops until browned on both sides. Remove the chops. Add the onion and garlic to the fat remaining in the pan and fry gently until just turning golden. Return the chops to the pan, add the rosemary, soup, water, beans and a little seasoning and mix really well.

Bring to the boil, stirring, cover and simmer for 1¼ hours, or until the meat is tender and the beans soft. Stir in the orange flesh and half the rind and adjust the seasoning if necessary. Cover again and cook for a further 10 minutes.

Transfer to a warm serving dish, sprinkle with the remaining rind and add the parsley sprig. **Serves 4**

Variation

Fruity beef stew Use 4 (100-g/4-oz) pieces of braising steak (U.S. chuck steak) instead of the lamb chops and substitute a can of condensed celery soup for the tomato soup. When the meat and beans are tender, stir in the drained fruit from a 225-g/8-oz can of pineapple chunks.

Above: Party beanpot. Below: Haricot lamb

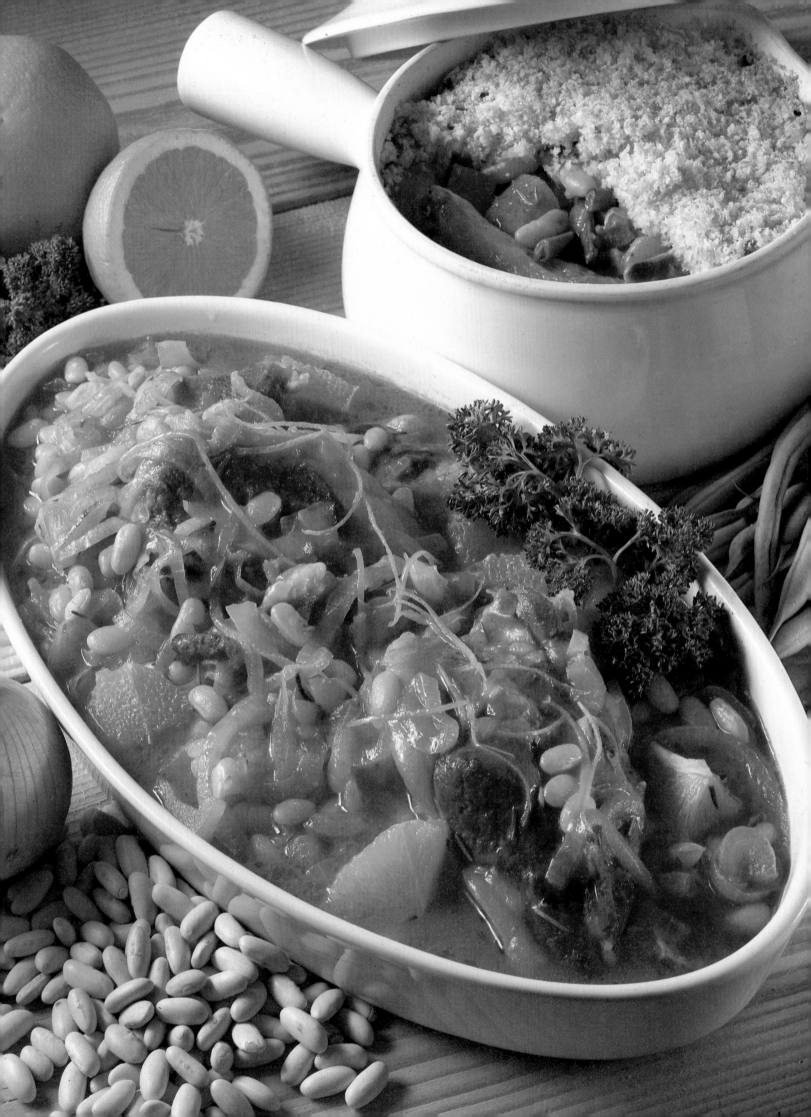

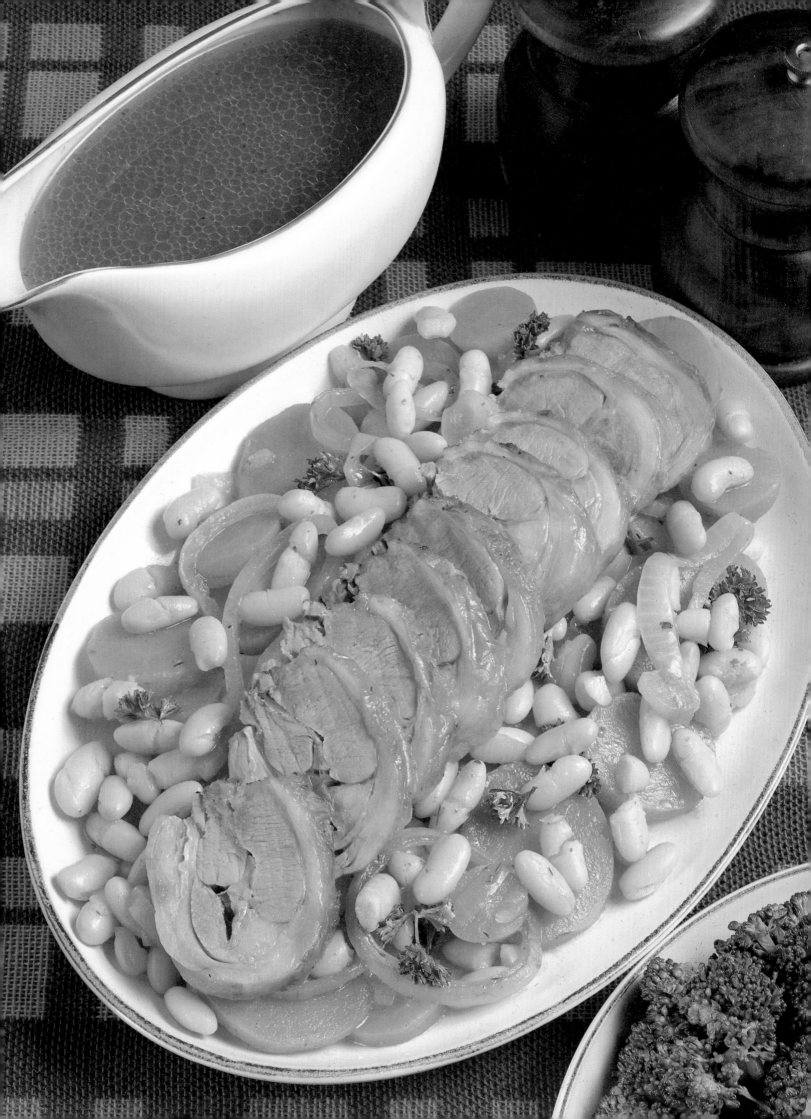

Duckling with green pea sauce

1 (2.3-kg/5-lb) duckling, completely defrosted
salt
600 ml/1 pint (U.S. 2½ cups) water
Sauce
25 g/1 oz (U.S. ¼ cup) flour
225 g/8 oz frozen peas (U.S. ½ lb green peas)
4 lettuce leaves, finely shredded
1 bouquet garni
large sprig of mint
1 teaspoon lemon juice
large pinch of ground nutmeg
2 tablespoons double cream (U.S. 3 tablespoons heavy cream)
salt and freshly ground black pepper
sprigs of mint to garnish

Heat the oven to 200°C/400°F, Gas Mark 6. Remove the giblets from the duck and dry it inside and out with absorbent kitchen towel. Prick the skin all over with a fork and sprinkle it with salt. Place on a rack over a roasting tin and cook for 1¾ hours. Meanwhile, put the giblets in a pan with the water. Bring to the boil and simmer for 45 minutes.

Drain the fat and juices from the roasting tin into a bowl and return the duck to the oven for a further 45 minutes. Take 2 tablespoons (U.S. 3 tablespoons) of the duck fat to make the sauce and place in a pan. Stir in the flour. Cook for 1 minute, stirring. Gradually add 450 ml/15 fl oz (U.S. scant 2 cups) of the strained giblet stock and bring to the boil, stirring constantly. Put in the peas, lettuce, bouquet garni, mint, lemon juice and nutmeg. Bring to the boil again, then simmer for 20 minutes. Liquidize in a blender or food processor and return to the rinsed pan. Stir in the cream, season to taste and reheat to boiling point. Keep hot.

Test that the duck is ready by piercing the thickest part of the thigh with a pointed knife. The juices which run should be clear with no hint of pinkness. Place the duck on a warm platter garnished with mint. Serve with boiled new potatoes and hand the sauce separately. **Serves 4**

Roast lamb with vegetable braise

(Illustrated opposite)

little lard or oil for frying
1 loin of lamb, boned and rolled (plus the bones)
2 large onions, peeled and sliced
2 large carrots, peeled and sliced
2 large sprigs of parsley
1 bay leaf
1 clove garlic
750 ml/1¼ pints (U.S. 3 cups) boiling water
1 lamb or beef stock cube (U.S. lamb or beef bouillon cube), crumbled
1 tablespoon tomato purée (U.S. paste)
1 teaspoon mixed dried herbs
150 ml/¼ pint (U.S. ⅔ cup) white wine
salt and freshly ground black pepper
1 (425-g/15-oz) can cannellini beans, drained

Heat the oven to 180°C/350°F, Gas Mark 4.

Grease a large frying pan (U.S. skillet) or strong roasting tin and seal the joint on all sides over moderately high heat. Remove the joint and add the bones, onion and carrot to the fat remaining in the pan. Add a little extra fat or oil if necessary. Fry, stirring frequently, until the onion is golden.

Arrange the joint in a roasting tin with the vegetables and bones around it. Reserve a few tiny parsley sprigs and add the rest to the tin with the bay leaf and unpeeled garlic. Mix together the water, stock cube, tomato purée, herbs and wine. Season lightly and pour into the tin. Cover with foil and cook for 1½ hours, turning the joint and basting the ingredients every 30 minutes.

Discard the bones and garlic clove. Stir the beans into the vegetable mixture and adjust the seasoning if necessary. Return the roasting tin to the oven, uncovered, for a further 30 minutes.

Slice the lamb and serve on a warm dish surrounded by the beans and vegetables. Sprinkle with the reserved parsley sprigs and hand the unthickened sauce separately in a jug. **Serves 6**

Roast lamb with vegetable braise

Fruited roast chicken

(Illustrated opposite)

75 g/3 oz dry wholemeal breadcrumbs (U.S. 1 cup
dry wholewheat bread crumbs)
6 spring onions (U.S. scallions), trimmed
and chopped
1 green pepper, seeds removed and chopped
15 g/½ oz (U.S. 1 tablespoon) butter or margarine,
melted
450 ml/¾ pint chicken stock (U.S. 2 cups chicken
bouillon)
1 (1.8-kg/4-lb) roasting chicken, fully defrosted
3 tablespoons (U.S. 4 tablespoons) clear honey
salt and freshly ground black pepper
1 teaspoon sweet paprika pepper
1 tablespoon cornflour (U.S. cornstarch)
finely grated rind and juice of 2 oranges
1 teaspoon horseradish sauce
Garnish
large sprig of watercress
1 lime or lemon, sliced

Heat the oven to 180°C/350°F, Gas Mark 4 and
grease a roasting tin.

First make the stuffing. Mix together the breadcrumbs, one third of the onion and a quarter of the
green pepper. Stir in the butter and about 150 ml/¼
pint (U.S. ⅔ cup) of the stock. Use to stuff the
chicken. Place it in the prepared tin. Combine the
honey, 1 teaspoon of salt and the paprika. Brush this
generously over the chicken. Roast for 2 hours,
basting frequently.

After 1½ hours, make the sauce. Moisten the
cornflour with a little orange juice. Put the remainder
in a pan with the rest of the stock, onion and green
pepper. Add the horseradish and orange rind, stir in
the cornflour mixture and bring to the boil, stirring
constantly. Simmer for 15 minutes, season to taste
and keep hot.

Check the chicken to make sure it is cooked by
piercing the thickest part of the thigh with a pointed
knife. The juices which run should be clear, with no
hint of pinkness. Place the chicken on a warm serving
dish and garnish with the watercress and lime or
lemon slices. Stir the pan juices into the sauce and
transfer to a serving boat. Serve the chicken with
oven-cooked carrots and hand the sauce separately.
Serves 6

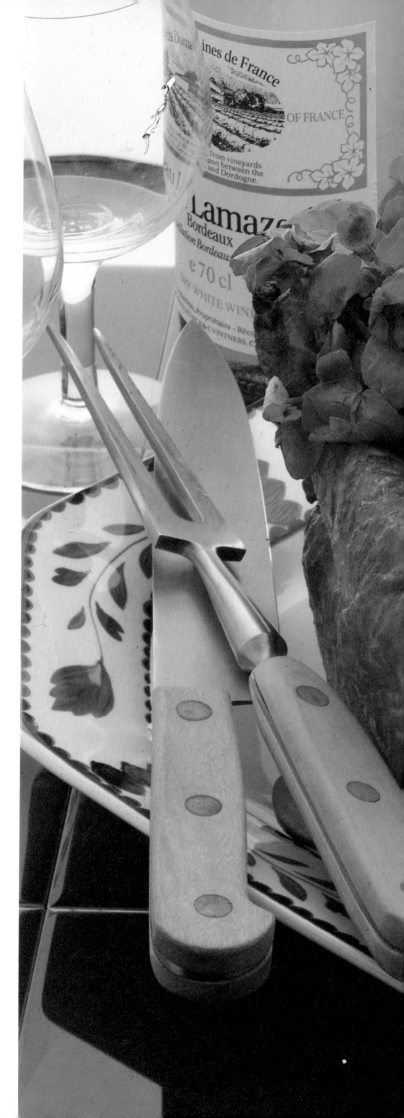

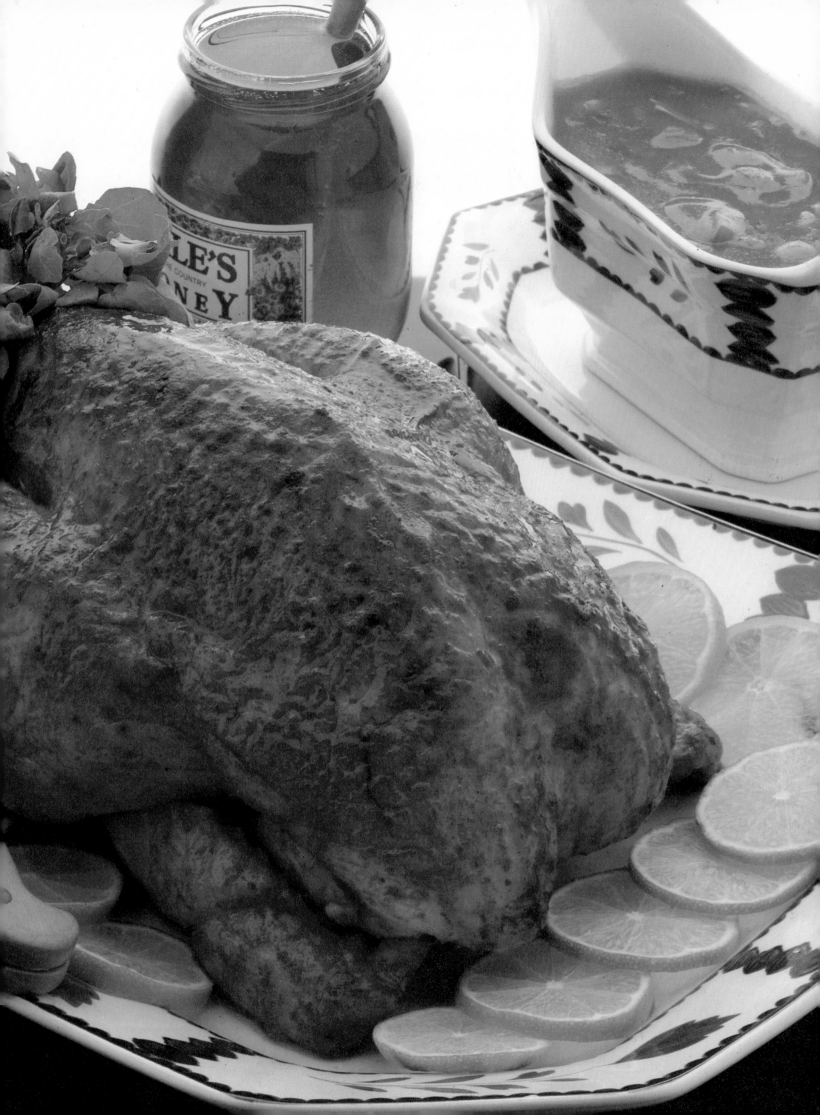

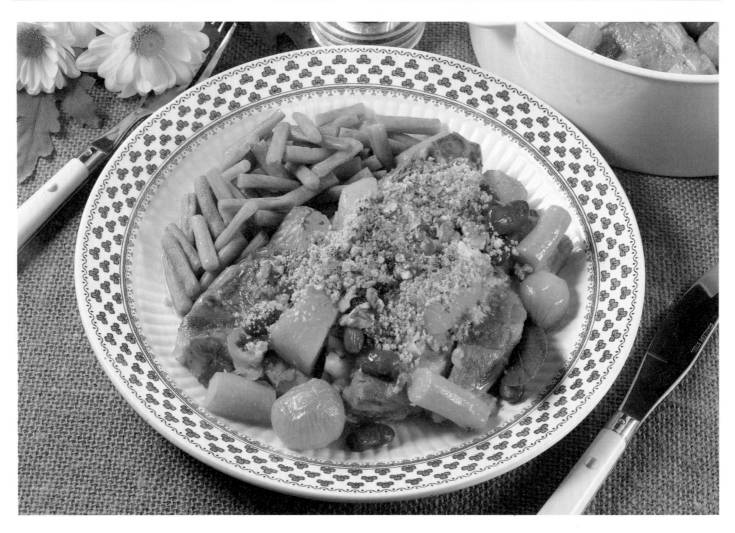

Tipsy lamb hotpot

(Illustrated above)

900 g/2 lb middle neck of lamb slices (U.S. lamb neck
slices)
12 pickling onions (U.S. tiny onions), peeled
2 medium-sized carrots, peeled and cut into chunks
225 g/8 oz swede (U.S. $\frac{1}{2}$ lb rutabaga), peeled and
diced
1 medium-sized potato, peeled and diced
2 bay leaves
300 ml/$\frac{1}{2}$ pint brown ale (U.S. $1\frac{1}{4}$ cups strong beer)
300 ml/$\frac{1}{2}$ pint lamb or chicken stock (U.S. $1\frac{1}{4}$ cups
lamb or chicken bouillon)
salt and freshly ground black pepper
1 (425-g/15-oz) can haricot or red kidney beans
Topping
50 g/2 oz fresh wholemeal breadcrumbs (U.S. 1 cup
fresh wholewheat bread crumbs)
2 tablespoons (U.S. 3 tablespoons) chopped parsley
25 g/1 oz (U.S. $\frac{1}{4}$ cup) chopped walnuts

Heat the oven to 160°C/325°F, Gas Mark 3.
    Place the lamb, onions, carrots, swede, potato and
bay leaves in a large pan. Add the ale, stock and a
little seasoning. Bring to the boil and skim any fat
from the surface. Transfer the mixture to a large
ovenproof dish and cover tightly.
    Cook in the oven for $1\frac{3}{4}$ hours, or until the lamb is
tender. Stir in the beans and liquid from the can.
Combine all the ingredients for the topping and
sprinkle over the hotpot. Return the hotpot to the
oven, uncovered, and cook for a further 30 minutes,
or until the top is crisp and golden. **Serves 4-6**

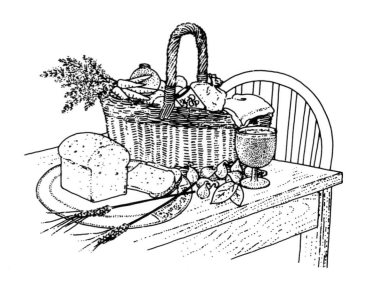

74

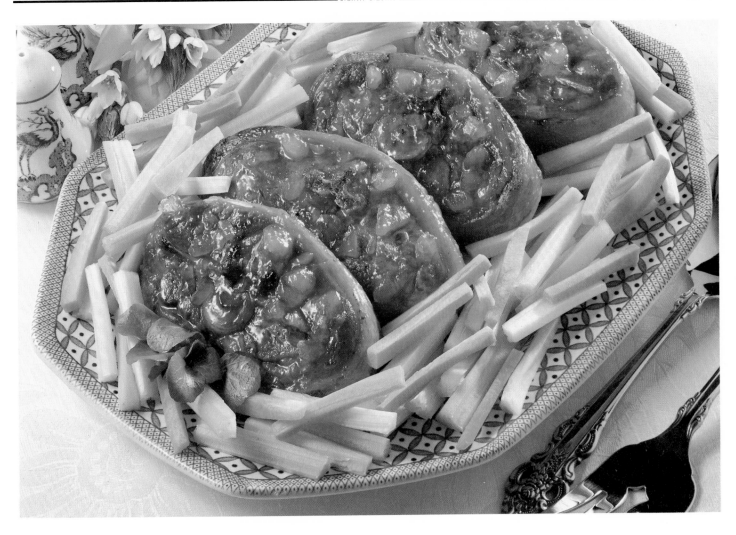

Gingery butterfly chops

(Illustrated above)

4 double loin or 'butterfly' lamb chops
salt and freshly ground black pepper
4 tablespoons (U.S. 6 tablespoons) ginger marmalade
or ginger preserve
Garnish
cucumber sticks
carrot sticks
sprigs of watercress

Trim the chops if necessary and season them lightly all over. Line a grill pan (U.S. broiler pan) with foil and put in the chops. Cook under moderate heat until just sealed. Turn and seal the second side.

Spread half the marmalade on the chops and cook for about 7 minutes, or until well browned and crispy round the edges. Turn the chops again, cover with the remaining marmalade and cook on for a further 5–7 minutes, or until again brown, crispy and cooked through.

Arrange the chops on a warm serving dish. Skim any fat from the pan juices and spoon the juices over the chops. Serve with a garnish of cucumber and carrot sticks and watercress sprigs. **Serves 4**

Variation

Butterfly chops with barbecue sauce Omit the marmalade and grill (U.S. broil) the chops plain for about 6 minutes on each side, or until cooked through. Meanwhile, peel and finely chop 1 large onion. Cook in 1 tablespoon oil in a pan until soft. Add 1 tablespoon tomato purée (U.S. tomato paste), 2 tablespoons (U.S. 3 tablespoons) brown sugar, 1 tablespoon wine vinegar, few drops of Tabasco pepper sauce and 2 teaspoons cornflour (U.S. 1 tablespoon cornstarch) blended with 150 ml/$\frac{1}{4}$ pint (U.S. $\frac{2}{3}$ cup) water. Bring to the boil, stirring constantly. Simmer for 3 minutes. Serve the chops on a bed of lightly cooked spinach and hand the sauce separately.

Turkey roast with plum sauce

675 g/1½ lb medium-sized parsnips, peeled
and quartered
1 turkey breast roll roast (about 550 g/1¼ lb), fully
defrosted
1 (550-g/20-oz) can red plums in syrup
50 g/2 oz (U.S. ¼ cup) margarine, melted
2 medium-sized cooking apples, peeled, cored and
quartered
1 tablespoon cornflour (U.S. cornstarch)
about 150 ml/¼ pint (U.S. ⅔ cup) apple juice
salt and freshly ground black pepper

Heat the oven to 180°C/350°F, Gas Mark 4 and grease a roasting tin.

Parboil the parsnips in a pan of boiling salted water for 3 minutes, then drain. Place the turkey in the centre of the prepared tin and surround with the parsnips. Drain the syrup from the plums into the margarine and mix well. Use this mixture to brush the turkey and parsnips. Cook in the oven for 30 minutes.

Add the apple to the parsnips and brush all the ingredients with the syrup mixture. Return the tin to the oven for a further 50 minutes, basting twice more with syrup mixture during this time, or until the turkey is cooked through.

Slice the turkey and arrange on a warm serving dish surrounded by the parsnips and apples. Keep hot.

Stir up the juices in the roasting tin and mix in any remaining baste. Stone (U.S. pit) the plums and purée the fruit. Blend the cornflour with the apple juice and add to the roasting tin with the plum purée. Stir constantly until the mixture comes to the boil then simmer for 3 minutes, adding extra apple juice if the sauce is too thick to pour easily. Season to taste, spoon a little sauce over the turkey on the dish and hand the rest separately in a jug. **Serves 4**

Note Fresh plums cooked in a little water with brown sugar can be substituted for the canned plums and syrup.

Braised lamb with fennel

(Illustrated opposite)

1 tablespoon oil
1 (1-kg/2-lb) half leg or shoulder of lamb
2 medium-sized carrots, peeled and sliced
2 stalks celery, sliced
1 large onion, peeled and chopped
1 (425-g/15-oz) can tomatoes
1 teaspoon fennel seeds
salt and freshly ground black pepper
2 heads fennel, quartered
150 ml/¼ pint lamb or chicken stock (U.S. ⅔ cup lamb
or chicken bouillon)
15 g/½ oz (U.S. 1 tablespoon) margarine
1 tablespoon redcurrant jelly

Heat the oil in a large heavy-based pan or flameproof casserole and fry the lamb over moderate heat for about 10 minutes, turning the joint occasionally, until browned on all sides. Remove the meat from the pan.

Add the carrots, celery and onion to the fat remaining in the pan and fry over moderate heat for 5 minutes, or until turning golden. Put in the tomatoes and liquid from the can, the fennel seeds and a little seasoning. Bring to the boil, return the lamb to the pan, cover tightly and simmer for 1½ hours, or until the lamb is tender.

Meanwhile, put the fennel quarters in a pan, pour the stock over and add the margarine. Bring to the boil, cover and cook for about 15 minutes, or until the fennel is just tender.

Transfer the lamb to a warm serving dish. Drain the fennel, reserving the cooking stock, and arrange the vegetable on the dish with the meat. Keep hot. Liquidize the tomato mixture or press through a sieve and return to the rinsed pan. Add the redcurrant jelly and heat the sauce, stirring briskly, until the jelly has dissolved. A little of the reserved fennel stock may be added if wished, to thin the sauce slightly. Adjust the seasoning, spoon a little sauce over the meat and hand the remainder separately in a sauce boat. **Serves 4-6**

Braised lamb with fennel

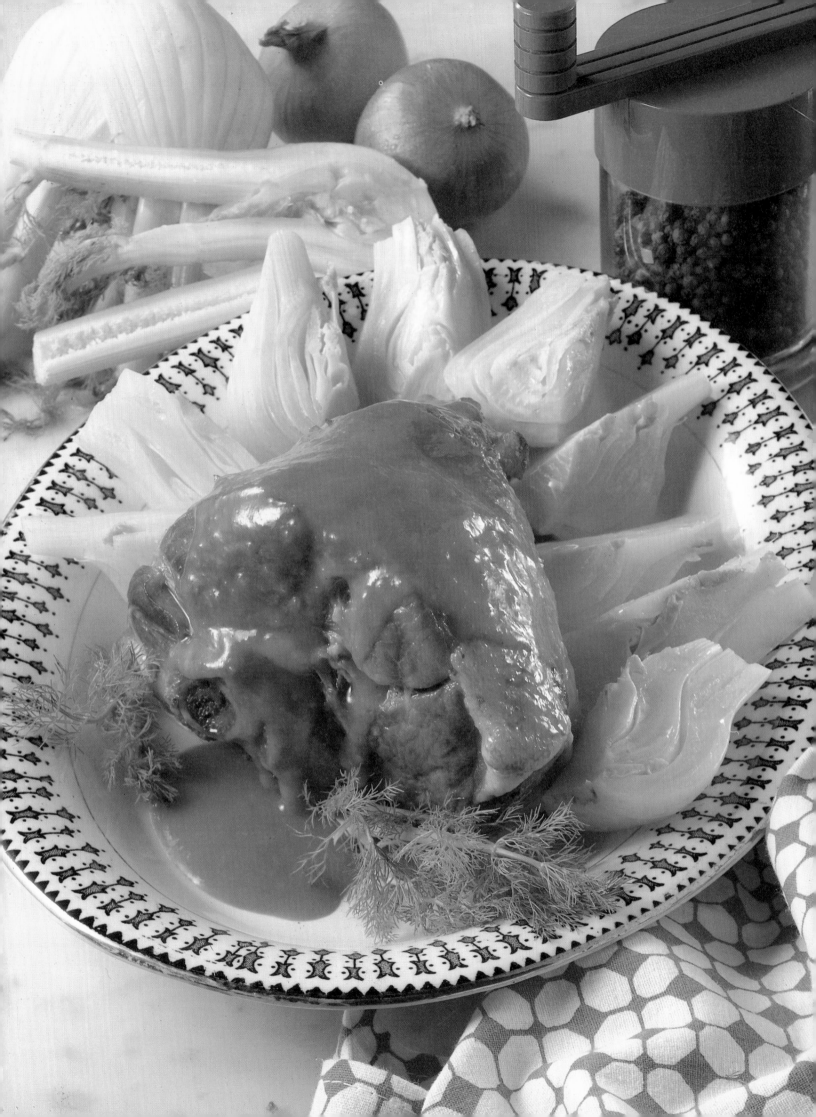

Crispy coated stuffed veal

(Illustrated opposite)

1 (1-kg/2¼-lb) shoulder of veal, boned
1 (213-g/7½-oz) can butter beans (U.S. lima beans),
drained
1 medium-sized onion, peeled and chopped
finely grated rind and juice of 1 lemon
2 tablespoons (U.S. 3 tablespoons) chopped fresh
herbs (such as parsley, chives, marjoram, mint)
2 cloves garlic, finely chopped
1 teaspoon ground ginger
salt and freshly ground black pepper
little oil
75 g/3 oz fresh wholemeal breadcrumbs (U.S. 1½
cups fresh wholewheat bread crumbs)
Garnish
lemon wedges
sprig of parsley

Heat the oven to 200°C/400°F, Gas Mark 6.
Lightly score the skin of the joint. Mix together the
beans, onion, lemon rind and juice, herbs, garlic,
ginger and a little seasoning. Pack inside the joint
then stand this in a roasting tin. Rub the skin with oil,
sprinkle with seasoning and press on the breadcrumbs.
Roast for 1 hour and 10 minutes. Transfer to a
warm serving dish and garnish with lemon wedges
and parsley sprig. Serve with lightly sautéed slices of
courgette (U.S. zucchini). **Serves 4-5**

Variations

Stuffed lamb roast Substitute a boned shoulder of
lamb for the veal, use a drained 225-g/8-oz can of
garden peas (U.S. green peas) in place of the beans,
and the rind and juice of 1 small orange instead of the
lemon. Cover with the breadcrumb coating and place
in the tin. Surround the joint with parboiled medium-
sized onions and potatoes, brushing them well with
oil, and roast for 1½ hours.

Sausage and bean bake Substitute 450 g/1 lb pork
sausages (U.S. pork links) for the veal. Brown the
sausages in a frying pan then place in an ovenproof
dish with the stuffing ingredients. Sprinkle with the
breadcrumbs and bake as above for 45 minutes, or
until brown.

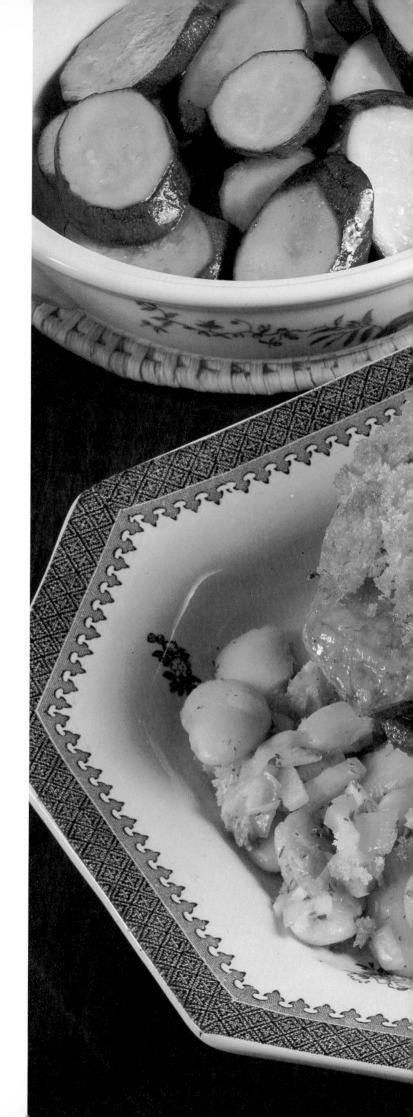

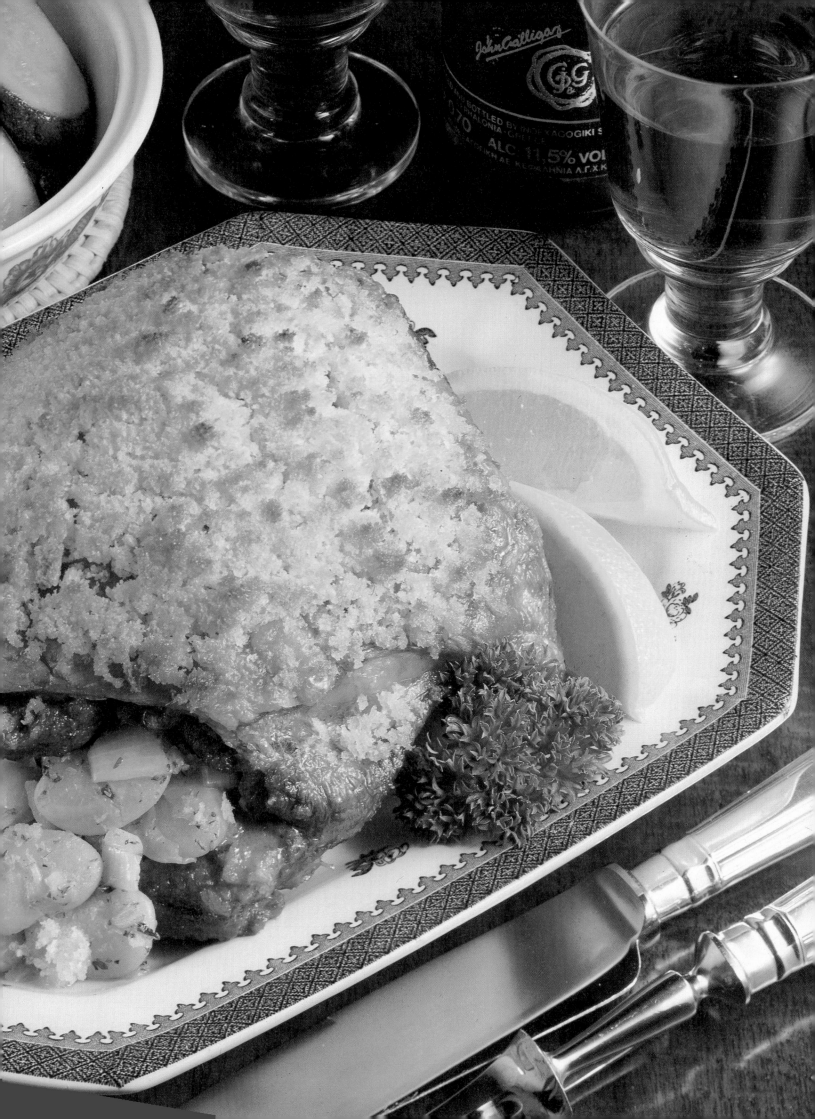

Almond-coated plaice

175 g/6 oz (U.S. generous $\frac{3}{4}$ cup) long grain brown
rice
1 egg, beaten
1 teaspoon water
100 g/4 oz (U.S. 1 cup) ground almonds
40 g/1$\frac{1}{2}$ oz dried wholemeal breadcrumbs
(U.S. $\frac{1}{2}$ cup dried wholewheat bread crumbs)
salt and freshly ground black pepper
8 (75-g/3-oz) plaice fillets (U.S. flounder fillets),
skinned
2 tablespoon (U.S. 3 tablespoons) oil
50 g/2 oz (U.S. $\frac{1}{4}$ cup) margarine
1 (198-g/7-oz) can corn kernels
about 100 ml/4 fl oz (U.S. $\frac{1}{2}$ cup) mayonnaise

Cook the rice in a pan of boiling salted water for 25
minutes, or until tender.

Meanwhile, mix together the egg and water in a
shallow dish and combine the almonds and breadcrumbs on a plate. Season the fish fillets, dip them in
egg, then coat all over in the almond mixture. Heat
the oil with half the margarine in a large frying pan
(U.S. skillet) and fry half the fish fillets briskly for
about 3 minutes on each side, until golden brown and
crisp. Drain on absorbent kitchen towel, arrange on a
serving dish and keep hot. Add the rest of the
margarine to the pan and cook the remainder of the
fish. Add to the dish.

Stir the corn into the rice in the pan and leave for 3
minutes. Drain well and transfer to a warm dish.
Serve hot with the fish and offer the mayonnaise
separately. **Serves 4**

Chicken schnitzel
with caper topping

4 boneless chicken breasts (about 450 g/1 lb total
weight)
salt and freshly ground black pepper
1 egg, beaten
finely grated rind and juice of $\frac{1}{2}$ lemon
about 175 g/6 oz fresh wholemeal breadcrumbs (U.S.
3 cups fresh wholewheat bread crumbs)
oil for shallow frying
Topping
50 g/2 oz (U.S. $\frac{1}{4}$ cup) margarine
finely grated rind and juice of $\frac{1}{2}$ lemon
1 tablespoon drained capers

Place the chicken breasts between sheets of greaseproof paper (U.S. waxed paper) and beat with a
rolling pin until evenly flat and twice the original size.
Try not to tear the slices. Season well.

Put the egg and lemon juice in a shallow dish and
the breadcrumbs and lemon rind on a plate. Carefully
dip the chicken slices in the egg, then coat them all
over in the breadcrumb mixture, making sure they
are completely covered. Place on a greased baking
sheet (U.S. cookie sheet) and chill for 10 minutes.

To make the topping, cream the margarine until
soft and gradually beat in the lemon rind and juice.
Stir in the capers. Transfer to a small serving dish and
swirl the top with a fork. Chill until required.

Heat a little oil in a large frying pan (U.S. skillet)
and cook the schnitzels, two at a time, for about 4
minutes on each side, until crisp and golden brown.
Keep hot until all are cooked. Serve very hot with
Brussels sprouts and hand the caper topping separately. **Serves 4**

Pork with rice
and peppers

3 tablespoons (U.S. 4 tablespoons) oil
1 large onion, peeled and sliced
350 g/12 oz (U.S. $\frac{3}{4}$ lb) boneless lean pork, cubed
200 g/7 oz (U.S. 1 cup) long grain brown rice
600 ml/1 pint chicken or lamb stock (U.S. 2$\frac{1}{2}$ cups
chicken or lamb bouillon)
salt and freshly ground black pepper
1 red pepper, seeds removed and cut into strips
1 green pepper, seeds removed and cut into strips
8 black olives, halved and stoned
(U.S. 8 ripe olives, halved and pitted)
1 tablespoon snipped chives to garnish

Heat the oven to 180°C/350°F, Gas Mark 4 and have
ready an ovenproof casserole.

Heat the oil in a large pan and gently cook the
onion until soft. Put in the pork and fry, stirring,
until sealed on all sides. Sprinkle in the rice and cook,
stirring gently now and then, for 3 minutes. Transfer
to the casserole. Pour the stock into the pan and heat
to boiling point. Add seasoning if necessary, then
pour into the casserole and stir well. Cover and cook
for 30 minutes.

Meanwhile, blanch the pepper strips in boiling
water for 2 minutes. Drain and stir into the pork
mixture with the olives. Cover the dish again and
return to the oven for a further 15 minutes, or until
the rice is tender and the liquid almost absorbed. Fluff
up the ingredients with a fork and serve hot,
sprinkled with chives. **Serves 4**

Stuffed pork chops

25 g/1 oz (U.S. 2 tablespoons) margarine
1 small cooking apple, peeled, cored and finely
chopped
1 small red or green pepper, seeds removed and finely
chopped
1 small onion, peeled and finely chopped
salt and freshly ground black pepper
4 thick pork chops
2 tablespoons (U.S. 3 tablespoons) oil
1 (425-g/15-oz) can baked beans in tomato sauce

Heat the oven to 180°C/350°F, Gas Mark 4 and grease a shallow ovenproof dish.

Melt the margarine in a frying pan (U.S. skillet) and fry the apple, pepper and onion over moderate heat, stirring occasionally, for 4 minutes. Season to taste.

Using a small sharp knife, remove the rind from the chops, then cut a 'pocket' in each one by slitting from the fat side in towards the bone. Fill the pockets with the apple mixture.

Heat the oil in the same pan and fry the chops over high heat until brown on both sides. Pour the beans into the prepared dish and arrange the chops on top. Cover and cook for 45 minutes. Remove the lid and return to the oven for a further 5 minutes. **Serves 4**

Beef and bean goulash

(Illustrated on the cover)

2 tablespoons (U.S. 3 tablespoons) oil
1 large onion, peeled and sliced
675 g/1½ lb lean stewing beef, cubed
25 g/1 oz wholemeal flour (U.S. ¼ cup wholewheat
flour)
4 teaspoons (U.S. 2 tablespoons) sweet paprika
pepper
½ teaspoon ground allspice
salt and freshly ground black pepper
1 (425-g/15-oz) can tomatoes, sieved
2 teaspoons tomato purée (U.S. 1 tablespoon tomato
paste)
1 beef stock cube (U.S. 1 beef bouillon cube),
crumbled
150 ml/¼ pint (U.S. ⅔ cup) water
1 (425-g/15-oz) can flageolet or borlotti beans
(U.S. fava or pinto beans), drained

Heat the oil and fry the onion gently until beginning to soften. Coat the beef with flour, add to the pan and fry over moderate heat, turning the cubes frequently, until golden on all sides.

Sprinkle in any remaining flour, the paprika, allspice and a little seasoning. Stir well. Add the tomato pulp, purée, stock cube and water and bring to the boil, stirring constantly. Cover and simmer for 1½ hours, stirring occasionally, or until the beef is tender.

Adjust the seasoning if necessary, stir in the beans and cook for a further 3 minutes. **Serves 4-6**

Beef stew with savoury dumplings

4 tablespoons wholemeal flour (U.S. 6 tablespoons
wholewheat flour)
salt and freshly ground black pepper
675 g/1½ lb braising steak (U.S. chuck steak), cubed
40 g/1½ oz (U.S. 3 tablespoons) margarine
300 ml/½ pint (U.S. 1¼ cups) beef stock (U.S. beef
bouillon)
4 medium-sized carrots, peeled and sliced
3 stalks celery, sliced
8 baby onions, peeled
1 tablespoon chopped parsley to garnish
Dumplings
100 g/4 oz wholemeal flour (U.S. 1 cup wholewheat
flour)
¼ teaspoon salt
½ teaspoon dry mustard powder
50 g/2 oz (U.S. ½ cup) shredded beef suet
2 tablespoons (U.S. 3 tablespoons) finely snipped
chives
2 tablespoons (U.S. 3 tablespoons) finely chopped
parsley
5 tablespoons (U.S. 7 tablespoons) water

Heat the oven to 160°C/325°F, Gas Mark 3.

Season the flour and use to coat the meat. Melt the margarine in a flameproof casserole and fry the meat cubes until brown on all sides. Stir in any remaining seasoned flour. Gradually add the stock and bring to the boil, stirring constantly. Put in the carrot, celery and onions, stir well, cover the dish and place in the oven for 2 hours.

Meanwhile, make the dumplings. Mix together the flour, salt, mustard, suet, chives and parsley in a bowl. Add the water to make a soft dough. Pat out on a floured surface, divide into 8 equal portions and shape each into a ball with floured hands.

Adjust the seasoning in the casserole, arrange the dumplings on top, cover the dish again and return to the oven for a further 15 minutes. Sprinkle with chopped parsley before serving from the dish. **Serves 4**

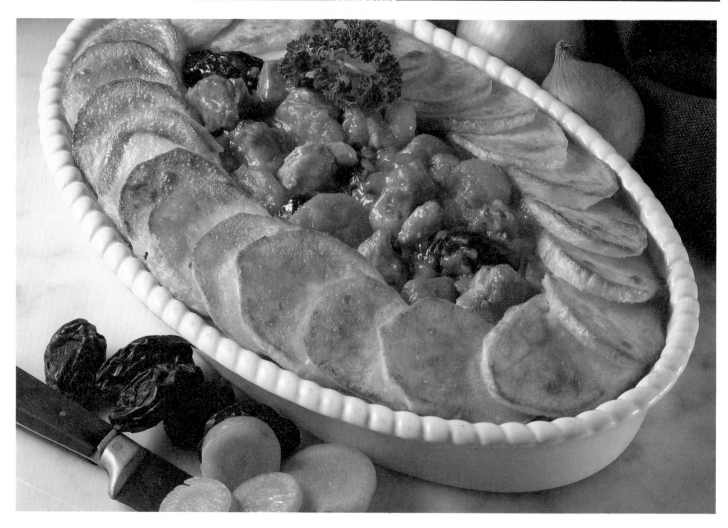

Pork and prune pie

(Illustrated above)

450 g/1 lb lean pork, cubed
1 large onion, peeled and sliced
2 large carrots, peeled and sliced
300 ml/½ pint stock (U.S. 1¼ cups bouillon)
salt and freshly ground black pepper
2 teaspoons cornflour (U.S. 1 tablespoon cornstarch)
2 medium-sized potatoes, peeled and thinly sliced
100 g/4 oz (U.S. ¼ lb) tender dried prunes, halved and stoned (U.S. pitted)
25 g/1 oz (U.S. 2 tablespoons) butter or margarine, melted
sprig of parsley to garnish

Heat the oven to 180°C/350°F, Gas Mark 4.

Arrange the pork, onion, carrot, stock and a little seasoning in an ovenproof dish. Cook for 1 hour, or until the meat is just tender. Adjust the seasoning if necessary. Moisten the cornflour with a little cold water, stir into the casserole and return to the oven for a further 10 minutes. Raise the oven temperature to 200°C/400°F, Gas Mark 6.

Put the potatoes in a pan with water to cover. Salt the water lightly, bring to the boil, cover and cook for 3 minutes. Drain well.

Transfer the meat mixture to an ovenproof pie dish and stir in the prunes. Arrange the potato slices, overlapping, round the top edge of the dish and brush with melted butter. Bake for about 30 minutes, or until the potato topping is golden brown. Garnish with the parsley sprig and serve hot. **Serves 4**

Variations

Pork and parsnip hotpot Use 1 large parsnip, peeled and diced, instead of the carrots and substitute 100 g/4 oz (U.S. ¼ lb) tender dried apricots for the prunes. Season the stock with a pinch of ground allspice before cooking the meat.

Beef cobbler Substitute cubed braising steak (U.S. chuck steak) for the pork. While the meat is cooking, make up a savoury cobbler topping (see page 145), omitting the sugar and coconut, and adding ½ teaspoon salt, ¼ teaspoon pepper and a pinch of mustard powder. Thicken the meat mixture and raise the oven heat. Arrange the cobbler in a ring on the meat and return the dish to the oven for 30 minutes, or until the topping is golden brown.

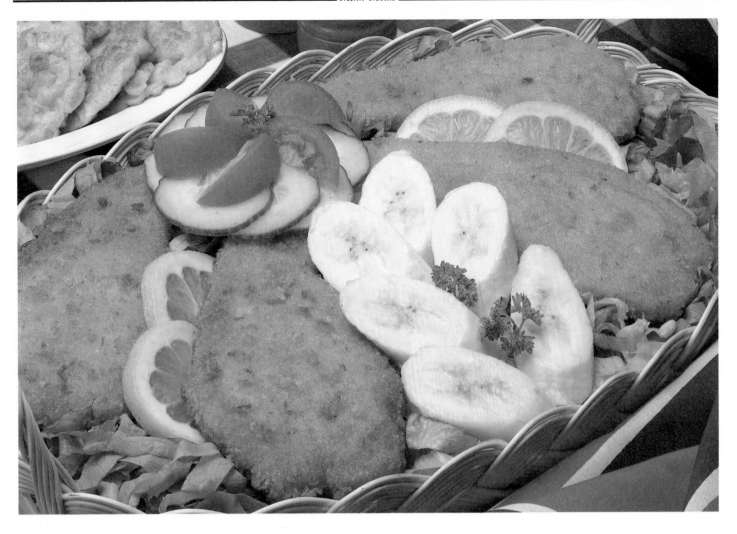

Danish Maryland

(Illustrated above)

4 bacon chops (U.S. thick slices Canadian bacon),
rind removed
wholemeal flour (U.S. wholewheat flour) for coating
1 egg, beaten
50 g/2 oz dried wholemeal breadcrumbs (U.S. $\frac{2}{3}$ cup
dried wholewheat bread crumbs)
50 g/2 oz (U.S. $\frac{1}{4}$ cup) butter
2 bananas, peeled
Fritters
100 g/4 oz wholemeal flour (U.S. 1 cup wholewheat
flour)
$\frac{1}{4}$ teaspoon salt
pinch of pepper
2 eggs
100 ml/4 fl oz (U.S. $\frac{1}{2}$ cup) milk
1 (340-g/12-oz) can corn kernels, drained
oil for shallow frying
Garnish
shredded lettuce
lemon slices
cucumber slices
tomato wedges
sprigs of parsley

Dust the chops with flour. Put the egg in a shallow bowl and the breadcrumbs on a plate. Dip the chops in egg and coat them all over in breadcrumbs, making sure they are completely covered. Chill.

Meanwhile, make the fritters. Put the flour, salt, pepper and eggs in a bowl. Add half the milk and whisk until the batter is smooth. Gradually whisk in the remaining milk and fold in the corn.

Heat a little oil in a frying pan (U.S. skillet) and make 8 fritters, using about 2 tablespoons (U.S. 3 tablespoons) mixture for each. Fry over moderately high heat for about 3 minutes on each side, or until cooked through and golden brown. Drain on absorbent kitchen towel, arrange on a heatproof plate and keep hot.

Add the butter to any oil remaining in the pan and fry the chops over moderately high heat for about 5 minutes on each side, until golden brown. Drain on absorbent kitchen towel.

Make a bed of shredded lettuce on a serving platter and top with the chops. Garnish with lemon and cucumber slices, tomato wedges and parsley sprigs. Cut the bananas into thick diagonal slices, add them to the platter and serve at once with the fritters.
Serves 4

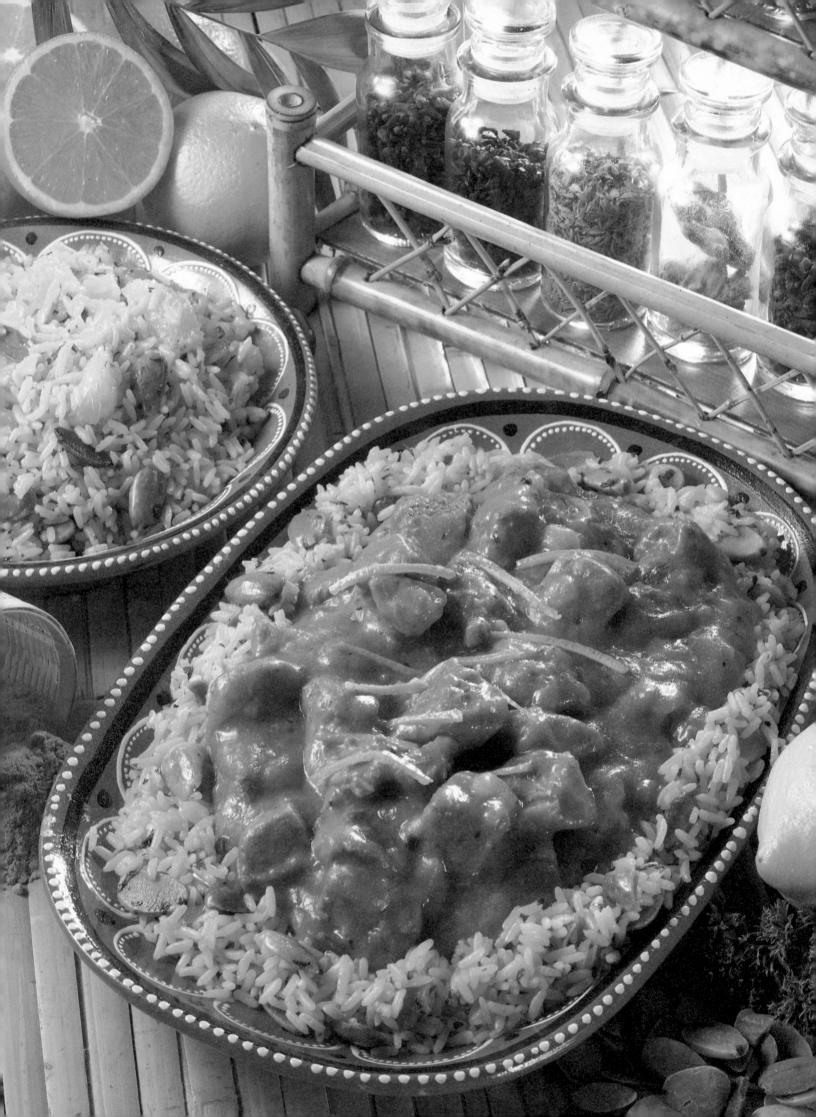

Spiced lamb casserole

(Illustrated opposite)

675 g/1½ lb lean boneless lamb, cut into 2.5-cm/1-inch cubes
¼ teaspoon ground ginger
2 tablespoons (U.S. 3 tablespoons) oil
1 large onion, peeled and sliced
1 tablespoon wholemeal flour (U.S. wholewheat flour)
1½ teaspoons (U.S. 2 teaspoons) ground coriander
1 tablespoon garam masala
1 teaspoon ground cumin
finely grated rind and juice of 1 lemon
finely grated rind and juice of 1 orange
salt
150 ml/¼ pint chicken stock (U.S. ⅔ cup chicken bouillon)
1 (225-g/8-oz) can tomatoes

Sprinkle the lamb cubes with ginger. Heat the oil in a large heavy pan and fry the lamb over moderately high heat until evenly brown on all sides. Remove with a slotted spoon and set aside.

Add the onion to the oil remaining in the pan and fry gently until soft. Return the meat, add the flour, spices, lemon rind, half the orange rind and a little salt. Stir really well and cook for 2 minutes. Pour in the stock, tomatoes and liquid from the can and the fruit juices. Bring to the boil, stirring constantly. Cover and simmer for about 1½ hours, or until the lamb is tender. Taste and add more salt if necessary.

Transfer to a warm dish and sprinkle with the remaining orange rind. Serve with Orange almond rice (see below). **Serves 4–5**

Orange almond rice

(Illustrated opposite)

1 orange
1 tablespoon oil
225 g/8 oz (U.S. generous 1 cup) long grain brown rice
600 ml/1 pint (U.S. 2½ cups) water
1 chicken stock cube (U.S. chicken bouillon cube), crumbled
½ teaspoon ground turmeric
salt and freshly ground black pepper
1 tablespoon blanched almonds, toasted

Grate the rind from the orange then divide the flesh into segments, discarding all pith, membranes and pips.

Spiced lamb casserole with Orange almond rice

Heat the oil in a pan and stir in the rice. Add the water, stock cube, turmeric and a little seasoning and bring to the boil. Stir once, cover and simmer for about 25 minutes, or until the rice is tender and has absorbed the liquid.

Adjust the seasoning and fork in the orange rind and segments and the almonds. Transfer to a warm serving dish, fluff up with a fork and serve hot. **Serves 4**

Crispy fish strips with herbed dip

150 ml/¼ pint (U.S. ⅔ cup) natural yogurt
150 ml/¼ pint (U.S. ⅔ cup) mayonnaise
7.5-cm/3-inch length cucumber, finely diced
4 tablespoons (U.S. 6 tablespoons) finely chopped fresh herbs (such as parsley, chives, marjoram, dill, fennel, mint)
450 g/1 lb plaice fillets (U.S. flounder fillets)
2 tablespoons wholemeal flour (U.S. 3 tablespoons wholewheat flour)
salt and freshly ground black pepper
1 egg
1 tablespoon water
100 g/4 oz fresh wholemeal breadcrumbs (U.S. 2 cups fresh wholewheat bread crumbs)
oil for deep frying
lemon wedges to garnish

Beat together the yogurt and mayonnaise, then fold in the cucumber and herbs. Transfer to a serving bowl and chill while cooking the fish.

Cut the large fillets of fish in half lengthways, then cut all fillets into 2-cm/¾-inch strips across the grain. Sprinkle the strips with the flour and a little seasoning, and toss lightly to coat. Beat together the egg and water and place in a shallow dish. Put the breadcrumbs in a plastic bag. Dip the fish strips, a few at a time, in the egg wash, then place in the crumbs, hold the bag closed and shake until the fish strips are coated. Remove the coated strips to a plate and repeat with the rest of the fish.

Heat oil to a temperature of 190°C/375°F or until cube of day-old bread turns golden brown in 40 seconds.

Deep fry the strips, in batches, for about 3 minutes, or until golden brown and crisp. Drain on absorbent kitchen towel and keep hot. When all the strips are cooked, transfer to a warm serving platter. Garnish with lemon wedges and stand the container of herbed dip in the centre. **Serves 4**

Herby bacon chops

(Illustrated opposite)

4 (100-g/4-oz) bacon chops (U.S. 4×¼-lb ½-inch
thick Canadian bacon slices)
50 g/2 oz dried wholemeal breadcrumbs (U.S. ⅔ cup
dried wholewheat bread crumbs)
½ teaspoon dried mixed herbs
1 egg, beaten
1 teaspoon water
wholemeal flour (U.S. wholewheat flour) for coating
50 g/2 oz (U.S. ¼ cup) butter

Trim the rind from the chops with scissors. Mix
together the breadcrumbs and herbs on a plate. Beat
the egg with the water in a shallow dish. Dust the
chops with flour, shaking off any excess. Dip each
one in the egg wash, then coat all over with
breadcrumbs.

Melt the butter in a large frying pan (U.S. skillet)
and fry the chops over moderate heat for about 5
minutes on each side, or until golden brown and
cooked through.

Transfer to a warm serving dish and garnish with
cucumber slices and wedges of lemon. These crispy-
coated bacon chops make a tasty hot meal with boiled
potatoes and mixed vegetables in a white sauce.
Serves 4

Oregon beef loaf

4 large slices wholemeal or granary bread
(U.S. wholewheat bread)
450 g/1 lb minced beef (U.S. ground beef)
100 g/4 oz (U.S. ¼ lb) button mushrooms, sliced
1 medium onion, peeled and chopped
1 teaspoon dried mixed herbs
1 tablespoon chopped parsley
1 tablespoon Worcestershire sauce
2 eggs, beaten
1 (296-g/10.5-oz) can condensed celery soup

Heat the oven to 160°C/325°F, Gas Mark 3 and line a
1-kg/2-lb loaf-shaped tin with greaseproof paper
(U.S. waxed paper).

Make the bread into breadcrumbs and mix with the
meat, mushrooms, onion, herbs, Worcestershire
sauce and eggs. When well blended, add the soup and
mix well. Transfer to the prepared tin and smooth the
top. Cover with foil, crimping it under rim of tin.

Bake for 2 hours. If required hot, leave the loaf in
the tin for 5 minutes, then turn out on a serving plate
and peel off the lining paper. If required to serve cold,
leave to cool completely in the tin then turn out,
remove the paper and chill well. **Serves 4**

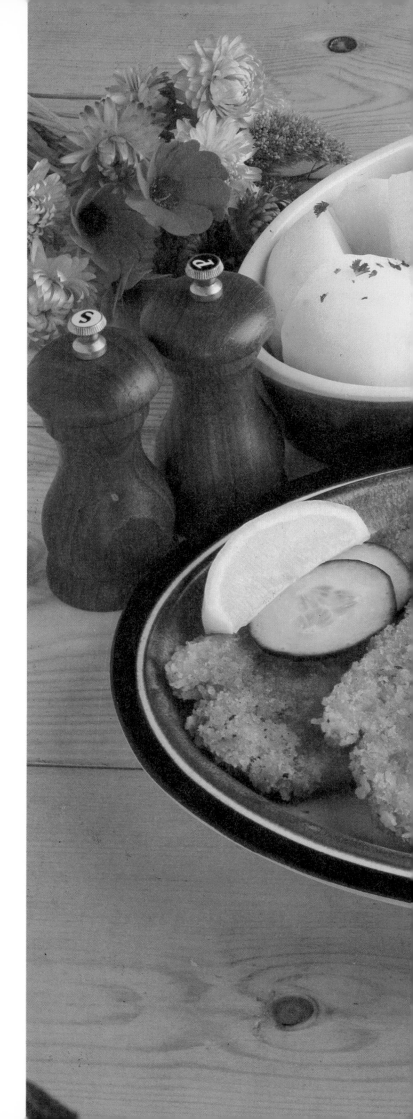

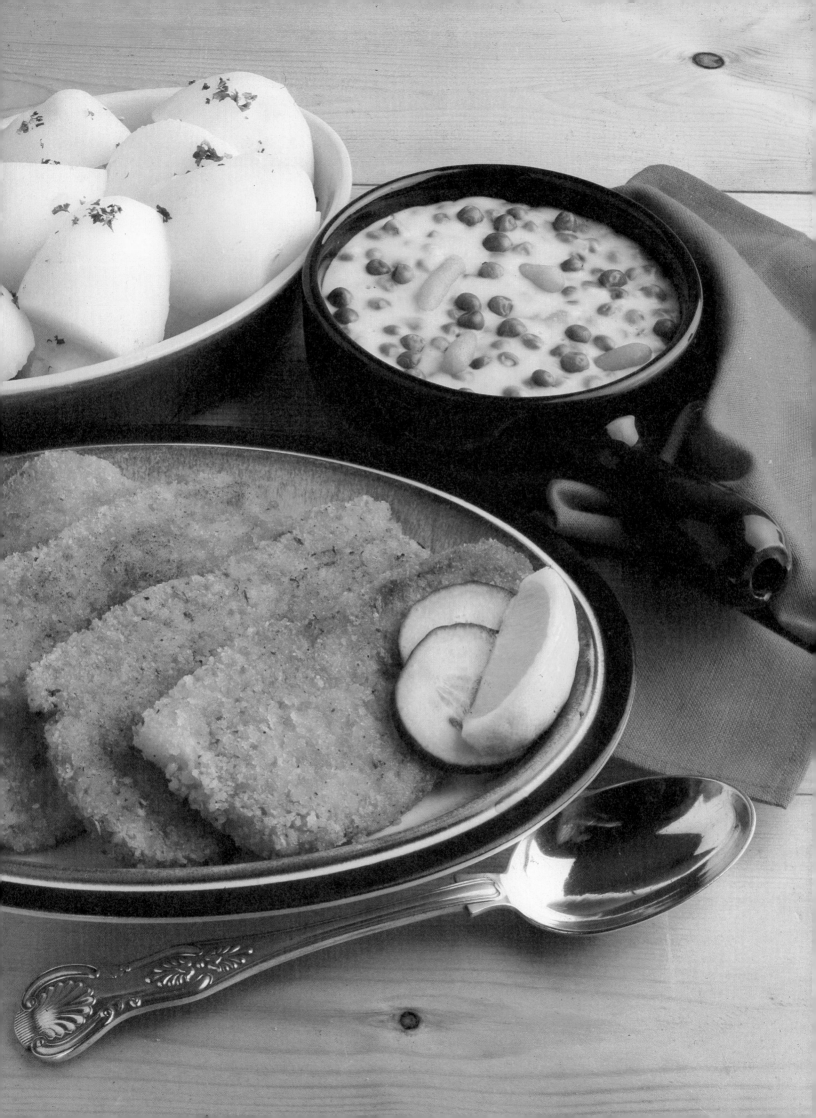

Pork steaks with spiced butter

40 g/1½ oz (U.S. 3 tablespoons) butter
2 tablespoons (U.S. 3 tablespoons) chopped parsley
1 teaspoon sweet paprika pepper
finely grated rind of ½ lemon
salt and freshly ground black pepper
4 (100-g/4-oz) boneless pork leg steaks
(U.S. 4×¼-lb boneless pork slices)
1 clove garlic, halved
large pinch of ground cumin
2 tablespoons (U.S. 3 tablespoons) oil or dripping
225 g/8 oz (U.S. ½ lb) Brussels sprouts, shredded
3-4 stalks celery, sliced
2 medium-sized carrots, peeled and cut in thin slivers

Cream the butter until soft. Beat in the parsley, paprika pepper, lemon rind and a little salt. Shape into a cylinder, wrap in cling film or foil and chill.

Place each steak between 2 sheets of cling film or dampened greaseproof paper (U.S. waxed paper) and beat with a cutlet bat or rolling pin until evenly thin. Rub all over with the cut surfaces of the garlic clove and sprinkle lightly with salt, pepper and cumin.

Heat the oil in a frying pan (U.S. skillet) and fry the steaks over moderately high heat for 3-4 minutes each side, until just cooked through.

Arrange the Brussels sprouts, celery and carrots on 4 serving plates and add a pork steak to each. Top with 1 or 2 slices of spiced butter. **Serves 4**

Nutty mackerel with fried cabbage

4 medium-sized mackerel, cleaned
2 eating apples, peeled and grated
75 g/3 oz (U.S. ¾ cup) chopped walnuts
salt and freshly ground black pepper
1 (295-g/10.5-oz) can condensed mushroom soup
2 tablespoons (U.S. 3 tablespoons) oil
1 medium-sized onion, peeled and sliced
2 medium-sized cooking apples, cored and sliced
450 g/1 lb white or green cabbage, finely shredded
150 ml/¼ pint (U.S. ⅔ cup) milk

Remove the heads from the fish and make 3 diagonal slashes on each side.

Mix together the apple and walnuts and season well. Stir in 2 tablespoons (U.S. 3 tablespoons) of the soup and use this mixture to stuff the fish. Lay them in a greased grill pan (U.S. broiler pan). Cook under high heat for about 5 minutes on each side, or until the flesh flakes easily when tested with a fork.

While the fish are cooking, heat the oil in a large pan, add the onion, apple slices, cabbage and a little seasoning and cook over moderately high heat, stirring frequently, for 7 minutes, or until the cabbage is tender but still slightly crunchy. Meanwhile, mix the remaining soup with the milk in a pan. Heat gently, stirring now and then, until the sauce is piping hot and smooth.

Serve the cabbage mixture in a warm dish topped with the fish, and hand the sauce separately. **Serves 4**

French bacon and broth

(Illustrated opposite)

1 small firm cabbage
1 medium-sized parsnip, peeled
3 tablespoons (U.S. 4 tablespoons) lard
1 large onion, peeled and thickly sliced
3 small carrots, peeled and cut in 5-cm/2-inch pieces
350-g/12-oz piece boiled bacon (U.S. ¾-lb piece boiled ham)
1 clove garlic, finely chopped
3 medium-sized potatoes, peeled and cut in 2.5-cm/1-inch cubes
1 (213-g/7½-oz) can cannellini beans
350-g/12-oz (U.S. ¾-lb) piece garlic sausage
1 chicken stock cube (U.S. 1 chicken bouillon cube), crumbled
2.5 litres/4 pints (U.S. 5 pints) water
salt and freshly ground black pepper

Remove the cabbage stalk and coarse outer leaves. Cut in half, from top to stalk end and blanch the halves in boiling water for 5 minutes. Drain. Meanwhile, cut the parsnip into pieces about the same size as the carrot. Slice any loose cabbage leaves. Cut each cabbage half into 3 equal sections.

Melt the lard in a large heavy pan and gently fry the onion until soft but not coloured. Add the carrot, parsnip and cabbage sections. Turn them in the fat until coated. Remove all the vegetables.

Add the bacon to the pan and brown lightly on all sides. Return the coated vegetables, adding the garlic, potatoes, beans and liquid from the can. Put in the sausage and add the stock cube and water. Bring to the boil, skim the surface well and add a little seasoning. Cover and simmer for about 30 minutes.

Lift out the bacon and sausage, slice them and arrange on a warm serving dish with the vegetables. Spoon over a little broth and keep hot. Adjust the seasoning of the broth and serve this as a first course, followed by the meat and vegetables. **Serves 6-8**

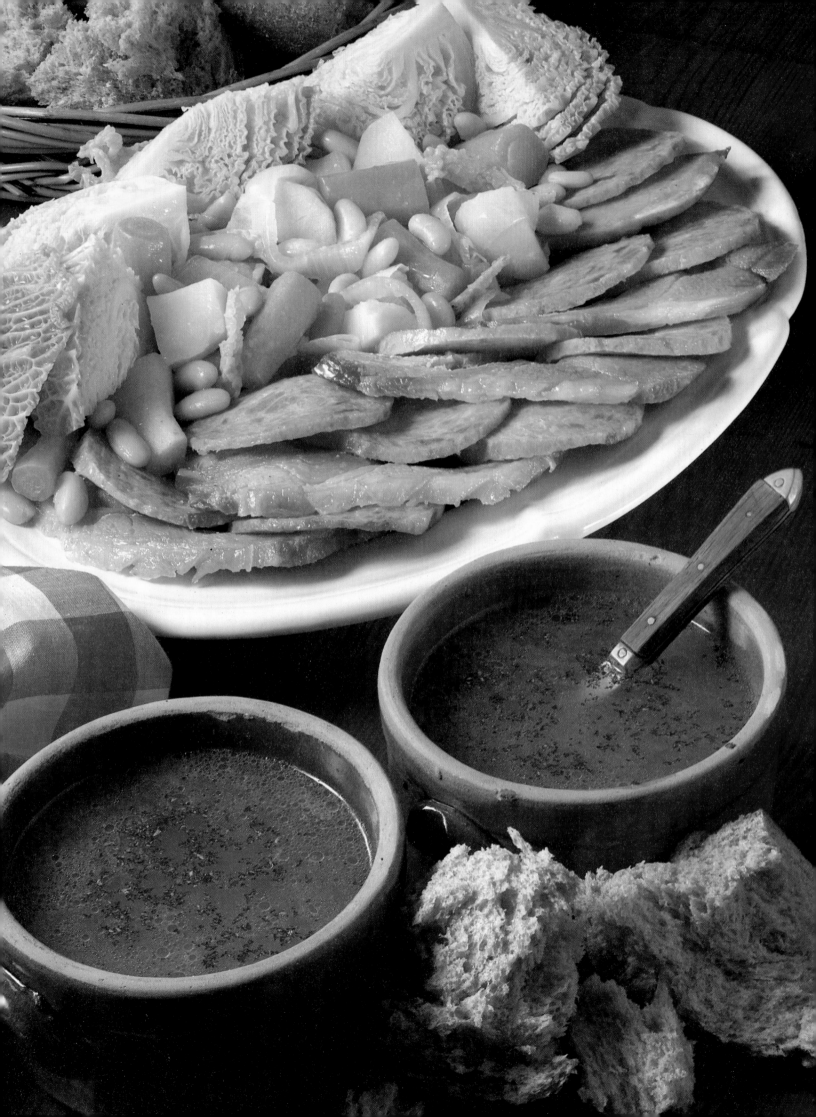

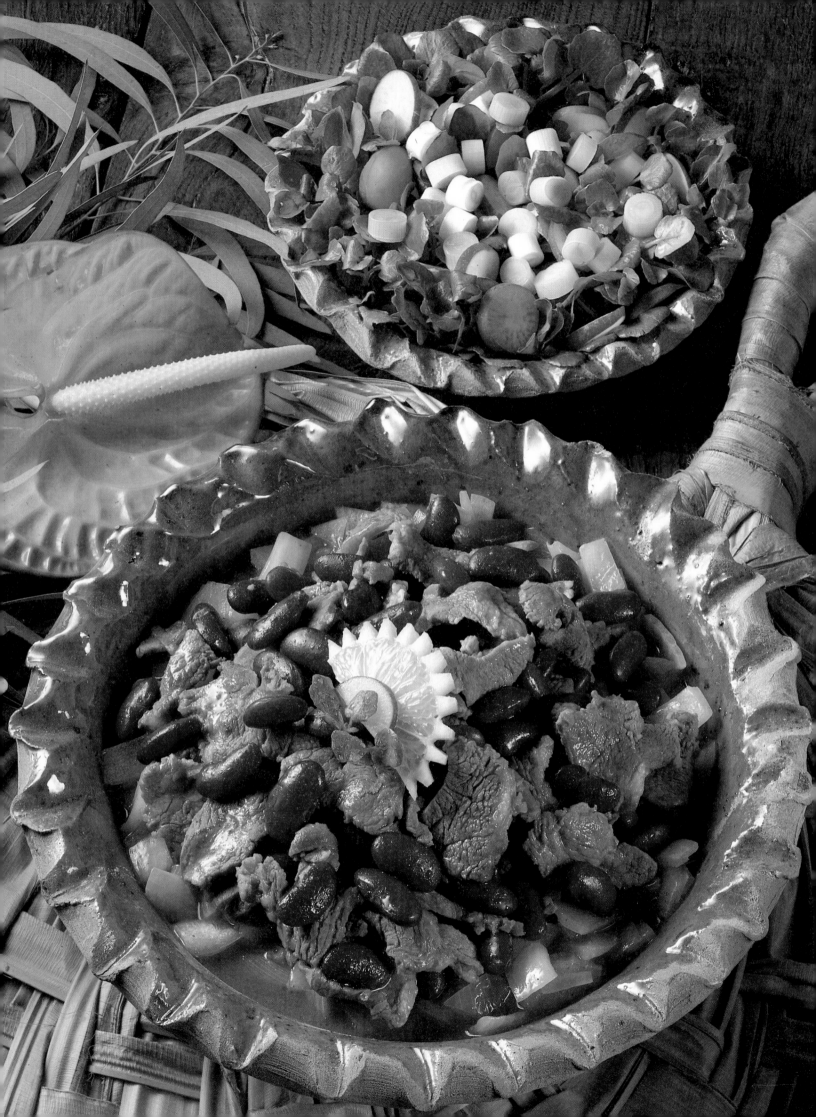

Baked fish on butter beans

4 tablespoons (U.S. 6 tablespoons) oil
4 medium-sized mackerel or herrings
juice of ½ lemon
1 (425-g/15-oz) can butter beans (U.S. lima beans),
drained
1 large onion, peeled and chopped
½ teaspoon dried basil
2 tablespoons (U.S. 3 tablespoons) chopped parsley
1 teaspoon light muscovado sugar (U.S. light brown
sugar)
1 teaspoon salt
¼ teaspoon ground black pepper
4 tablespoons (U.S. 6 tablespoons) white wine or
apple juice

Heat the oven to 200°C/400°F, Gas Mark 6 and use some of the oil to generously grease an ovenproof dish.

Cut the heads and tails from the fish. Slit the undersides and remove the entrails. Wash the fish and dry with absorbent kitchen towel. Open the fish out on a board with the skin side upwards, then press along the backbones to loosen them. Turn the fish over and remove the bones. Sprinkle the insides with lemon juice, then reform the fish. Slash one side of each 3 times with a sharp knife.

Put the beans, onion and herbs into the prepared dish. Stir the mixture then spread it flat. Arrange the fish on top, pressing them slightly. Combine the sugar, salt, pepper, wine or apple juice and the remaining oil and lemon juice. Spoon over the fish.

Cover with lid or foil and bake for 40 minutes. Serve hot from the dish. **Serves 4**

Broccoli bolognaise

40 g/1½ oz (U.S. 3 tablespoons) margarine
1 large onion, peeled and chopped
1 medium-sized carrot, peeled and coarsely grated
450 g/1 lb minced beef (U.S. ground beef)
1 tablespoon wholemeal flour
(U.S. wholewheat flour)
1 (425-g/15-oz) can tomatoes, roughly chopped
1 teaspoon dried oregano
½ teaspoon dried basil
salt and freshly ground black pepper
450 g/1 lb broccoli spears
1 teaspoon oil
75 g/3 oz fresh wholemeal breadcrumbs (U.S. 1½
cups fresh wholewheat bread crumbs)

Polynesian beef

Melt half the margarine in a large pan and gently cook the onion and carrot until the onion is soft. Add the meat and cook, stirring, until brown and crumbly. Sprinkle on the flour, stir well then gradually add the tomatoes and liquid from the can, the oregano and basil. Season lightly, bring to the boil, stirring constantly. Cover and simmer for 20 minutes.

Meanwhile, cook the broccoli in a pan of boiling salted water for about 10 minutes, or until tender but not breaking.

While the broccoli is cooking, heat the remaining margarine with the oil in a frying pan (U.S. skillet) and fry the breadcrumbs over moderately high heat, stirring, until golden.

Adjust the seasoning in the meat sauce if necessary. Drain the broccoli well and arrange round the outside of a warm serving dish. Pour the bolognaise into the centre and sprinkle the fried crumbs over the broccoli. Serve hot. **Serves 4**

Polynesian beef

(Illustrated opposite)

1 (200-g/7-oz) can bamboo shoot
1 beef stock cube (U.S. beef bouillon cube), crumbled
2 teaspoons (U.S. 1 tablespoon) oil
1 large onion, peeled and chopped
1 tablespoon grated fresh ginger (U.S. fresh ginger
root)
225 g/8 oz (U.S. ½ lb) rump steak, very thinly sliced
1 teaspoon cornflour (U.S. cornstarch)
1 tablespoon dry sherry
2 tablespoons (U.S. 3 tablespoons) soy sauce
1 (425-g/15-oz) can red kidney beans, drained
salt and freshly ground black pepper
Garnish
½ slice lemon, vandyked
radish slice
tiny sprig of watercress

Drain the liquid from the bamboo shoot into a small pan. Heat and use to dissolve the stock cube. Cut the bamboo shoot into small dice.

Heat the oil in a wok or large shallow frying pan (U.S. skillet) and gently fry the onion and ginger until transparent. Push to the sides of the pan and put the beef in the centre. Stir fry briskly until the meat is sealed but not brown. Mix the cornflour with the sherry and soy sauce, and add to the pan with the bamboo shoot, beans and stock. Stir all the ingredients over moderate heat until boiling. Cook for 1 minute and season to taste.

Transfer to a warm serving dish and garnish with the lemon, radish and watercress. Serve with brown rice and a salad of watercress, sliced radishes and spring onions (U.S. scallions). **Serves 4**

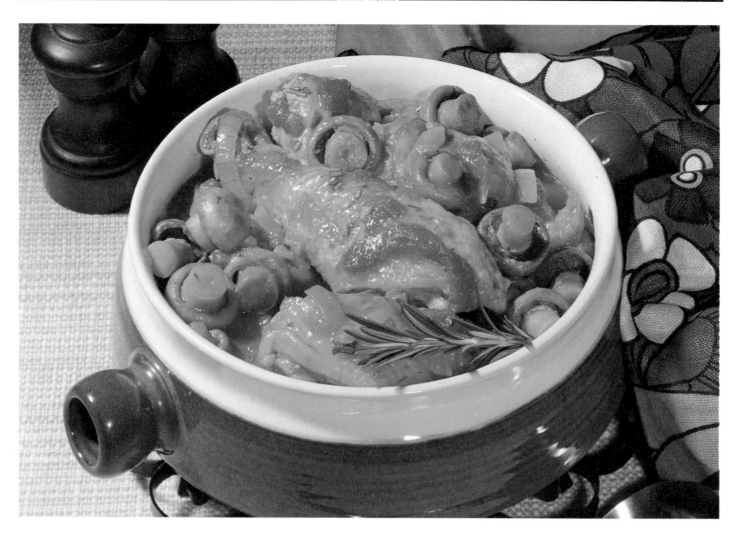

Chicken and mushroom pot

(Illustrated above)

50 g/2 oz (U.S. ¼ cup) butter or margarine
50 g/2 oz (U.S. ⅓ cup) diced bacon
1 (1.4-kg/3-lb) chicken, divided into 6 pieces
175 g/6 oz small onions, peeled
175 g/6 oz (U.S. 1½ cups) button mushrooms
1 tablespoon brandy
1 clove garlic, crushed
2 tablespoons wholemeal flour (U.S. 3 tablespoons wholewheat flour)
150 ml/¼ pint (U.S. ⅔ cup) red wine
150 ml/¼ pint strong chicken stock (U.S. ⅔ cup strong chicken bouillon)
1 (425-g/15-oz) can tomatoes
1 bay leaf
2 sprigs of parsley
2 sprigs of rosemary
salt and freshly ground black pepper

Melt the butter in a flameproof casserole or heavy pan and fry the bacon until pale golden. Remove with a slotted spoon. Add the chicken pieces to the pan, brown them quickly on all sides then remove. Put the onions and mushrooms into the pan and fry, stirring frequently, until the onions are golden.

Spoon off about half the fat, add the brandy to the pan and ignite. As soon as the flames die down, put in the garlic and flour, and stir over the heat until the flour begins to brown then gradually add the wine, stock, tomatoes and liquid from the can and bring to the boil, stirring constantly.

Return the chicken and bacon to the pan, and add the bay leaf, parsley and one sprig of rosemary. Season lightly with pepper and bring back to boiling point. Stir, then cover and simmer for 45 minutes.

Remove the herbs, adjust the seasoning if necessary and serve garnished with the remaining sprig of rosemary. **Serves 6**

Variation

Family chicken and bean casserole Omit the brandy and wine, increase the quantity of stock to 350 ml/12 fl oz (U.S. 1½ cups chicken bouillon) and use a can of baked beans in tomato sauce in place of the tomatoes. Serve with a mixture of freshly cooked potato and carrot dice.

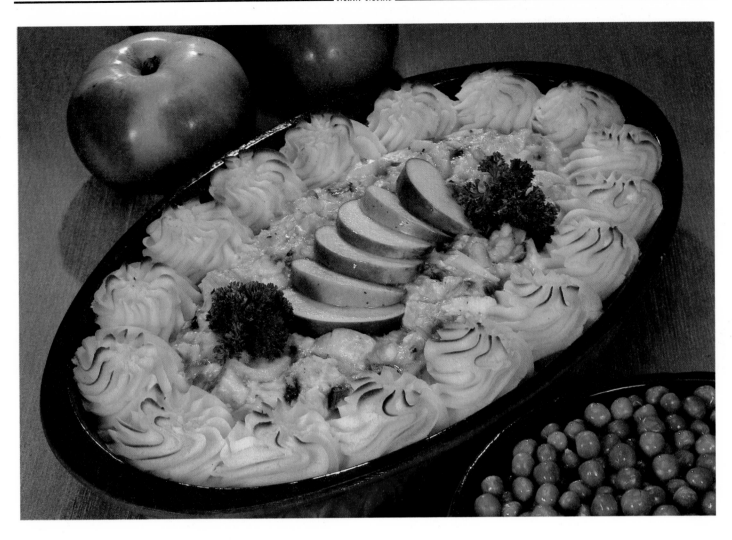

Bramley scalloped fish

(Illustrated above)

900 g/2 lb potatoes, peeled and sliced
675 g/1½ lb white fish fillets, skinned
about 300 ml/½ pint (U.S. about 1¼ cups) milk
1 tablespoon lemon juice
2 bay leaves
salt and pepper
75 g/3 oz (U.S. ⅓ cup) butter or margarine
1 small onion, peeled and finely chopped
100 g/4 oz (U.S. ¼ lb) mushrooms, chopped
25 g/1 oz wholemeal flour (U.S. ¼ cup wholewheat
flour)
225 g/8 oz Bramley cooking apples (U.S. ½ lb
cooking apples), peeled, cored and sliced
3 tablespoons single cream (U.S. 4 tablespoons light
cream)
Garnish
few slices Bramley apple (U.S. cooking apple)
little lemon juice
2 sprigs of parsley

Cook the potatoes in a pan of boiling salted water
until tender. Meanwhile, put the fish in a pan with
300 ml/½ pint (U.S. 1¼ cups) milk, the lemon juice,

bay leaves and plenty of seasoning. Cover and poach
for about 10 minutes, until the fish is cooked. Heat
the oven to 200°C/400°F, Gas Mark 6 and have ready
a shallow ovenproof dish.

Drain the potatoes, mash until smooth with half
the butter and season to taste. Measure the cooking
liquid from the fish and make up to 300 ml/½ pint
(U.S. 1¼ cups) again with more milk. Discard the bay
leaves and roughly flake the fish.

Melt the remaining butter in a pan and fry the
onion gently until soft. Stir in the mushrooms and
cook for a further 2 minutes. Sprinkle on the flour,
stir well and cook for 1 minute. Gradually add the
milk liquid and bring to the boil, stirring constantly.
Add the apple slices and cook for 2 minutes, then
blend in the cream and fold in the fish. Adjust the
seasoning and transfer to the dish. Spread or pipe the
potato decoratively round the edge.

Bake for about 30 minutes, or until the potato
edging is browned. Dip the apple slices in lemon juice
before using them and the parsley sprigs to garnish
the scallop. Serve hot with green peas. **Serves 4-5**

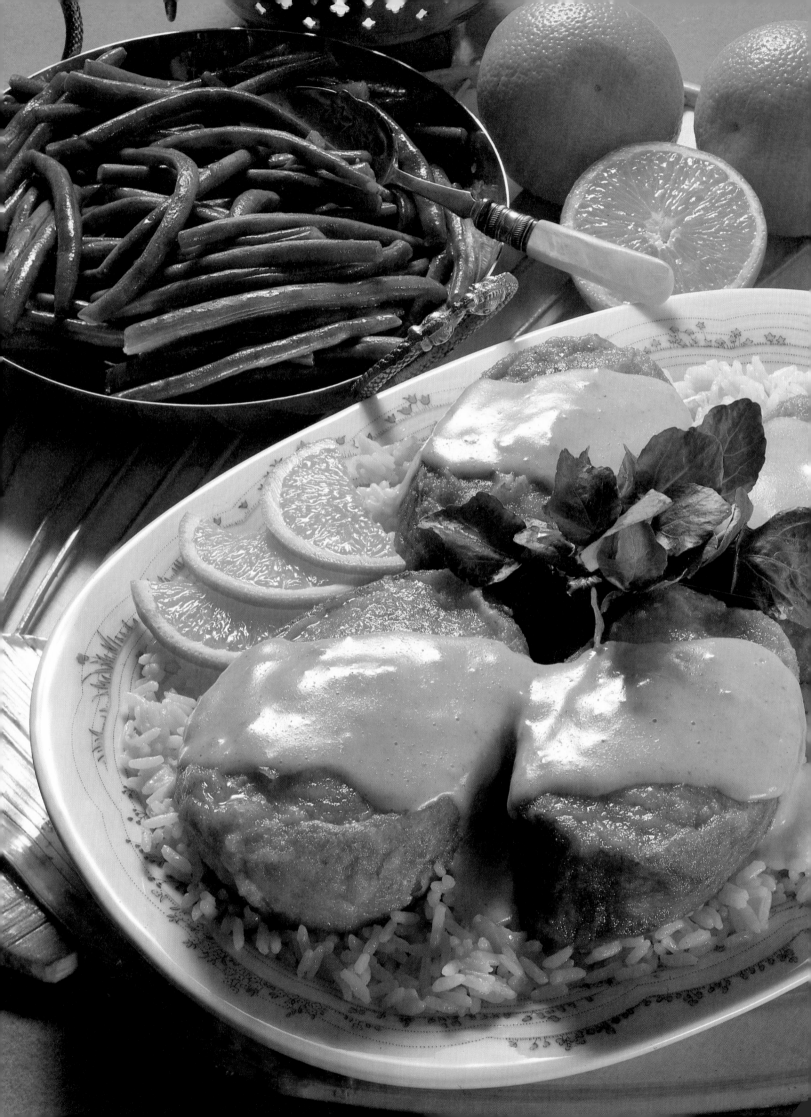

Spicy orange cod steaks with rice

(Illustrated opposite)

350 g/12 oz (U.S. 1⅔ cups) long grain brown rice
2 tablespoons wholemeal flour (U.S. 3 tablespoons
wholewheat flour)
1 teaspoon ground cumin
1 teaspoon ground turmeric
salt and freshly ground black pepper
6 (175-g/6-oz) cod steaks
4 tablespoons (U.S. 6 tablespoons) oil for frying
1 small onion, peeled and finely chopped
finely grated rind of 1 orange
Sauce
25 g/1 oz (U.S. 2 tablespoons) butter or margarine
2 tablespoons (U.S. 3 tablespoons) oil
150 ml/¼ pint chicken stock (U.S. ⅔ cup chicken
bouillon)
finely grated rind of 2 oranges
juice of 3 oranges
150 ml/¼ pint single cream (U.S. ⅔ cup light cream)
Garnish
orange slices
sprigs of watercress

Cook the rice in a pan of lightly salted water for about
25 minutes, or until tender. Meanwhile, put the flour,
cumin, turmeric and a little seasoning on a board.
Use to coat the cod steaks and reserve remaining flour
mixture.

Heat the oil in a frying pan (U.S. skillet) and fry the
onion until soft. Remove with a slotted spoon and
reserve. Add the cod steaks to the oil and fry for 4
minutes on each side.

While the fish is cooking, make the sauce. Heat the
butter and oil in a pan and stir in the reserved flour
mixture. Cook for 1 minute, stirring. Remove from
the heat and gradually add the chicken stock and the
orange rind and juice. Bring to the boil, stirring
constantly, until thick. Blend in the cream, adjust the
seasoning and remove from the heat. Keep hot.

Drain the rice and fork in the orange rind and fried
onion. Cover the pan and leave to stand for 3
minutes. Arrange the rice mixture on a warm serving
dish, top with the cod steaks and spoon over a little of
the sauce. Garnish with orange slices and watercress
sprigs and hand the rest of the sauce separately. Serve
with French beans (U.S. green beans). **Serves 6**

Turkey fillets with mixed beans

(Illustrated on title page)

175 g/6 oz dried flageolet beans
(U.S. 1 cup dried fava beans)
100 g/4 oz (U.S. ⅔ cup) dried red kidney beans
salt and freshly ground black pepper
4 turkey breast fillets
4 tablespoons (U.S. 6 tablespoons) oil
finely grated rind of 1 large lemon
4 tablespoons (U.S. 6 tablespoons) lemon juice
300 ml/½ pint chicken stock (U.S. 1¼ cups chicken
bouillon)
2 teaspoons cornflour (U.S. 1 tablespoon cornstarch)
1 medium-sized onion, peeled and chopped
1 tablespoon chopped mixed herbs
sprigs of fresh herbs to garnish

Place the beans in separate pans and cover with cold
water. Leave to soak overnight. Drain the beans, still
keeping them separate, cover with fresh water and
place over high heat. Boil rapidly for 10 minutes then
cover the pans and simmer for about 1 hour, or until
tender, adding a little salt to each pan just before the
beans are ready.

Meanwhile, season the turkey fillets lightly. Heat
half the oil in a frying pan (U.S. skillet) and gently fry
the turkey until golden on both sides. Add the lemon
rind and half the juice and the stock. Bring to the boil
and simmer for about 20 minutes, turning the fillets
once or twice, until the turkey is tender. Remove the
fillets from the pan and keep hot. Season the pan
juices to taste. Moisten the cornflour with a little cold
water, add to the pan and stir until boiling. Simmer
for 2 minutes.

At the same time, heat the remaining oil in a pan
and gently fry the onion until soft. Add the rest of the
lemon juice, the herbs and seasoning to taste, and heat
through. Drain the beans thoroughly and combine
with the onion mixture. Transfer to a warm serving
dish, top with the turkey fillets and spoon the sauce
over them. Garnish with herbs. **Serves 4**

Spicy orange cod steaks with rice

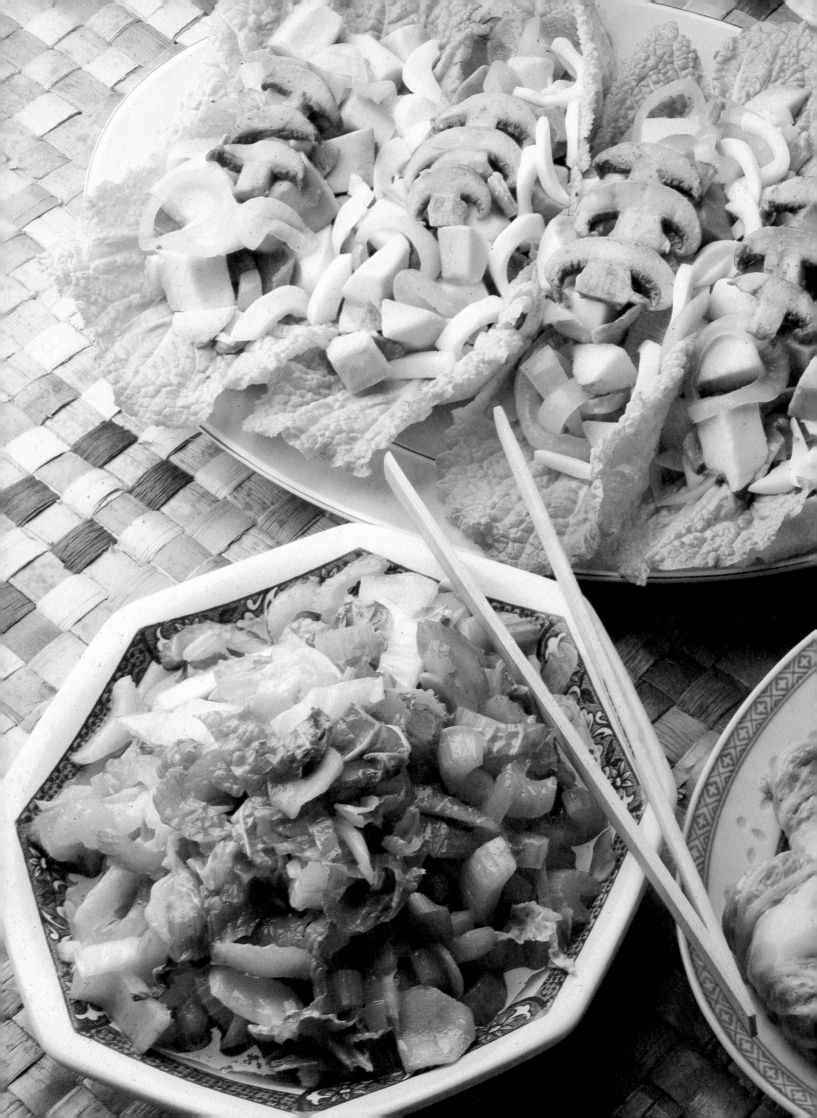

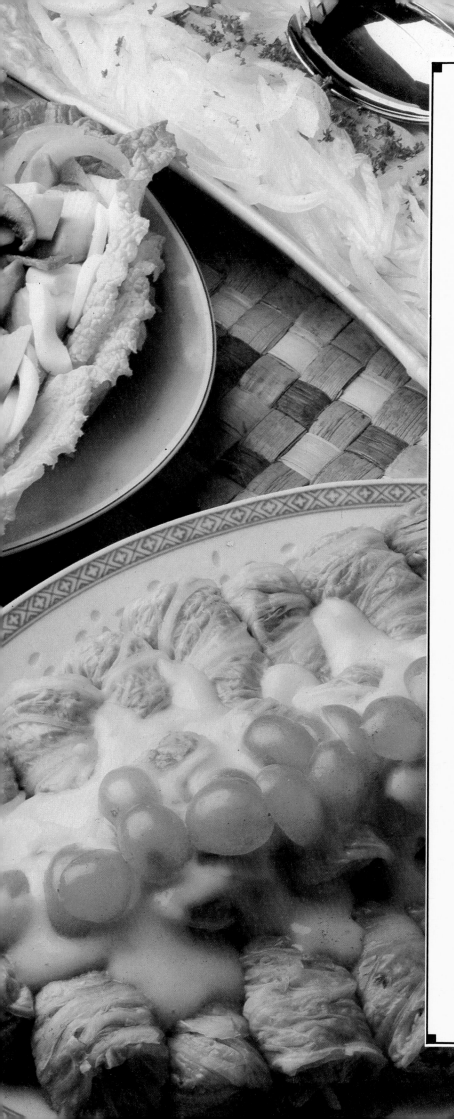

Salads and Vegetable Dishes

The selection available in the fresh produce department of any supermarket is quite frankly fabulous compared with the limited choice of a few years back. Specialist greengrocers nowadays have scarcely space to display all the goods they regularly keep in stock. Careful growing and marketing by big producers have made it possible for us to buy exotic items, such as avocados, during almost any season. If a vegetable is freezable, it can be a year-round delight.

The myth that salads or vegetable dishes are dreary can be forgotten. They come in all guises; light and crisp, just a whisper of a side salad; or filling enough to be the only dish needed. There are wonderfully tempting mixtures to be made including nourishing beans, rice and pasta, which take so well to salad dressings of all kinds. If the salad has to be your main source of fibre in the meal, this is a great advantage. Fresh and dried fruit, and nuts, make up very tasty dishes with crunchy greenstuffs and lightly cooked root vegetables or grated raw ones. You will find that I have included many combinations of ingredients, mixing and matching them, with great success.

These dishes, served in small individual portions, make very good meal starters. Or, try a soup-and-salad meal. Served with fresh wholemeal bread and a wedge of cheese, you have a perfectly balanced repast.

Above left: Chinese bacon and avocado cups
(recipe page 103).
Above right: Stir-fried Chinese leaves (recipe page 98).
Below right: Chinese leaf parcels (recipe page 98).
Below left: Spicy tossed vegetables (recipe page 106).

Chinese leaf parcels

(Illustrated on pages 96-97)

1 head Chinese leaves
275 g/10 oz (U.S. scant 1½ cups) long grain brown rice
1 clove garlic, finely chopped
2 teaspoons (U.S. 1 tablespoon) sweet paprika pepper
2 teaspoons (U.S. 1 tablespoon) dill or caraway seeds
3 tablespoons tomato purée (U.S. 4 tablespoons tomato paste)
1 tablespoon light muscovado sugar (U.S. light brown sugar)
salt and freshly ground black pepper
225 g/8 oz green grapes, halved and seeds removed (U.S. ½ lb green grapes, halved and pitted)
150 ml/¼ pint chicken stock (U.S. ⅔ cup chicken bouillon)
Sauce
15 g/½ oz (U.S. 1 tablespoon) butter or margarine
1 tablespoon wholemeal flour (U.S. wholewheat flour)
2 tablespoons (U.S. 3 tablespoons) lemon juice
extra grapes, halved and seeds removed (U.S. halved and pitted) to garnish

Heat the oven to 190°C/375°F, Gas Mark 5 and grease a shallow ovenproof dish.

Separate the leaves and cut out the hard centre triangle at the base of each. (Reserve these triangles for stir-frying, see opposite.) Blanch the leaves by dropping them into a pan of boiling water for 1 minute or by steaming for 5 minutes. Drain well and spread out on a board to cool and dry.

Meanwhile, cook the rice in a pan of boiling salted water for about 25 minutes, or until tender. Drain well and mix with the garlic, paprika, dill or caraway seeds, tomato purée, sugar and seasoning to taste. Stir in the grapes. Divide among the blanched leaves, fold the sides in over the filling and roll up. Pack the rolls into the prepared dish and pour the stock over. Cover and cook for 20 minutes.

Transfer the parcels to a warm serving dish and keep hot. Melt the butter in a pan and blend in the flour. Cook for 1 minute, stirring, then gradually add the liquid from the ovenproof dish and the lemon juice. Stir until boiling and simmer for 3 minutes. Adjust the seasoning if necessary and pour over the parcels. Serve hot, garnished with a few grapes. **Serves 8**

Stir-fried Chinese leaves

(Illustrated on pages 96-97)

triangular bases cut from about 8 large Chinese leaves
2 tablespoons (U.S. 3 tablespoons) oil
1 teaspoon lemon juice
salt and freshly ground black pepper
Garnish
2 tablespoons (U.S. 3 tablespoons) chopped parsley
1 lemon slice, twisted into a curl

Cut the leaf bases diagonally into 3-mm/⅛-inch thick strips.

Heat the oil in a frying pan (U.S. skillet) over moderate heat. Toss in the strips and fry and stir for about 2 minutes. Add the lemon juice and seasoning. Serve at once in a warm dish, sprinkled with parsley and garnished with the lemon curl. **Serves 4**

Vegetarian pasta salad

(Illustrated opposite)

350 g/12 oz (U.S. ¾ lb) pasta spirals or shells
5 stalks celery, chopped
1 medium-sized red pepper, seeds removed and diced
1 bunch spring onions (U.S. scallions), trimmed and chopped
1 (340-g/12-oz) can corn kernels, drained
4 tablespoons French dressing (U.S. 6 tablespoons Italian dressing)
salt and freshly ground black pepper
100 g/4 oz (U.S. ¼ lb) button mushrooms, sliced

Cook the pasta in a pan of boiling salted water as directed. Drain, rinse under running cold water and drain really well.

Place the cold pasta in a bowl and add the celery, pepper, onion and corn. Pour the dressing over, season to taste and mix well.

Transfer to a serving plate and arrange mushroom slices all round the edge. **Serves 6**

Vegetarian pasta salad

98

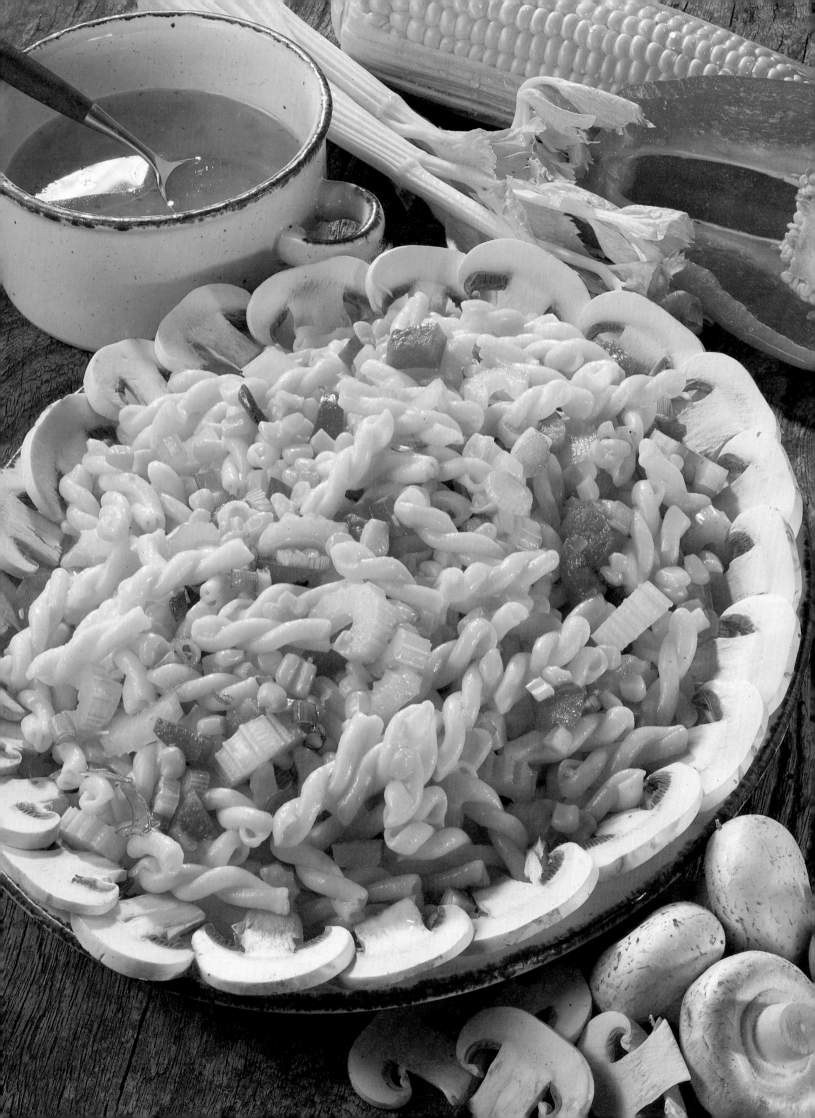

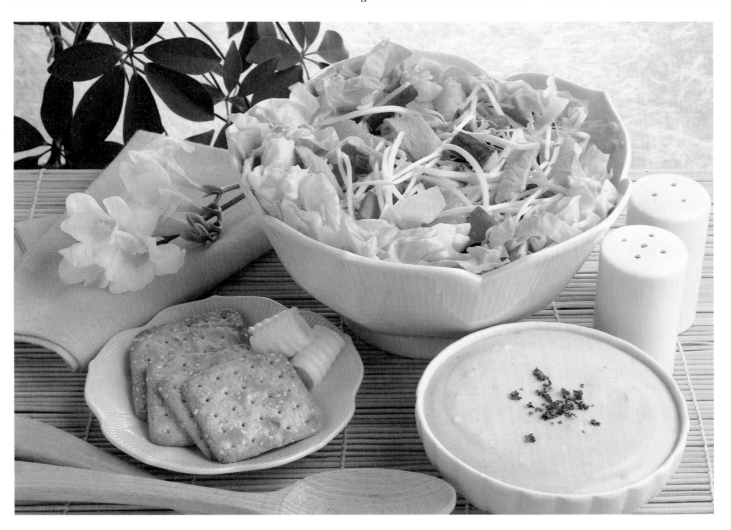

Crispy bacon and beansprout salad

(Illustrated above)

225 g/8 oz rashers back bacon (U.S. $\frac{1}{2}$ lb Canadian bacon slices), rind removed
7.5-cm/3-inch length cucumber, cut into thin strips
1 small red pepper, seeds removed and diced
1 small green pepper, seeds removed and diced
225 g/8 oz (U.S. 4 cups) beansprouts
2 small oranges, peeled and segmented
shredded lettuce
Dressing
50 g/2 oz (U.S. $\frac{1}{2}$ cup) crumbled Danish blue cheese
150 ml/$\frac{1}{4}$ pint (U.S. $\frac{2}{3}$ cup) natural yogurt
2 tablespoons (U.S. 3 tablespoons) white wine vinegar
pinch of pepper
1 tablespoon grated onion
$\frac{1}{2}$ teaspoon light muscovado sugar (U.S. light brown sugar)

First make the dressing. Put the cheese in a bowl and mash with a fork. Gradually blend in the yogurt, then whisk in remaining ingredients. Chill the dressing.

Cook the bacon rashers under a hot grill (U.S. broiler) until the fat is golden. Leave until cold, then cut into strips. Put the bacon and all salad ingredients, except the lettuce, into a bowl and toss lightly. Arrange the lettuce around the rim of the bowl. Hand the dressing separately with the salad and serve with wholewheat crackers and butter. **Serves 4**

Potatoes in spiced hollandaise sauce

Boil 1 kg/2 lb even-sized new potatoes until tender. Meanwhile, soften 175 g/6 oz (U.S. $\frac{3}{4}$ cup) unsalted butter. Finely chop 1 clove of garlic and place in a bowl with 2 egg yolks. Stand the bowl over a pan of simmering water and stir constantly until the eggs just begin to thicken. Add the butter in small pieces, whisking the sauce vigorously after each addition. Whisk in 2 tablespoons (U.S. 3 tablespoons) natural yogurt, $\frac{1}{4}$ teaspoon ground coriander and seasoning. Spoon over the drained potatoes and sprinkle with chopped parsley. **Serves 4**

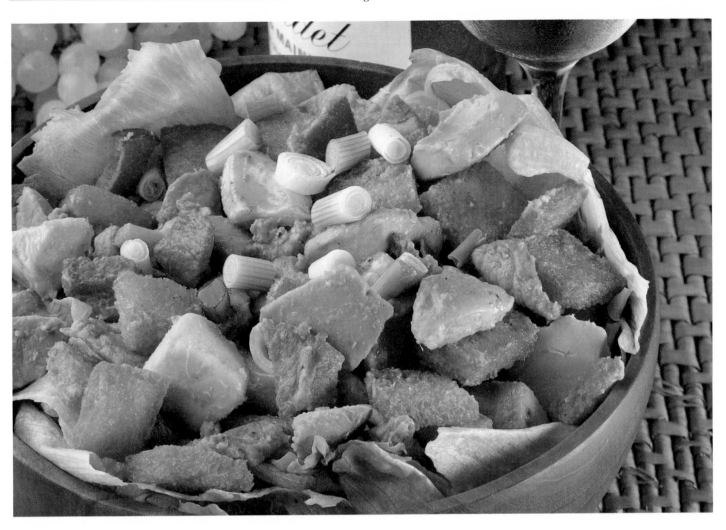

Avocado and smoked bacon salad

(Illustrated above)

450 g/1 lb thickly sliced smoked bacon
(U.S. smoked Canadian bacon), rind removed
2 thick slices wholemeal bread
(U.S. wholewheat bread), cubed
oil for frying
2 ripe avocado pears, halved and stoned
(U.S. halved and pitted)
lemon juice
1 bunch of spring onions (U.S. scallions), trimmed
and chopped
few leaves Iceberg lettuce, shredded
Dressing
1 clove garlic, crushed
$\frac{1}{2}$ teaspoon salt
$\frac{1}{2}$ teaspoon freshly ground black pepper
$\frac{1}{2}$ teaspoon sweet paprika pepper
2 tablespoons (U.S. 3 tablespoons) lemon juice
5 tablespoons (U.S. 7 tablespoons) olive oil

Grill (U.S. broil) the bacon until crisp and drain on absorbent kitchen towel. When cool, cut into bite-sized pieces. Shallow fry the bread cubes in oil until golden brown. Drain these on kitchen towel in the same way.

Cut the avocado flesh into chunks and toss in a little lemon juice to prevent discolouration. Combine the bacon, croûtons, onion and avocado and place on a bed of lettuce in serving bowl.

Put all the dressing ingredients into a screw-topped container and shake vigorously. Spoon over the salad at serving time and toss lightly. Serve with crusty bread. **Serves 4**

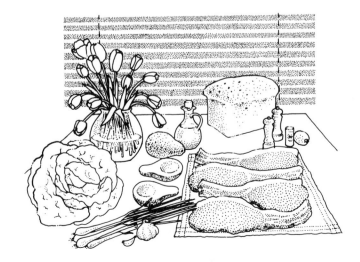

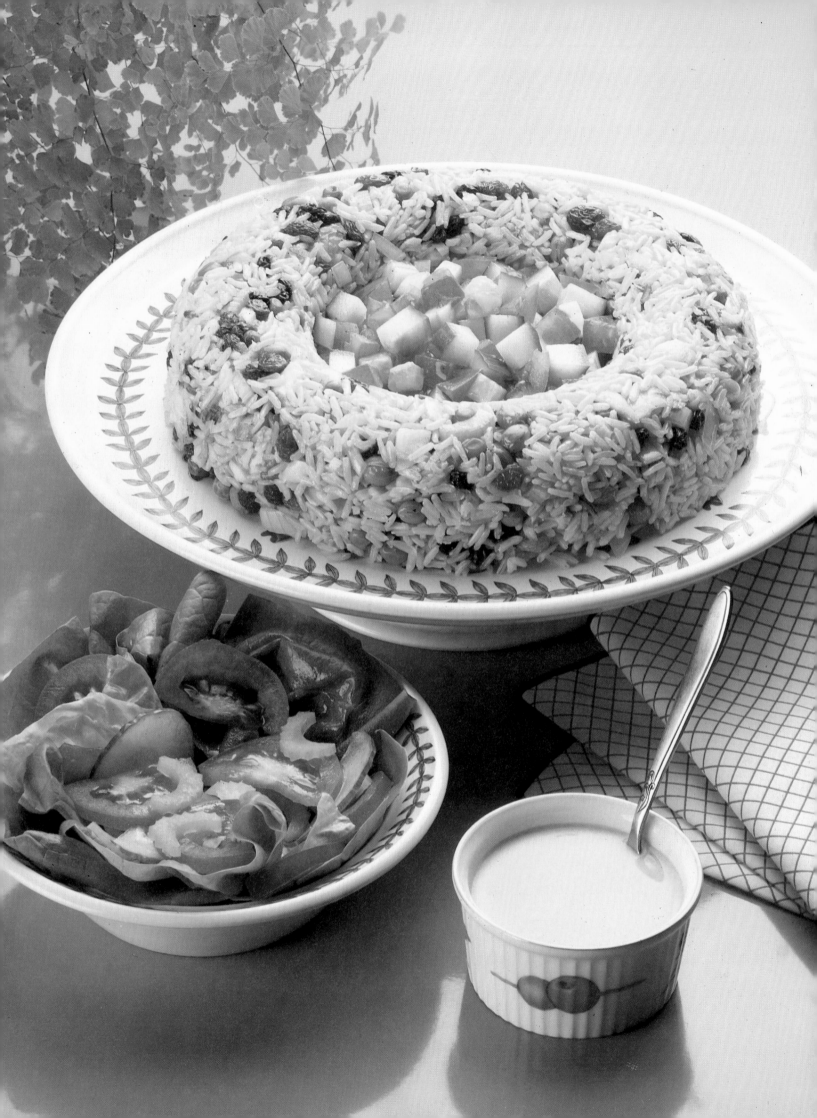

Fennel and grapefruit salad

2 grapefruits
1 large head of fennel, sliced
1 bunch spring onions (U.S. scallions), trimmed and chopped
1 lettuce, divided into leaves
100 g/4 oz (U.S. ¼ lb) Emmenthal cheese, cut into strips
½ small red pepper, seeds removed and cut into strips
Dressing
3 tablespoons (U.S. 4 tablespoons) olive oil
1 tablespoon wine vinegar
½ teaspoon light muscovado sugar (U.S. light brown sugar)
large pinch of salt
small pinch of freshly ground black pepper
1 teaspoon mild continental mustard

Peel and segment the grapefruits, removing all pith and membranes. Put most of the segments in a bowl and add the fennel, onion and lettuce.

Make the dressing. Put all the ingredients in a screw-topped container and shake well. Pour the dressing over the grapefruit salad and toss thoroughly.

Transfer to a salad bowl and garnish with the cheese and pepper strips and the reserved grapefruit segments. **Serves 4**

Chinese bacon and avocado cups

(Illustrated on pages 96-97)

about ½ head Chinese leaves, divided into 8 even-sized leaves
squeeze of lemon juice
2 avocado pears, peeled and diced
2 tablespoons (U.S. 3 tablespoons) oil
100 g/4 oz streaky bacon (U.S. ¼ lb bacon), rind removed and chopped
2 medium-sized onions, peeled, sliced into rings
4 medium-sized mushrooms, sliced
freshly ground black pepper
2 hard-boiled (U.S. hard-cooked) egg whites, cut into strips

Fit the leaves together in pairs to give 4 double 'cups'. Arrange on a serving dish. Squeeze the lemon juice over the avocado and divide it among the 'cups'.

Heat the oil in a frying pan (U.S. skillet) and fry the bacon, onion and mushroom until the onion is tender. Season with pepper and spoon the mixture over the avocado, arranging the slices of mushroom on the top. Garnish with egg white. **Serves 4**

Note The hard-boiled egg yolks can be used at another meal, or sieved and beaten into 150 ml/¼ pint French dressing (U.S. ⅔ cup Italian dressing) to give a thick creamy texture.

Haddock and rice moulded salad

(Illustrated opposite)

225 g/8 oz (U.S. 1⅛ cups) long grain brown rice
sweet paprika pepper
225 g/8 oz smoked haddock fillet (U.S. ½ lb finnan haddie), cooked
1 small onion, peeled and finely chopped
50 g/2 oz (U.S. ⅓ cup) seedless raisins
2 tablespoons (U.S. ¼ cup) currants
50 g/2 oz (U.S. generous ¼ cup) peanuts
50 g/2 oz (U.S. ½ cup) cooked green peas
2 small stalks celery, sliced
2 large tomatoes, diced
10-cm/4-inch length cucumber, diced
Dressing
150 ml/¼ pint (U.S. ⅔ cup) natural yogurt
75 ml/3 fl oz (U.S. ⅓ cup) tomato juice
1 teaspoon Worcestershire sauce
pinch of dry mustard powder
celery salt

Cook the rice in boiling salted water for about 25 minutes, or until tender. Drain well and sprinkle generously with paprika. Leave to cool.

Flake the fish, discarding any skin and bones. Mix with the rice, onion, raisins, currants, peanuts, peas and celery. Press into an oiled 1-litre/1¾-pint (U.S. 4½-cup) ring mould. Mix together the ingredients for the dressing with celery salt to taste. Transfer to a small serving dish. Cover the ring and the dressing and chill for 1 hour.

Unmould the ring salad on to a serving dish and fill the centre with tomato and cucumber. Hand the dressing separately. **Serves 4**

Haddock and rice moulded salad

Mitzi's favourite salad
(Illustrated opposite)

2 small courgettes (U.S. 2 small zucchini)
100 g/4 oz (U.S. ¼ lb) Caramelle or pasta shells, cooked
100 g/4 oz (U.S. ¼ lb) red cabbage, finely shredded
8 radishes, finely sliced
225 g/8 oz silverside of beef
(U.S. ½ lb corned beef), cut in julienne strips
1 tablespoon French dressing (U.S. Italian dressing)
4 large sprigs of watercress
2 tablespoons (U.S. 3 tablespoons) natural yogurt
2 tablespoons (U.S. 3 tablespoons) mayonnaise
1 tablespoon pumpkin seeds
2 lettuce leaves, roughly chopped

Top and tail the courgettes and slice them thinly.
Place in a bowl with the pasta, cabbage, radishes and
beef. Add the French dressing and toss lightly.

Very finely chop 2 of the watercress sprigs and mix
with the yogurt and mayonnaise. Transfer to a dish.

Arrange the beef mixture in a serving dish and
sprinkle with the pumpkin seeds. Divide the remaining watercress into tiny sprigs and tuck these round
the salad, alternating them with bits of shredded
lettuce. Serve with the dressing. **Serves 4**

Corn and spinach pasta plate
(Illustrated opposite)

225 g/8 oz (U.S. ½ lb) wholewheat pasta spirals
225 g/8 oz (U.S. ½ lb) fresh spinach, stalks removed
and leaves torn into large pieces
1 (340-g/12-oz) can baby corn
25 g/1 oz (U.S. 2 tablespoons) butter or margarine
1 (50-g/2-oz) can anchovies
100 g/4 oz (U.S. ¼ lb) feta cheese, crumbled

Cook the pasta in boiling salted water as directed.

Meanwhile, wash the spinach, drain well and place
in a pan with just the water clinging to the leaves.
Cover and cook over moderately high heat for about
2 minutes, shaking the pan frequently, until the
spinach is limp. Heat the corn in the can liquid.

Drain the pasta well and return it to the hot pan
with the butter and oil from the anchovies. Toss until
the pasta is coated. Add the spinach with any juices
from the pan. Chop the anchovies and add to the
mixture with the cheese. Fold in lightly and transfer
to a warm serving dish. Cut each baby corn into 3
and arrange round the edge of the dish. **Serves 4**

*Above: Corn and spinach pasta plate. Below: Mitzi's favourite
salad*

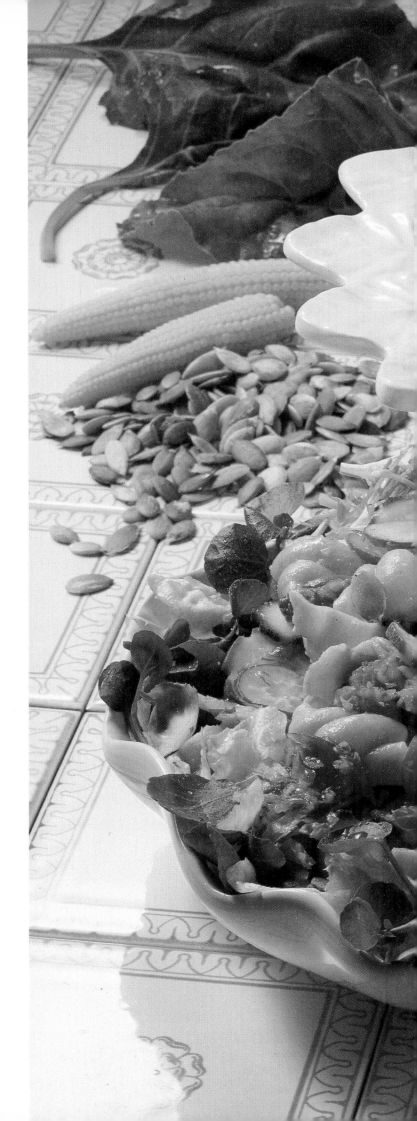

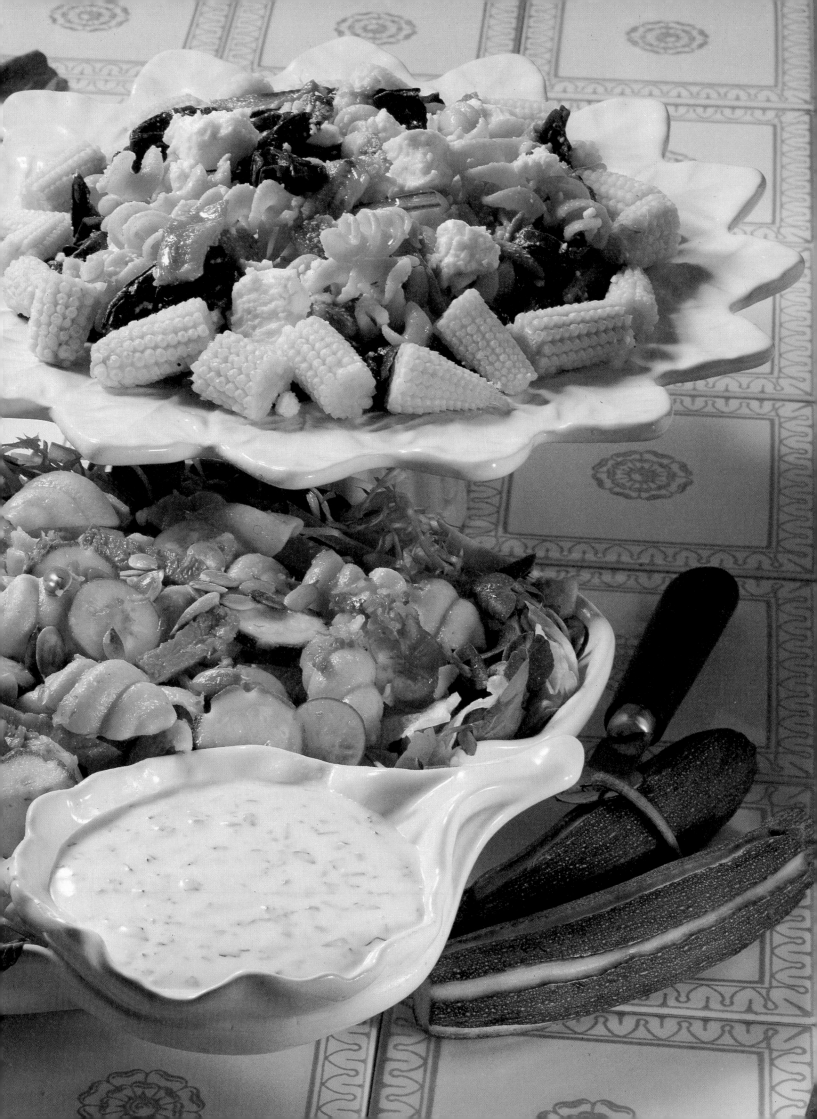

Spicy tossed vegetables

(Illustrated on pages 96-97)

1 teaspoon finely chopped fresh root ginger or
½ teaspoon ground ginger
¼ head Chinese leaves, shredded
2 stalks celery, finely chopped
1 small onion, peeled and sliced
1 clove garlic, very finely chopped
2 tablespoons (U.S. 3 tablespoons) oil
salt and freshly ground black pepper
Glaze
1 chicken stock cube (U.S. 1 chicken bouillon cube)
4 tablespoons (U.S. 6 tablespoons) boiling water
4 teaspoons cornflour (U.S. 2 tablespoons cornstarch)
1 tablespoon sherry
pinch of aniseed powder or 5-spice powder

Mix together the ginger, Chinese leaves, celery, onion and garlic. Make the glaze, mix the stock cube with the water. Blend the cornflour with the sherry and spice, and gradually mix in the stock. Set aside.

Heat the oil in a wok or large frying pan (U.S. skillet). Add the vegetable mixture and stir-fry over moderately high heat for about 1½ minutes, or until the leaves are barely wilted. Pour in the glaze and continue stir-frying until it is glossy and coats the vegetables. Add seasoning if necessary. **Serves 2-4**

Cauliflower in batter

1 medium-sized cauliflower, divided into florets
Batter
50 g/2 oz wholemeal flour (U.S. ½ cup wholewheat flour)
50 g/2 oz plain flour (U.S. ½ cup flour)
pinch of salt
½ teaspoon ground nutmeg
1 tablespoon oil
1 egg, separated
150 ml/¼ pint (U.S. ⅔ cup) lukewarm water
oil for deep frying

Blanch the cauliflower florets in a pan of boiling salted water for 3 minutes. Drain in a colander while making the batter.

Place the flours, salt and nutmeg in a bowl. Add the oil, egg yolk and half the water. Whisk until smooth. Gradually add the remaining water. Whisk the egg white until stiff and fold into the batter.

Heat the oil to a temperature of 190°C/375°F or until a cube of day-old bread turns golden brown in 40 seconds. Dip pieces of vegetable in the batter and fry in the oil a few at a time for about 3 minutes, or until golden brown. Drain and keep hot. Serve as soon as all the balls are cooked. **Serves 4**

Moulded Mexican salad

225 ml/8 fl oz (U.S. 1 cup) tomato juice
1 tablespoon gelatine (U.S. 1 envelope unflavored gelatin)
100 ml/4 fl oz (U.S. ½ cup) sieved fresh tomato pulp
1 tablespoon vinegar
½ teaspoon salt
pinch of black pepper
few drops Tabasco (U.S. hot pepper) sauce
1 small green pepper, seeds removed and finely chopped
2 stalks celery, finely chopped
10-cm/4-inch length cucumber, finely chopped

Put the tomato juice in a pan, sprinkle the gelatine over the surface and leave to stand for 5 minutes. Heat gently, stirring, until the gelatine has completely dissolved. Leave to cool but not set.

Stir the tomato pulp, vinegar, salt, pepper and Tabasco sauce into the gelatine mixture. Combine the chopped vegetables in an oiled 900-ml/1½-pint (U.S. 3¾-cup) mould and pour the tomato mixture over. Leave to set.

Turn out on a serving plate or scoop out portions with a spoon. **Serves 4**

Summer orange potato salad

(Illustrated opposite)

1 kg/2 lb small even-sized new potatoes
4 oranges
150 ml/¼ pint (U.S. ⅔ cup) mayonnaise
salt and pepper
1 tablespoon snipped chives

Scrub the potatoes. (Halve or quarter larger potatoes.) Cook in boiling salted water until tender. Drain well and leave to cool.

Finely grate the rind from 2 of the oranges and mix almost all of it into the mayonnaise. Add seasoning if desired. Divide all the oranges into segments, discarding any pith, membranes and pips.

Gently combine the potatoes, most of the orange segments and half the orange mayonnaise and transfer to a serving platter. Garnish with the remaining orange segments and sprinkle them with chives. Put the rest of the orange mayonnaise into a small dish and top with the reserved orange rind. **Serves 6**

Summer orange potato salad

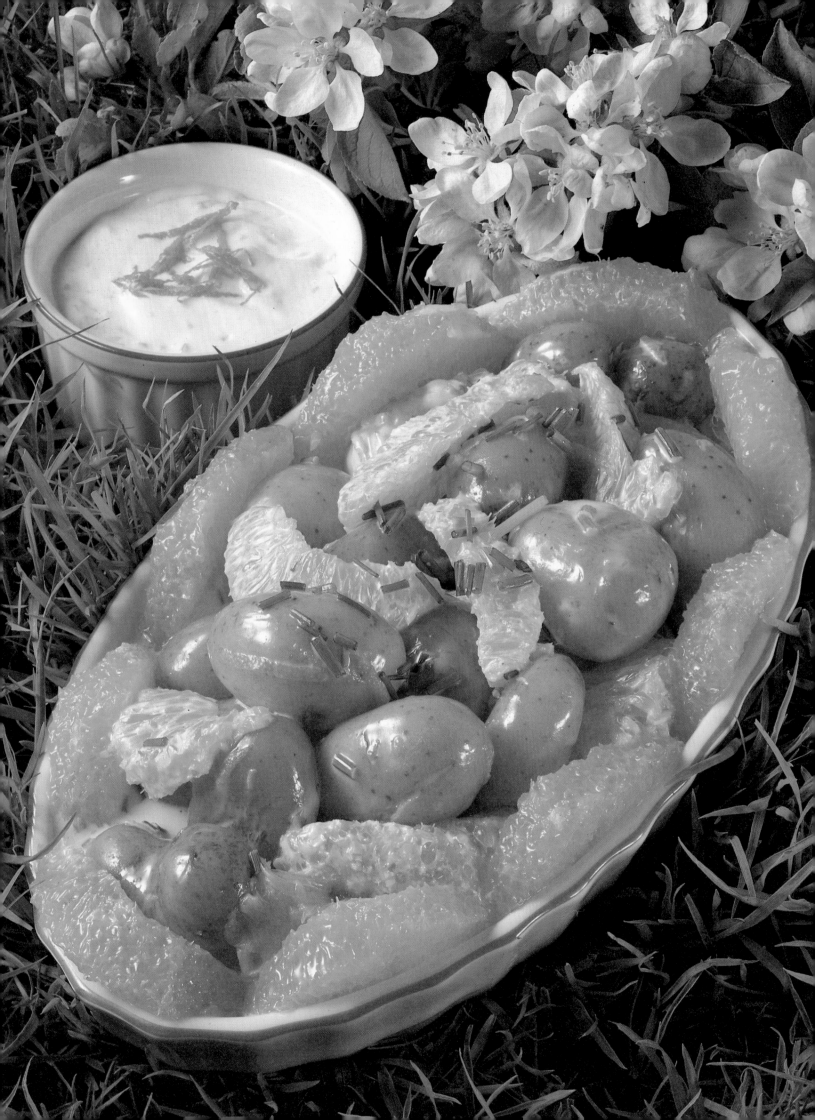

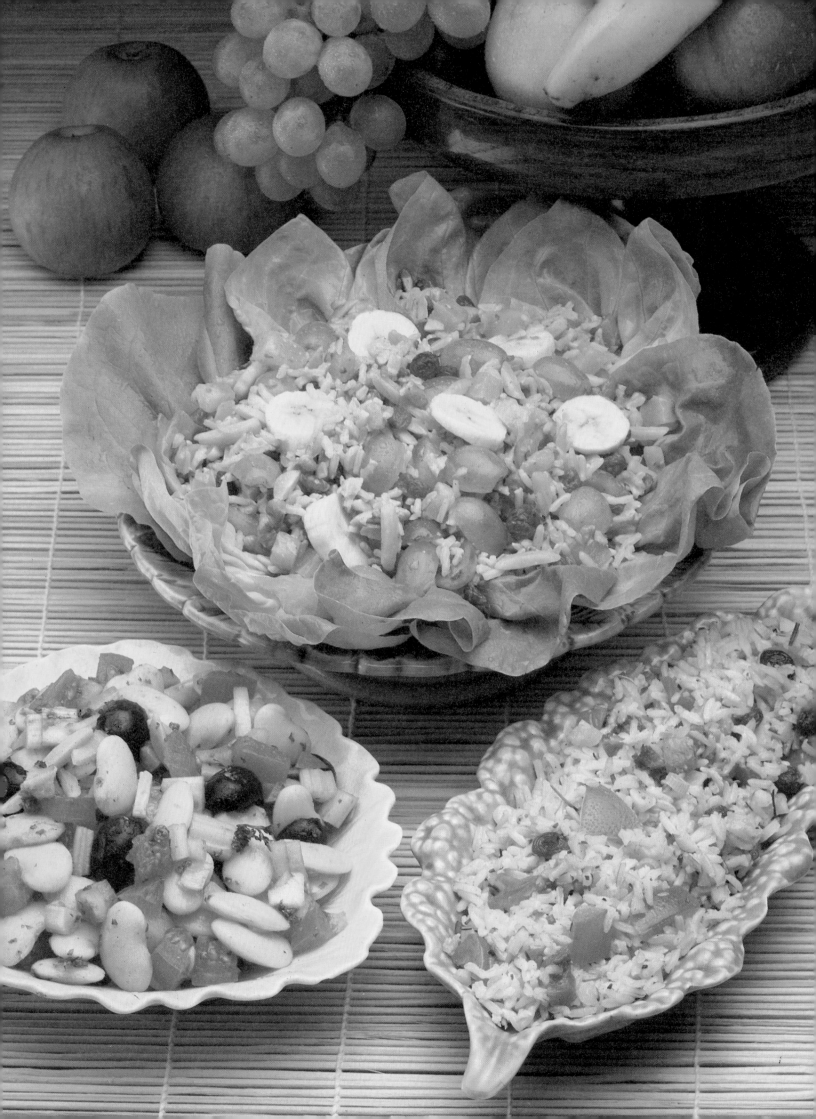

Tropical fruit and nut salad

(Illustrated opposite)

4 bananas, peeled and sliced
1 red-skinned eating apple, cored and chopped
2 tablespoons (U.S. 3 tablespoons) lemon juice
100 g/4 oz (U.S. generous $\frac{1}{2}$ cup) long grain brown rice, cooked and cooled
100 g/4 oz green grapes, halved and pips removed (U.S. $\frac{1}{4}$ lb green grapes, halved and pitted)
75 g/3 oz (U.S. $\frac{1}{3}$ cup) chopped canned or fresh pineapple
50 g/2 oz sultanas (U.S. $\frac{1}{3}$ cup seedless white raisins)
50 g/2 oz (U.S. $\frac{1}{2}$ cup) chopped walnuts
50 g/2 oz flaked almonds (U.S. $\frac{1}{2}$ cup slivered almonds)
lettuce leaves

Put the banana slices and apple in a bowl, add the lemon juice and toss well. Combine with the rice, grapes, pineapple, sultanas, walnuts and almonds.

Use lettuce leaves to line a serving bowl and pile the salad in the centre. Chill before serving. **Serves 8**

Beans Provençal

(Illustrated opposite)

225 g/8 oz dried butter beans (U.S. $\frac{1}{2}$ lb dried large limas), soaked overnight and cooked as directed
4 medium-sized tomatoes, chopped
1 large mild onion, peeled and chopped
50 g/2 oz flaked almonds (U.S. $\frac{1}{2}$ cup slivered almonds)
2 stalks celery, chopped
1 clove garlic, finely chopped
50 g/2 oz black olives, stoned (U.S. $\frac{1}{3}$ cup pitted ripe olives), halved
2 tablespoons (U.S. 3 tablespoons) chopped parsley
salt and freshly ground black pepper
Dressing
4 tablespoons (U.S. 6 tablespoons) tomato juice
1 tablespoon lemon juice
1 tablespoon Worcestershire sauce

Combine the beans, tomato, onion, almonds, celery, garlic, olives and parsley in a serving dish.

Place the dressing ingredients in a small screw-topped container and shake well. Pour over the salad, toss lightly and add seasoning to taste.

Cover and chill for at least 30 minutes before serving. **Serves 4**

Above: Tropical fruit and nut salad. Below right: Nutty fruit and rice salad. Below left: Beans Provençal

Nutty fruit and rice salad

(Illustrated opposite)

225 g/8 oz (U.S. $1\frac{1}{8}$ cups) long grain brown rice
75 g/3 oz (U.S. $\frac{1}{2}$ cup) chopped ready-to-eat figs
25 g/1 oz (U.S. scant $\frac{1}{4}$ cup) seedless raisins
3 spring onions (U.S. scallions), thinly sliced
50 g/2 oz (U.S. $\frac{1}{2}$ cup) coarsely chopped Brazil nuts
2 small firm tomatoes, chopped
1 tablespoon finely chopped rosemary
Dressing
2 tablespoons (U.S. 3 tablespoons) oil
1 tablespoon orange juice
$\frac{1}{4}$ teaspoon ground nutmeg
salt and freshly ground black pepper

Cook the rice in a pan of boiling salted water for 25 minutes, or until just tender. Drain and mix with the figs, raisins, onion, nuts, tomato and rosemary.

Put the oil, orange juice and nutmeg in a small screw-topped container and season well. Shake, pour over the rice and toss well. Chill. **Serves 4**

Lettuce, orange and almond salad

1 Cos lettuce (U.S. romaine lettuce)
1 bunch of watercress
3 small oranges
25 g/1 oz flaked almonds (U.S. $\frac{1}{4}$ cup silvered almonds)
Dressing
$\frac{1}{4}$ teaspoon salt
pinch of freshly ground black pepper
pinch of sugar
1 tablespoon chopped shallot or spring onion (U.S. green onion or scallion)
1 tablespoon orange juice
1 tablespoon lemon juice
3 tablespoons (U.S. 4 tablespoons) olive oil

Cut the lettuce leaves across in 2.5-cm/1-inch strips and put into a salad bowl. Pinch off the tender sprigs of watercress and scatter over the lettuce. Peel the oranges carefully, reserving the juice. Lay the orange slices over the green salad, scatter over almonds.

To make the dressing, put the salt, pepper, sugar, shallot, fruit juices and oil into a screw-topped container. Shake well. Pour over the salad and toss the ingredients lightly. **Serves 4-6**

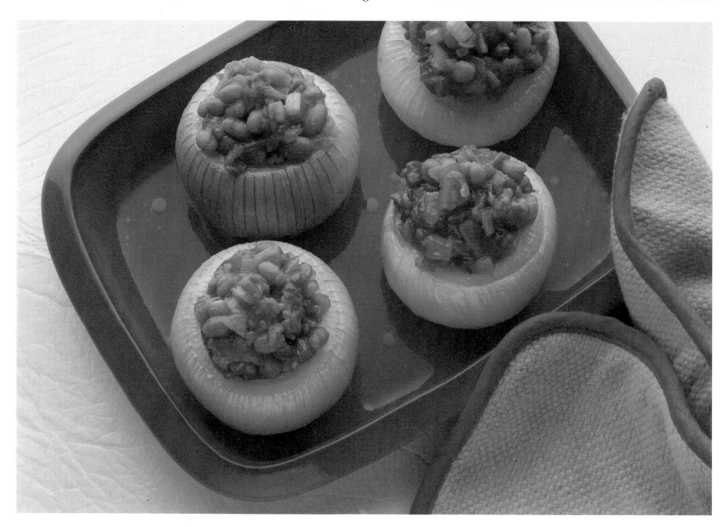

Ritzy baked onions

(Illustrated above)

4 large onions, peeled
I large rasher bacon(U.S. 2 bacon slices), chopped
4 chicken livers, roughly chopped
I (225-g/8-oz) can curried beans with sultanas
2–3 tablespoons mango chutney, chopped
I5 g/½ oz (U.S. I tablespoon) butter or margarine
2 tablespoons (U.S. 3 tablespoons) water

Put the onions in a large pan and cover with cold water. Bring to the boil, cover and simmer for about 30 minutes, or until just tender. Drain and leave to cool. Cut a slice from one end of each onion so that it will stand firmly. Scoop out the centre onion pulp, leaving 2 layers as an 'outside wall'. Roughly chop the pulp. Heat the oven to 200°C/400°F, Gas Mark 6.

Heat the bacon in a frying pan (U.S. skillet) until the fat begins to run. Add the chopped onion and chicken liver and fry over moderate heat, stirring, for 3 minutes. Stir in the beans and chutney.

Stand the onions in a greased ovenproof dish, spoon the bean mixture into the centres and dot with butter. Add the water to the dish. Cover cook for 30 minutes. Serve with brown rice. **Serves 4**

Waldorf cabbage salad

2 red-skinned eating apples, cored
I teaspoon lemon juice
225 g/8 oz (U.S. 2 cups) finely shredded white or green cabbage
50 g/2 oz (U.S. ½ cup) chopped walnuts
75 g/3 oz (U.S. ½ cup) seedless raisins
6 stalks celery, very finely chopped
I00 g/4 oz (U.S. ¼ lb) Cheddar cheese, diced
Dressing
75 ml/3 fl oz (U.S. ⅓ cup) mayonnaise
75 ml/3 fl oz (U.S. ⅓ cup) natural yogurt
2 tablespoons (U.S. 3 tablespoons) snipped chives

Cut the apples into neat dice and toss with the lemon juice to prevent discolouration. Combine the apple dice with the cabbage, walnuts, raisins, celery and cheese in a salad bowl, and toss lightly.

Beat together the ingredients for the dressing and transfer to a small jug or sauce boat. Hand separately with the salad. **Serves 4**

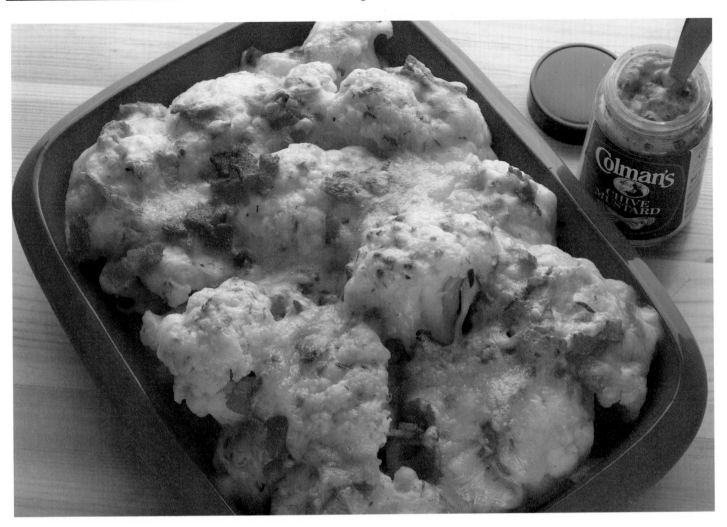

Cauliflower bake

(Illustrated above)

1 large cauliflower, trimmed and cut into florets
25 g/1 oz (U.S. 2 tablespoons) butter
175 g/6 oz rashers streaky bacon (U.S. 6 bacon
slices), rind removed and cut in strips
2 tablespoons (U.S. 3 tablespoons) wholewheat flour
300 ml/½ pint (U.S. 1¼ cups) milk
2–3 tablespoons chive mustard
175 g/6 oz (U.S. 1½ cups) grated Cheddar cheese

Cook the cauliflower in salted water for 5 minutes, until just tender. Drain, reserving 150 ml/¼ pint (U.S. ⅔ cup) cooking water. Keep cauliflower hot.

Melt the butter in a pan and fry the bacon over moderate heat until crisp. Remove the bacon pieces with a slotted spoon. Stir the flour into the fat remaining in the pan and cook for 1 minute. Gradually add the reserved water, the milk and mustard. Simmer, stirring, for 3 minutes. Remove from the heat and stir in ⅔ of the cheese.

Arrange the cauliflower in a heatproof dish, spoon the sauce over and sprinkle with the bacon and remaining cheese. Place under a hot grill (U.S. broiler) until bubbling and golden. **Serves 3–4**

Cannellini salad

1 red-skinned eating apple, cored
few drops of lemon juice
4 large frankfurters
1 (425-g/15-oz) can cannellini beans, drained
4 spring onions (U.S. 4 scallions), sliced
2 tablespoons (U.S. 3 tablespoons) chopped parsley
1 tablespoon peanut butter
2 teaspoons oil
1 teaspoon vinegar
salt and freshly ground black pepper

Slice the apple thinly and sprinkle the slices with lemon juice to prevent discolouration. Cut the sausages into diagonal slices. Combine the beans, apple, frankfurters, onion and parsley. Beat together the peanut butter, oil and vinegar until blended, then season. Pour over the bean mixture and toss lightly.
Serves 4

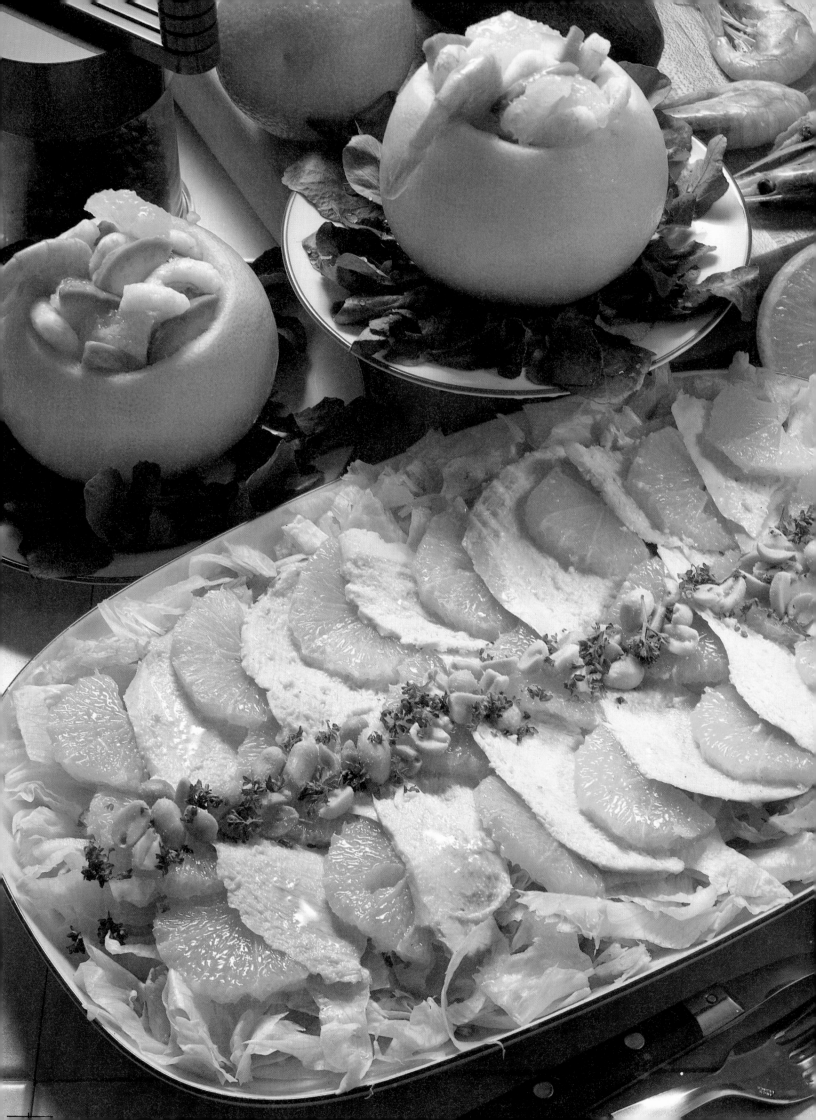

Grapefruit and prawn cocktail

(Illustrated opposite)

4 grapefruits
100 g/4 oz peeled prawns (U.S. ¼ lb shelled cooked shrimp)
2 stalks celery, chopped
1 large avocado, peeled, stoned (U.S. pitted) and sliced
2 tablespoons (U.S. 3 tablespoons) oil
1 tablespoon wine vinegar
1 teaspoon light muscovado sugar (U.S. light brown sugar)
½ teaspoon made mustard
salt and freshly ground black pepper
4 whole prawns (U.S. whole shrimp) to garnish (optional)

Slice the tops off the grapefruits and scoop out the flesh. Place the grapefruit segments in a bowl with the prawns, celery and avocado.

Combine the oil, wine vinegar, sugar and mustard in a small screw-topped container. Shake well. Pour over the grapefruit mixture and season to taste. Turn the ingredients carefully in the dressing.

Spoon the cocktail into the grapefruit shells and serve garnished with a prawn as a starter, or on a bed of watercress as a side salad. **Serves 4**

Chicken and orange salad

(Illustrated opposite)

3 chicken breasts, cooked
3 oranges
1 lettuce
juice of ½ orange
1 tablespoon oil
salt and freshly ground black pepper
75 g/3 oz (U.S. scant ½ cup) roasted peanuts
1 tablespoon chopped parsley to garnish

Slice the meat thinly from the chicken breasts. Remove the peel and pith from the oranges and slice them thinly. Discard any pips. Roughly chop the lettuce and make a bed of it on a serving dish. Arrange alternate layers of chicken and orange slices over the lettuce.

Mix the orange juice and oil together and season to taste. Spoon over the chicken. Sprinkle peanuts down the centre of the dish and top with parsley. **Serves 4**

Above: Grapefruit and prawn cocktail. Below: Chicken and orange salad

Pineapple rice side salad

5 tablespoons (U.S. 7 tablespoons) oil
1 medium-sized onion, peeled and finely chopped
200 g/7 oz (U.S. 1 cup) long grain brown rice
400 ml/14 fl oz chicken stock
(U.S. 1¾ cups chicken bouillon)
1 teaspoon dried mixed herbs
1 (350-g/12-oz) can pineapple pieces in natural juice
1 green pepper, seeds removed and finely chopped
4 tablespoons (U.S. 6 tablespoons) white wine vinegar

Heat the oil in a large pan and gently fry the onion until soft. Stir in the rice and cook for 1 minute. Add the stock, herbs and juice from the pineapple. Bring to the boil. Stir once, cover and simmer for 25 minutes, or until the rice is tender and has absorbed the liquid.

Remove the pan from the heat, fork in the pineapple, pepper and vinegar, and toss the ingredients lightly. Leave to cool then chill well before serving with any cold meat. **Serves 4**

Note Left-over Pineapple rice side salad makes a delicious light meal used as a filling for halved avocados or tomato cups. (Tomato pulp from the cups can be used in Moulded Mexican salad (see page 106).)

Hot tuna and bean salad

225 g/8 oz shelled broad beans (U.S. ½ lb fava or lima beans)
675 g/1½ lb potatoes, peeled and cubed
1 (198-g/7-oz) can tuna, drained
4 tablespoons (U.S. 6 tablespoons) mayonnaise
1 red-skinned eating apple, cored and diced
2 teaspoons (U.S. 1 tablespoon) lemon juice
4 spring onions (U.S. 4 scallions), chopped

Cook the beans and potatoes in separate pans of boiling salted water until tender. Meanwhile, drain the liquid from the tuna into the mayonnaise and stir well. Flake the fish. Drain the potatoes and beans. Add the tuna to the potato in the pan and put the beans on top. Cover the pan again. Leave to stand for 5 minutes. Toss the apple dice with the lemon juice. Transfer the tuna mixture to a serving dish and fork in the onion and apple. Pour the mayonnaise dressing over and toss the ingredients lightly until coated. Serve while still warm. **Serves 4**

Gouda and courgette bread

(Illustrated opposite)

100 g/4 oz courgettes (U.S. $\frac{1}{4}$ lb zucchini)
50 g/2 oz plain flour (U.S. $\frac{1}{2}$ cup all-purpose flour)
1$\frac{1}{2}$ teaspoons (U.S. 2 teaspoons) baking powder
1 teaspoon ground cinnamon
175 g/6 oz wholemeal flour (U.S. 1$\frac{1}{2}$ cups
wholewheat flour)
2 eggs
100 g/4 oz light muscovado sugar
(U.S. $\frac{1}{2}$ cup light brown sugar)
100 g/4 oz (U.S. $\frac{1}{2}$ cup) unsalted butter, melted
50 g/2 oz (U.S. $\frac{1}{3}$ cup) currants
100 g/4 oz (U.S. 1 cup) grated Gouda cheese
50 g/2 oz (U.S. $\frac{1}{2}$ cup) chopped walnuts or pecans
1 teaspoon vanilla essence (U.S. vanilla extract)
2 tablespoons (U.S. 3 tablespoons) milk

Heat the oven to 160°C/325°F, Gas Mark 3 and
grease a 1-kg/2-lb loaf-shaped tin.

Top and tail the courgettes and grate them
coarsely. Sift the white flour with the baking powder
and cinnamon, then stir in the brown flour. Place the
eggs and sugar together in a bowl and whisk until
pale and creamy. Gradually add the butter, whisking
well after each addition. Stir in the flour mixture,
then the remaining ingredients. When well combined, transfer to the prepared tin.

Bake for about 1$\frac{1}{4}$ hours. Turn the loaf out of the
tin and tap the base with the knuckles. If ready, the
loaf will sound hollow and the bottom crust will be
hard. If necessary, lay the loaf on its side on a baking
sheet (U.S. cookie sheet) and return to the oven for a
few minutes.

Serve warm or cold, sliced and spread with butter.
Makes 1 loaf, about 10 slices

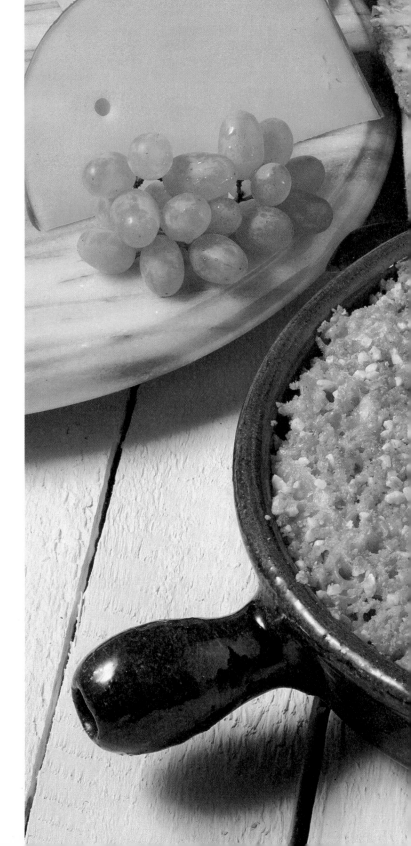

*Above: Gouda and courgette bread. Below: Baked vegetarian
pasta (recipe page 61)*

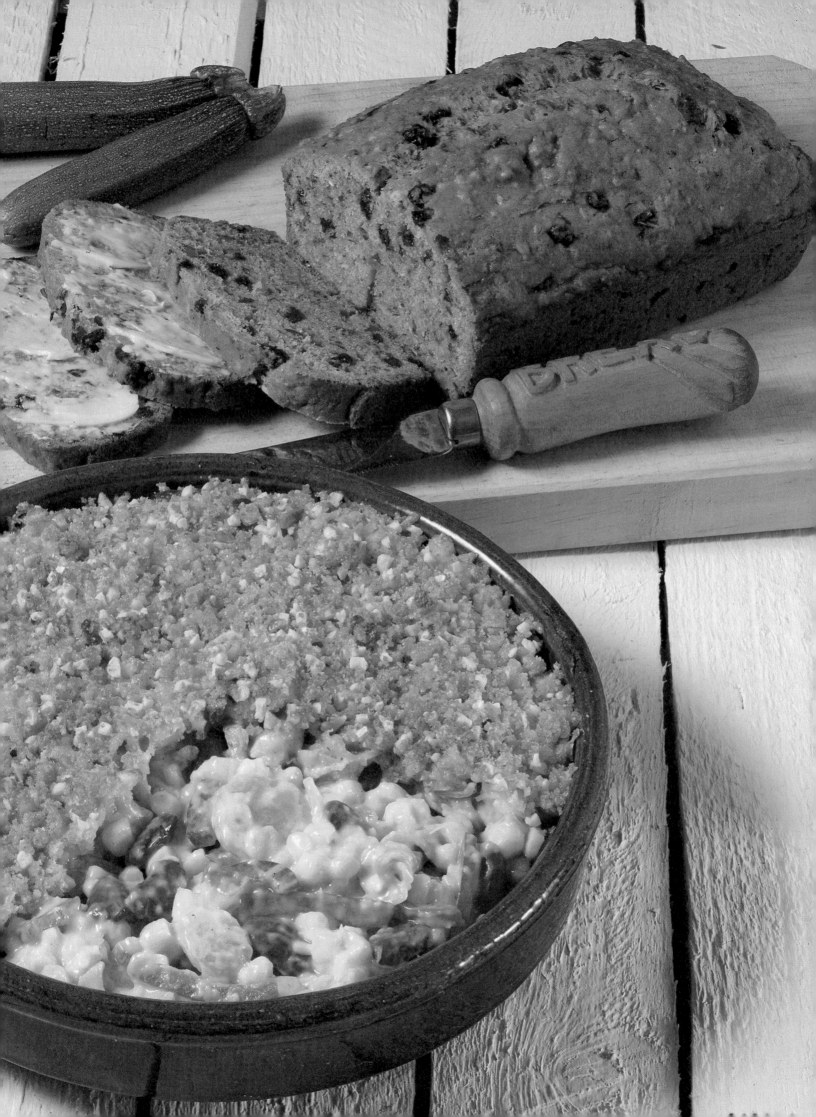

Tuna stuffed aubergines

(Illustrated opposite)

2 (225-g/8-oz) aubergines
(U.S. 2×½-lb eggplants)
2 tablespoons (U.S. 3 tablespoons) oil
1 large onion, peeled and chopped
1 clove garlic, crushed
1 (425-g/15-oz) can tomatoes, drained
½ teaspoon dried mixed herbs
1 tablespoon tomato purée (U.S. tomato paste)
salt and freshly ground black pepper
1 (200-g/7-oz) can tuna, drained and flaked
100 g/4 oz (U.S. 1 cup) grated Cheddar cheese

Heat the oven to 190°C/375°F, Gas Mark 5 and grease a shallow ovenproof dish.

Cut the aubergines in half lengthways. Using a grapefruit knife, carefully remove the inside flesh leaving a thin shell. Chop the flesh roughly.

Heat the oil in a pan and fry the onion gently until golden. Add the garlic, tomatoes, herbs, tomato purée and chopped aubergine. Season lightly, bring to the boil and cook gently for about 15 minutes, or until the aubergine is tender. Fold in the tuna and adjust the seasoning if necessary.

Pile the mixture into the aubergine shells, stand them in the prepared dish and sprinkle over the cheese.

Bake for about 30 minutes, or until golden brown on top and the aubergine shells are tender. **Serves 4**

Tomato and onion bake

1 (425-g/15-oz) can cannellini beans
1 teaspoon salt
finely grated rind of ½ lemon
75 g/3 oz (U.S. ⅓ cup) butter or margarine
2 medium-sized onions, peeled and chopped
1 teaspoon dried rosemary
4 medium-sized tomatoes, thinly sliced
100 g/4 oz (U.S. 1 cup) grated Cheddar cheese
1 tablespoon chopped parsley
sprig of parsley to garnish

Heat the oven to 190°C/375°F, Gas Mark 5 and grease a 1-litre/1¾-pint (U.S. 4½-cup) ovenproof dish.

Turn the beans and liquid from the can into a pan. Add the salt and bring to the boil. Simmer for 3 minutes. Drain the beans and sprinkle them with the lemon rind.

Melt 50 g/2 oz (U.S. ¼ cup) of the butter in a frying pan (U.S. skillet) and cook the onion and rosemary, stirring, over low heat until the onion is soft and pale golden. Remove from the heat, add the beans and mix well. Put half the bean mixture in an even layer in the bottom of the prepared dish and cover with half the tomato slices. Sprinkle with half the cheese. Repeat the layers once, using all the ingredients and finishing with cheese mixed with the chopped parsley. Melt the remaining butter and sprinkle over top.

Bake for 20 minutes, or until piping hot and the crust is golden. Garnish with a sprig of parsley and serve hot from the dish. **Serves 4**

Vegetable fritters au gratin

100 g/4 oz wholemeal flour (U.S. 1 cup wholewheat flour)
½ teaspoon salt
¼ teaspoon pepper
1 teaspoon dried thyme
½ teaspoon ground nutmeg
½ teaspoon light muscovado sugar (U.S. light brown sugar)
½ teaspoon mild Continental mustard
1 tablespoon oil
1 egg, separated
150 ml/¼ pint (U.S. ⅔ cup) water
1 large onion, peeled and finely chopped
100 g/4 oz (U.S. 1¼ cups) coarsely grated carrot
100 g/4 oz (U.S. 1¼ cups) coarsely grated parsnip
oil for shallow frying
100 g/4 oz (U.S. 1 cup) grated Cheddar cheese

Combine the flour, salt, pepper, thyme, nutmeg, sugar, mustard, oil and egg yolk in a large bowl. Add half the water and whisk until the batter is smooth. Gradually whisk in the remaining water. Leave to stand for 20 minutes.

Add the vegetables to the batter and mix well. Just before frying, whisk the egg white in a clean bowl and fold into the fritter mixture.

Heat a little oil in a heavy frying pan (U.S. skillet) and, using 1 heaped tablespoon of mixture for each fritter, fry a few at a time over moderate heat for about 3 minutes on each side, until golden brown. Drain quickly on absorbent towel and arrange in a flameproof serving dish. Keep hot until all the fritters are cooked and in the dish.

Sprinkle the cheese over the fritters and grill (U.S. broil) under high heat until the cheese is golden. **Serves 4**

Tuna stuffed aubergines

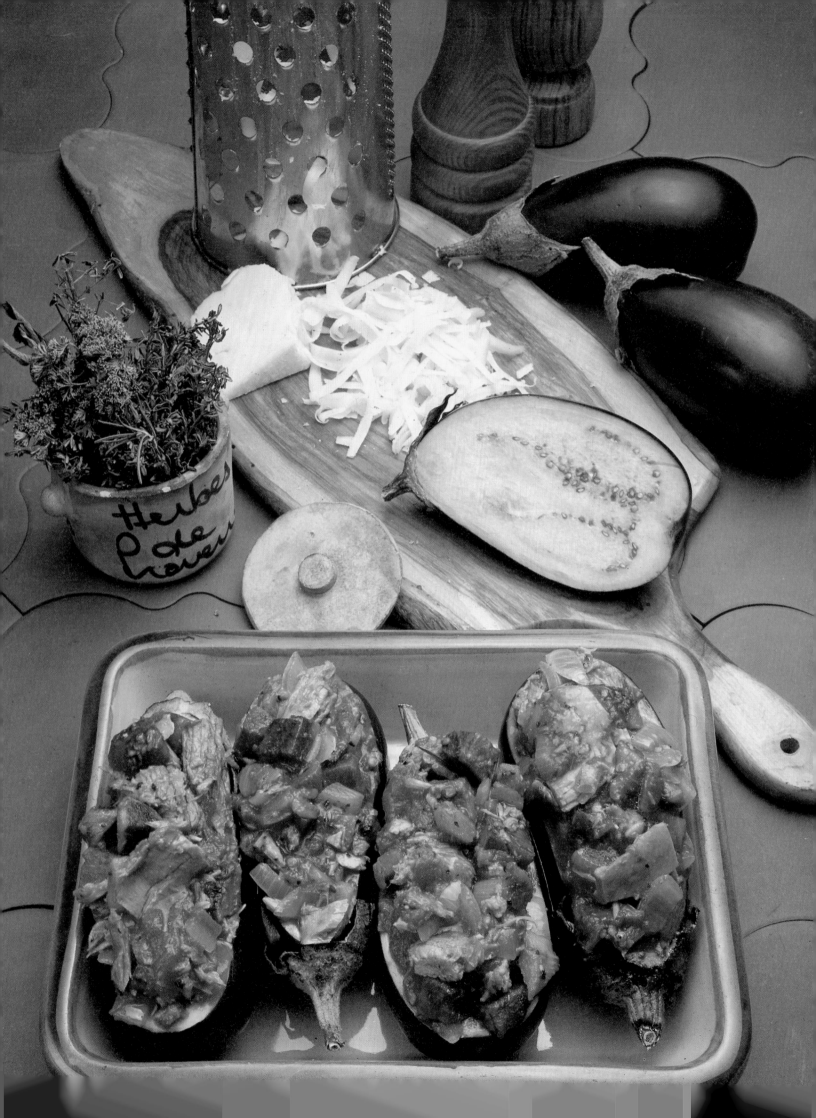

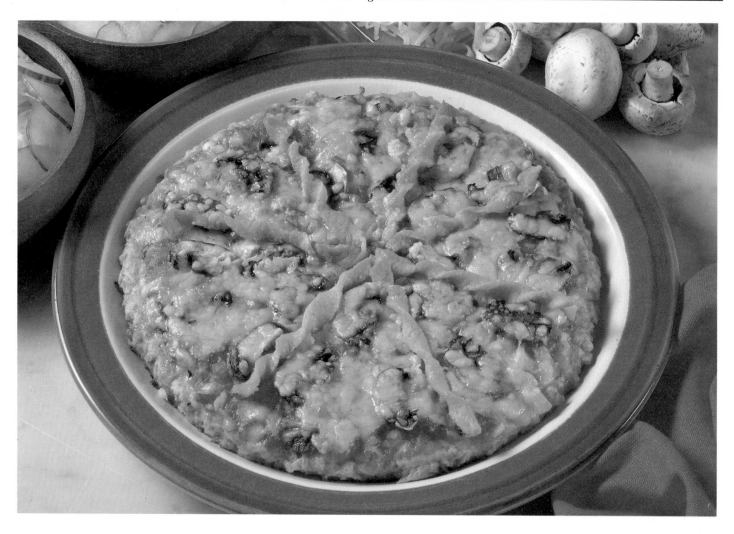

Mushroom and bacon pizza

(Illustrated above)

75 g/3 oz plain flour (U.S. $\frac{3}{4}$ cup all-purpose flour)
1 tablespoon (U.S. 4 teaspoons) baking powder
75 g/3 oz wholemeal flour (U.S. $\frac{3}{4}$ cup wholewheat flour)
40 g/1$\frac{1}{2}$ oz (U.S. 3 tablespoons) butter
100 ml/4 fl oz (U.S. $\frac{1}{2}$ cup) milk
Topping
1 small onion, peeled and finely chopped
1 (425-g/15-oz) can tomatoes, drained and roughly chopped
$\frac{1}{2}$ teaspoon dried oregano
salt and freshly ground black pepper
100 g/4 oz (U.S. $\frac{1}{4}$ lb) button mushrooms, sliced
175 g/6 oz (U.S. 1$\frac{1}{2}$ cups) grated Edam cheese
2 rashers streaky bacon (U.S. 2 bacon slices), rind removed and cut into thin strips

Heat the oven to 230°C/450°F, Gas Mark 8 and grease a baking sheet (U.S. cookie sheet).

Sift the white flour and baking powder into a bowl and stir in the brown flour. Rub or cut in the butter until the mixture resembles breadcrumbs. Add the milk and mix to a soft dough. Knead lightly and roll out to a round about 20 cm/8 inches in diameter. Place on the prepared sheet.

Combine the onion, tomato, oregano and a little seasoning. Cover the pizza base with the mushrooms, sprinkle over half the cheese, then spread the tomato mixture over this and top with the remaining cheese. Finally arrange the strips of bacon decoratively on top.

Bake for 20 minutes, reduce the oven temperature to 200°C/400°F, Gas Mark 6 and continue cooking for further 10 minutes. Serve hot or cold with a salad.
Serves 4-6

Variation

Mushroom and bean pizza Omit the bacon. Combine 1 (200-g/7-oz) can baked beans with the tomato mixture and spread on the pizza base. Top with grated Gouda cheese instead of the Edam and grind a little black pepper over just before serving.

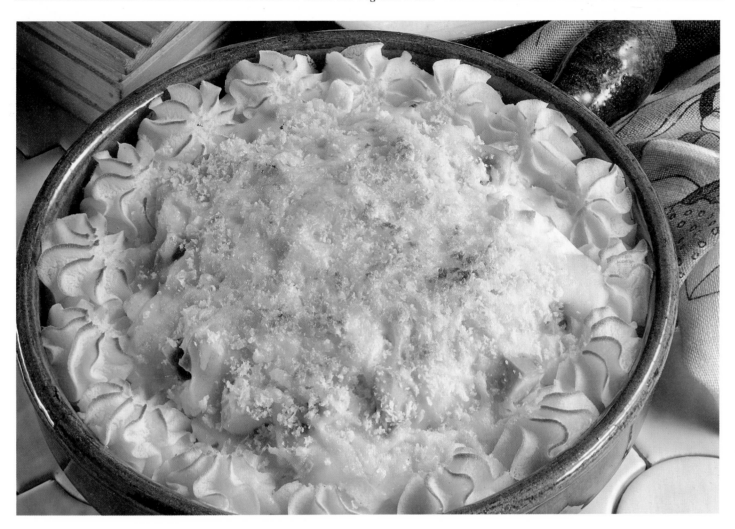

Avocado gratinée

(Illustrated above)

1 kg/2¼ lb potatoes, peeled
65 g/2½ oz (U.S. generous ¼ cup) butter or margarine
salt and freshly ground black pepper
1 (99-g/3½-oz) can pink salmon, drained, boned and
flaked
1 ripe avocado pear, peeled and diced
4 eggs, hard-boiled (U.S. hard-cooked), shelled and
roughly chopped
40 g/1½ oz wholemeal flour
(U.S. scant ⅓ cup wholewheat flour)
450 ml/¾ pint (U.S. 2 cups) milk
1 teaspoon Continental mustard
2 tablespoons (U.S. 3 tablespoons) wine vinegar
100 g/4 oz (U.S. 1 cup) finely grated Cheddar cheese

Cook the potatoes in a pan of boiling salted water
until tender. Heat the oven to 220°C/425°F, Gas
Mark 7 and grease a shallow ovenproof dish.

Drain the potatoes and mash with 25 g/1 oz (U.S. 2
tablespoons) of the butter until smooth. Season to
taste. Pipe or fork the potatoes around the edge of the
prepared dish. Bake for 20 minutes, or until beginning to turn golden.

Meanwhile, combine the salmon, avocado and
egg. Melt the remaining butter in a pan and blend in
the flour. Cook for 1 minute, stirring. Gradually add
the milk and bring to the boil, stirring constantly.
Season well and add the mustard and vinegar.
Simmer for 3 minutes and stir in half the cheese.

Spoon the avocado mixture into the centre of the
potato ring and pour the sauce over. Sprinkle with
the rest of the cheese and return to the oven for a
further 20 minutes. Serve hot. **Serves 4**

Variations

Chicken and avocado in a potato nest Omit the
salmon and eggs and substitute 225 g/8 oz (U.S. 2
cups) chopped cooked chicken and 25 g/1 oz (U.S. ¼
cup) chopped garlic sausage. Sprinkle the avocado
with 1 teaspoon lemon juice before mixing it with the
chicken and sausage to make the filling.

Smoked haddock and avocado gratinée Omit the
salmon and reduce the eggs to 2. Sprinkle the
avocado with 1 teaspoon lemon juice as above. Poach
225 g/8 oz smoked haddock fillet (U.S. ½ lb finnan
haddie) then remove any skin and bones, flake the fish
and combine with the avocado and egg for the filling.

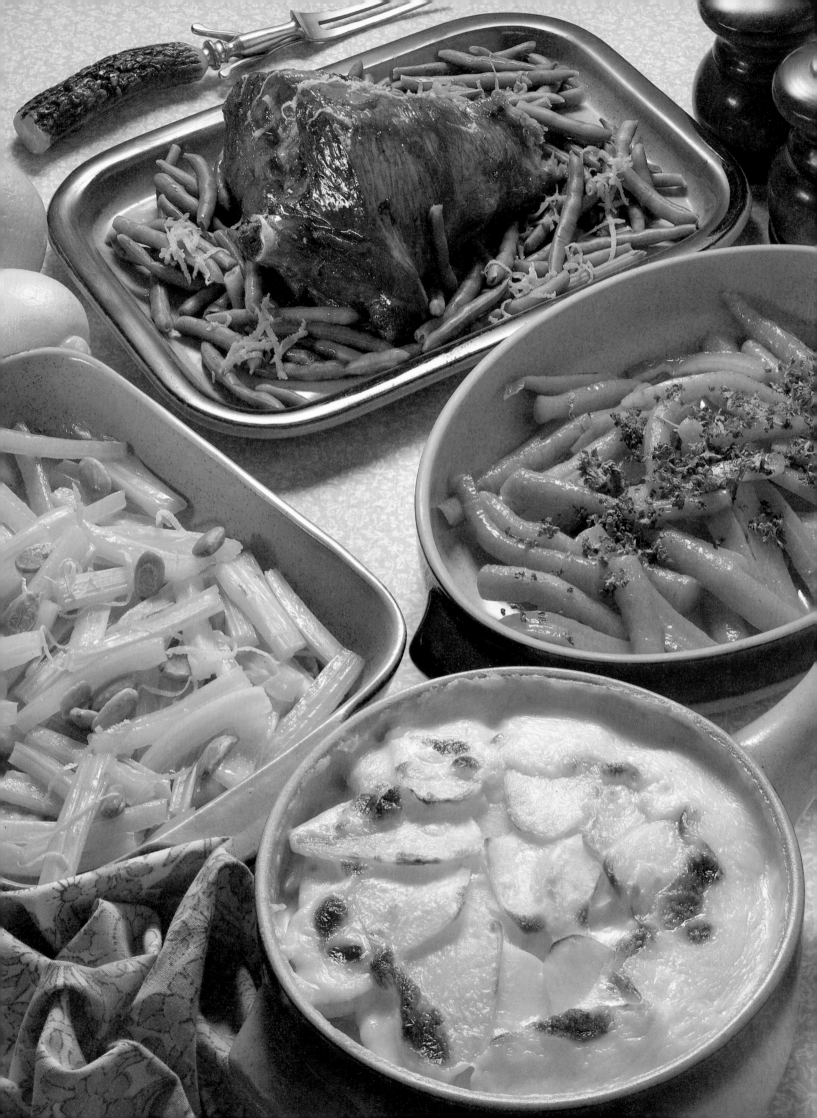

Orange tossed green beans

(Illustrated opposite)

450 g/1 lb frozen whole green beans
salt
finely grated rind and juice of 1 orange
15 g/½ oz (U.S. 1 tablespoon) butter or margarine

Cook the beans in a pan of boiling salted water as directed on the pack. Drain well and return to the hot pan. Add the orange juice and butter, cover and shake the pan briskly until the beans are coated with the orange mixture. Serve on a warm dish, sprinkled with the orange rind, round a joint of roast lamb or pork. **Serves 4**

Celery with lemon and almonds

(Illustrated opposite)

1 head of celery (U.S. 1 bunch of celery)
50 ml/2 fl oz (U.S. ¼ cup) water
juice of 2 lemons
75 g/3 oz (U.S. ⅓ cup) butter or margarine
1 tablespoon light muscovado sugar (U.S. light brown sugar)
finely grated rind of 1 lemon
50 g/2 oz flaked almonds (U.S. ½ cup slivered almonds), toasted

Cut the celery into strips 10 cm/4 inches long and 1.25 cm/½ inch wide. Put the water, lemon juice, butter and sugar in a pan. Add the celery, bring to the boil, cover and simmer for about 10 minutes, or until the celery is tender.

Remove the lid and shake the pan over moderate heat until the celery is glossy and the liquid almost evaporated. Transfer to a warm dish, sprinkle with the lemon rind and almonds. Serve hot. **Serves 4**

Lemon and garlic potatoes

(Illustrated opposite)

900 g/2 lb potatoes, peeled and thinly sliced
salt and freshly ground black pepper
25 g/1 oz (U.S. 2 tablespoons) margarine
20 g/¾ oz wholemeal flour (U.S. scant ¼ cup whole-wheat flour)
300 ml/½ pint (U.S. 1¼ cups) milk
1 clove garlic, very finely chopped
finely grated rind and juice of 1 lemon

Heat the oven to 160°C/325°F, Gas Mark 3 and generously grease a large ovenproof dish.

Layer up the potato slices in the prepared dish, sprinkling with a little seasoning between the layers. Put the margarine, flour and milk in a pan and whisk over moderate heat until the sauce boils and thickens. Whisk in the garlic and lemon rind and juice. Pour the sauce over the potatoes.

Bake for 1½ hours, or until the potatoes are tender and the top is turning golden. This dish is an ideal accompaniment to roast meat and can be cooked in the oven alongside the joint. **Serves 6**

Orange glazed carrots

(Illustrated opposite)

450 g/1 lb carrots, peeled
50 ml/2 fl oz (U.S. ¼ cup) water
juice of 2 oranges
75 g/3 oz (U.S. ⅓ cup) butter or margarine
1 tablespoon light muscovado sugar (U.S. light brown sugar)
1 tablespoon chopped parsley to garnish

Cut the carrots into strips about 1.25 cm/½ inch wide. Put the water, orange juice, butter and sugar in a pan. Add the carrots, bring to the boil, cover and simmer for about 10 minutes, or until the carrots are tender.

Remove the lid and shake the pan over moderate heat until the carrots are fully glazed. Transfer to a warm dish, sprinkle with parsley. Serve hot. **Serves 4**

Above: Orange tossed green beans. Centre left: Celery with lemon and almonds. Centre right: Orange glazed carrots. Below: Lemon and garlic potatoes

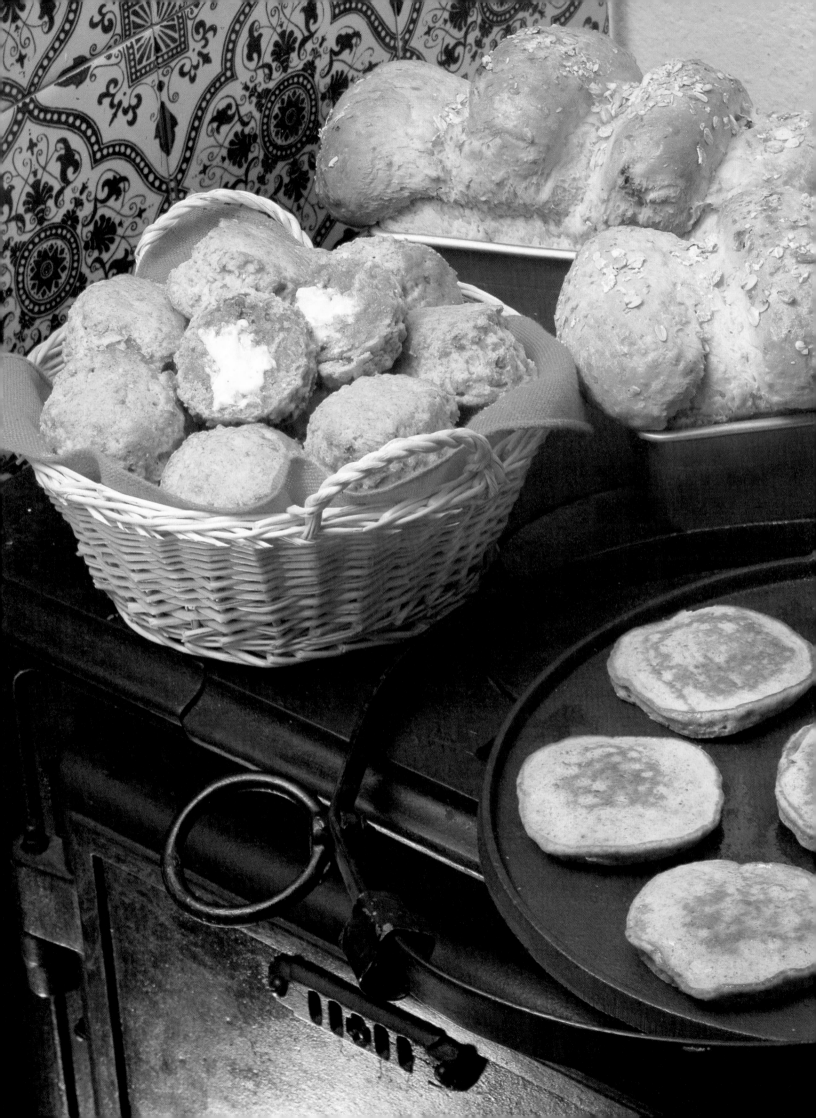

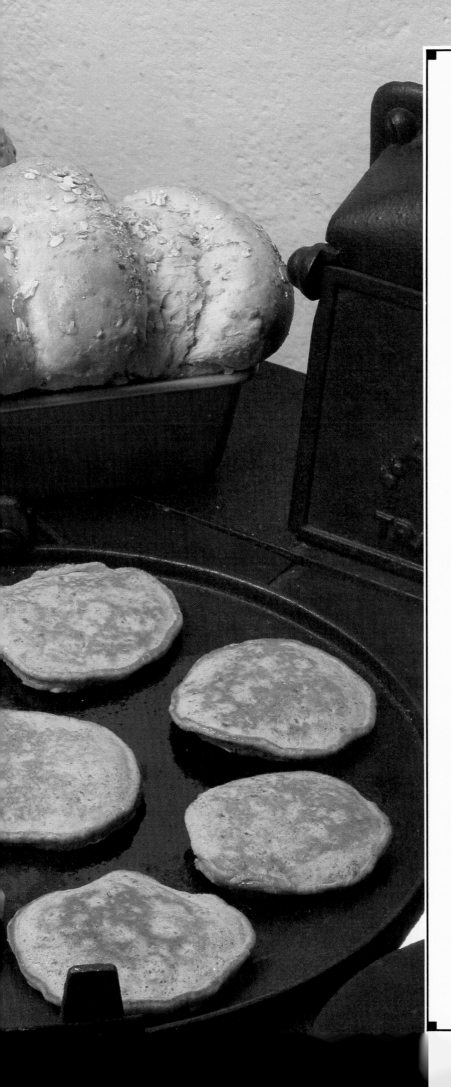

Breads, Pastries and Teatime Favourites

The kitchen scene has completely changed with the introduction of many new ingredients to make our daily bread part of a healthy hi-fi diet. The same rules happily apply to making pastry and many other baked goods. You may wish to try your hand at making your own bread. Use traditional fresh yeast, handy dried yeast or the easy blend variety, which is mixed directly with the flour. The addition of a vitamin C tablet speeds up the rising process. If you want to proceed cautiously, begin with yeasted recipes for a dough that's half white and half wholemeal flour, and can even include muesli. Our own bread chain for loaves, rolls, pizza bases and plaits is based on 100% wholewheat flour. Never be confused by references in cookbooks to wholewheat or wholemeal, because they both mean the same thing. Carry on from there and extend your hi-fi cook's repertoire to include pastry. My brown pastries have fascinating ingredients – wheat flakes, ground nuts and granary flour.

My drop scones, very quickly cooked by pouring the batter on a heated griddle, are positively bursting with healthy ingredients. If you have no griddle, a heavy-based frying pan (U.S. skillet) will do admirably instead. Baking powder breads and scones (U.S. biscuits) can be sweet or savoury, which I find greatly extends their appeal. A development of the basic scone recipe is the cobbler topping for fruit, which can easily be adapted to a savoury topping for stews. Cookies and several other small fillers are catered for in this section too, and some of them use oaty flour which can be made by grinding down oats in a blender or food processor.

Above: Muesli bumpy loaves (recipe page 137). Left: Rich original scones (recipe page 129). Centre: Wholewheat drop pancakes (recipe page 137)

Herby ham round

(Illustrated opposite)

450 g/1 lb wheatmeal flour
(U.S. 4 cups wholewheat flour)
$\frac{1}{2}$ teaspoon salt
25 g/1 oz (U.S. 2 tablespoons) lard
1 sachet easy blend yeast
200 ml/7 fl oz (U.S. scant 1 cup) cold water
100 ml/3$\frac{1}{2}$ fl oz (U.S. $\frac{1}{3}$ cup) boiling water
1 (113-g/4-oz) pack sliced ham, diced
1 tablespoon dried mixed herbs
1 egg, beaten

Put the flour and salt into a bowl and rub or cut in the lard. Stir in the yeast and make a well in the centre. Combine the cold and boiling water, add to the bowl and mix to a dough. Turn out on a floured surface and knead for 10 minutes. Grease the bowl, return the ball of dough to it and turn once to coat. Cover and leave in a warm place until double in bulk.

Turn the dough out again on a floured surface and knead for 2 minutes, working in the ham and herbs at the same time. Shape into a 20-cm/8-inch round and place on a greased baking sheet (U.S. cookie sheet). Cut a deep cross in the top with a sharp knife. Cover with greased cling film and leave in a warm place for about 30 minutes, or until puffy. Meanwhile, heat the oven to 230°C/450°F, Gas Mark 8.

Uncover the loaf, brush with egg and bake for 15 minutes, then reduce the oven temperature to 200°C/400°F, Gas Mark 6 and continue baking for a further 20 minutes, or until browned. The loaf is cooked if it sounds hollow when tapped on the base with the knuckles. **Makes 1 medium-sized loaf**

Cheese, onion and celery bread

(Illustrated opposite)

50 g/2 oz (U.S. $\frac{1}{4}$ cup) butter or margarine
1 medium-sized onion, peeled and chopped
2 stalks celery, chopped
450 g/1 lb (U.S. 4 cups) wholewheat flour
1 teaspoon salt
1 sachet easy blend yeast
75 g/3 oz mature Cheddar cheese, grated
(U.S. $\frac{3}{4}$ cup grated sharp Cheddar cheese)
200 ml/7 fl oz (U.S. scant 1 cup) cold water
100 ml/3$\frac{1}{2}$ fl oz (U.S. $\frac{1}{2}$ cup) boiling water

Melt half the butter in a pan and fry the onion and celery gently until soft but not brown. Set aside.

Mix together the flour and salt in a bowl and rub or cut in the rest of the butter. Sprinkle the yeast over.

Add the cheese, mix again, then add the onion mixture. Make a well in the centre. Combine the cold and boiling water, add to the bowl and mix to a dough. Turn out on a floured surface and knead for 10 minutes. Grease the bowl, return the ball of dough to it and turn once to coat. Cover and leave in a warm place until double in bulk.

Turn the dough out again on to a floured surface and knead for 2 minutes. Shape into an oblong to fit a greased 1-kg/2-lb) loaf-shaped tin. Placed in the tin with the smoothest side uppermost. Cover with greased cling film and leave in a warm place until the dough is about 1.25 cm/$\frac{1}{2}$ inch above the top of the tin. Heat the oven to 230°C/450°F, Gas Mark 8.

Uncover the loaf, sprinkle with flour and bake for about 40 minutes. The loaf is cooked if it sounds hollow when tapped on the base with the knuckles. Cool on a wire rack. **Makes 1 large loaf**

Caraway lager loaf

(Illustrated opposite)

350 g/12 oz strong white flour
(U.S. 3 cups white bread flour)
350 g/12 oz wheatmeal flour
(U.S. 3 cups wholewheat flour)
1 teaspoon salt
25 g/1 oz (U.S. 2 tablespoons) lard
1 sachet easy blend yeast
2 tablespoons (U.S. 3 tablespoons) caraway seeds
1 (440-ml/15-fl oz) can lager (U.S. light beer)
1 egg, beaten

Mix together the white flour, brown flour and salt in a bowl. Rub or cut in the lard. Sprinkle in the yeast and seeds and make a well in the centre. Gently heat the lager in a pan until lukewarm. Add to the dry ingredients and mix to a dough. Turn the dough out on a floured surface and knead for 10 minutes. Grease the bowl, return the ball of dough to it and turn once. Cover and leave in a warm place until double in bulk.

Turn the dough out again on a floured surface and knead for 2 minutes. Shape into a smooth oval about 25 cm/10 inches long and place on a greased baking sheet (U.S. cookie sheet). Slash the top of the loaf at 2.5-cm/1-inch intervals. Cover with greased cling film and leave in a warm place to rise until puffy. Heat the oven to 230°C/450°F, Gas Mark 8.

Uncover the loaf, brush with egg and bake for about 35 minutes, or until golden brown. The loaf is cooked if it sounds hollow when tapped on the base with the knuckles. **Makes 1 large loaf**

Above: Herby ham round. Centre: Cheese, onion and celery bread. Below: Caraway lager loaf

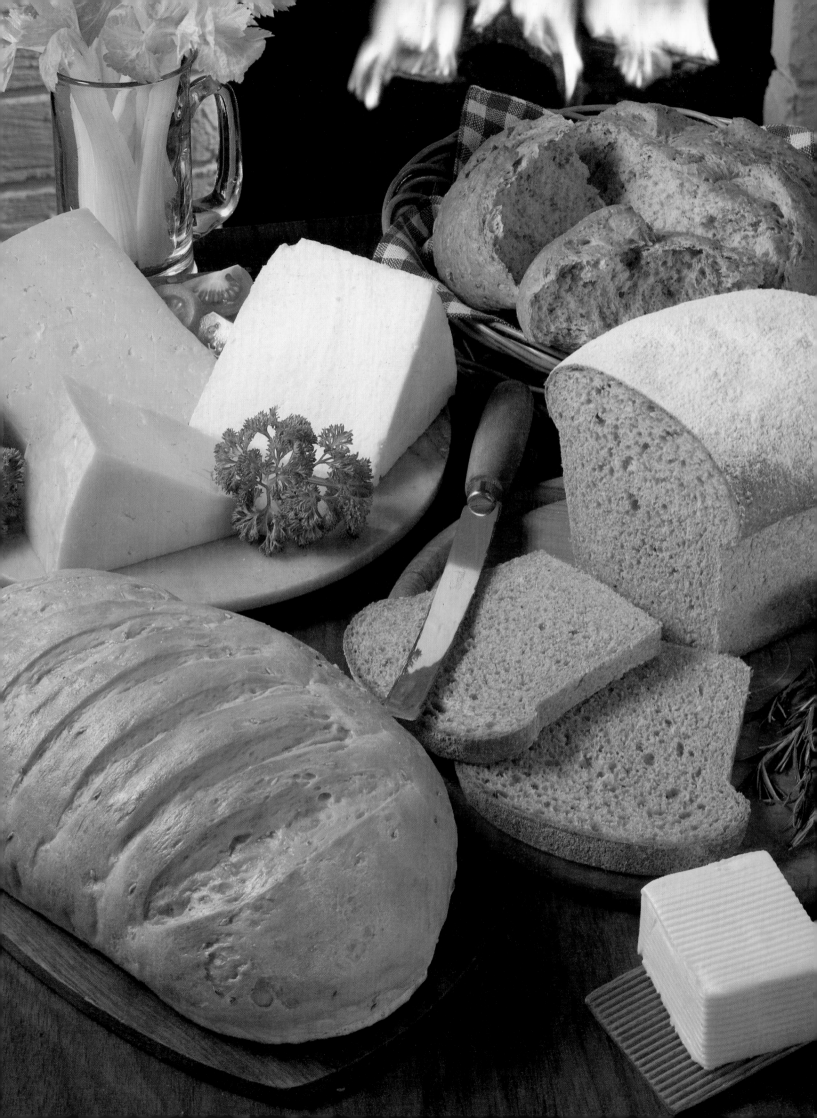

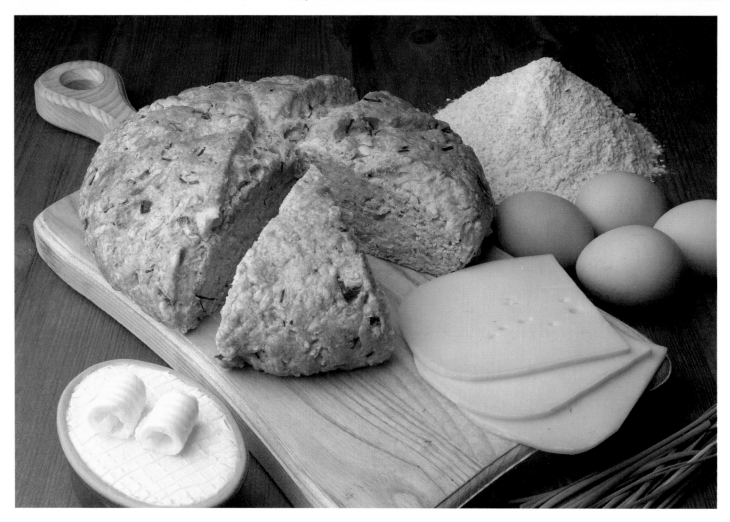

Cheese and chive bread

(Illustrated above)

225 g/8 oz plain flour (U.S. 2 cups all-purpose flour)
1 teaspoon salt
2 teaspoons dry mustard powder
4 teaspoons (U.S. 2 tablespoons) baking powder
225 g/8 oz (U.S. 2 cups) wholewheat flour
100 g/4 oz (U.S. $\frac{1}{2}$ cup) butter
225 g/8 oz (U.S. 2 cups) finely grated Gouda cheese
1 small onion, peeled and finely chopped
1 tablespoon snipped chives
2 eggs, lightly beaten
175 ml/6 fl oz (U.S. $\frac{3}{4}$ cup) milk

Heat the oven to 190°C/375°F, Gas Mark 5 and grease a baking sheet (U.S. cookie sheet).

Sift the white flour, salt, mustard and baking powder into a bowl. Stir in the brown flour then rub or cut in the butter until the mixture resembles breadcrumbs. Add the cheese, onion, chives, eggs and milk, and mix well to a soft dough. Shape into a large round, transfer to the prepared tin and score the top into 8 wedges with a knife. Brush with egg.

Bake for 1 hour, until risen and golden. Cool on a wire rack. Serve cut into wedges, split and buttered.
Makes 1 loaf, 8 portions

Brown muffins

1 egg
225 ml/8 fl oz (U.S. 1 cup) milk
50 ml/2 fl oz (U.S. $\frac{1}{4}$ cup) oil
100 g/4 oz plain flour (1 cup all-purpose flour)
4 teaspoons (U.S. 2 tablespoons) baking powder
$\frac{1}{2}$ teaspoon salt
100 g/4 oz wholemeal flour (U.S. 1 cup wholewheat flour)
2 tablespoons light muscovado sugar
(U.S. 3 tablespoons light brown sugar)

Heat the oven to 200°C/400°F, Gas Mark 6 and well grease 12 deep bun tins (U.S. muffin pans).

Lightly whisk the egg with the milk and oil. Sift the white flour with the baking powder and salt into a bowl. Stir in the brown flour and sugar and make a well in the centre. Pour in the egg liquid and stir with a fork until the dry ingredients are just moist. Do not beat the mixture although it will be somewhat lumpy. Divide equally among the prepared tins.

Bake for 20-25 minutes, or until golden brown. A wooden cocktail stick (U.S. toothpick) inserted in the centre should come out clean if the muffins are ready. Turn out and serve fresh with butter. **Makes 12**

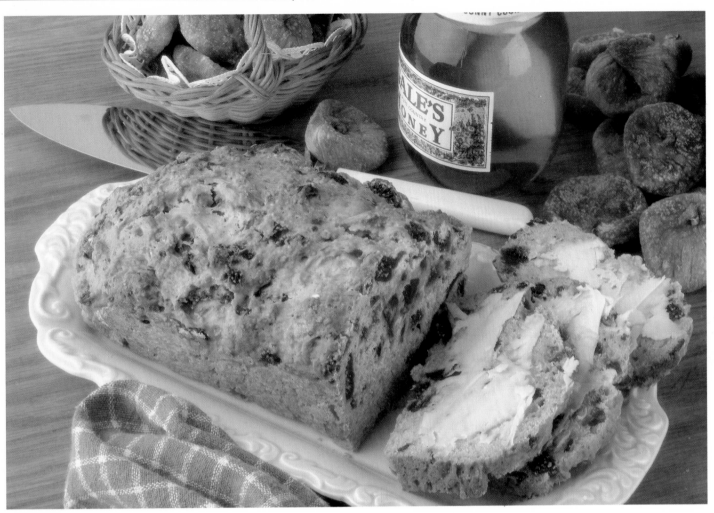

Honeyed fig loaf
(Illustrated above)

100 g/4 oz plain flour (U.S. 1 cup all-purpose flour)
2 teaspoons (U.S. 1 tablespoon) baking powder
150 g/5 oz wholemeal flour
(U.S. 1¼ cups wholewheat flour)
25 g/1 oz (U.S. 2 tablespoons) butter or margarine
75 g/3 oz muscovado sugar (U.S. ⅓ cup brown sugar)
100 g/4 oz (U.S. ⅔ cup) chopped dried figs
50 g/2 oz (U.S. ½ cup) chopped walnuts or pecans
2 tablespoons (U.S. 3 tablespoons) clear honey
1 egg
150 ml/¼ pint (U.S. ⅔ cup) milk

Sift the white flour with the baking powder into a
bowl. Stir in the brown flour then rub or cut in the
butter. Add the sugar, figs and walnuts. Mix together
the honey, egg and milk, add to the dry ingredients
and mix to a dough. Transfer to a greased 450-g/1-lb
loaf-shaped tin and leave to stand for 15 minutes.
Heat the oven to 180°C/350°F, Gas Mark 4.

Bake for about 50 minutes, or until the centre is
firm to the touch. Remove from the tin and cool
slightly on a wire rack. Serve warm, thinly sliced and
buttered. **Makes 1 loaf, about 8 slices**

Honey and ginger nuts
(Illustrated on page 139)

150 g/5 oz plain flour (U.S. 1¼ cups all-purpose flour)
pinch of salt
2 teaspoons (U.S. 1 tablespoon) baking powder
1 teaspoon ground ginger
75 g/3 oz (U.S. ¾ cup) wholewheat flour
100 g/4 oz (U.S. ½ cup) butter or margarine
1 tablespoon set honey
1 egg, beaten
100 g/4 oz light muscovado sugar
(U.S. ½ cup light brown sugar)
25 g/1 oz (U.S. ¼ cup) pine nuts, ground

Heat the oven to 180°C/350°F, Gas Mark 4 and grease
about 3 baking sheets (U.S. cookie sheets).

Sift the white flour with the salt, baking powder
and ginger. Stir in the brown flour and rub or cut in
the butter. Blend the honey with the egg and add to
the bowl with the sugar and nuts. Mix to a stiff
dough.

Turn out on a lightly floured surface and shape
into a roll about 4 cm/1½ inches in diameter. Cut the
roll into 40 slices and arrange these on the prepared
sheets about 2.5 cm/1 inch apart.   Bake for 10-12
minutes, or until golden round the edges. **Makes 40**

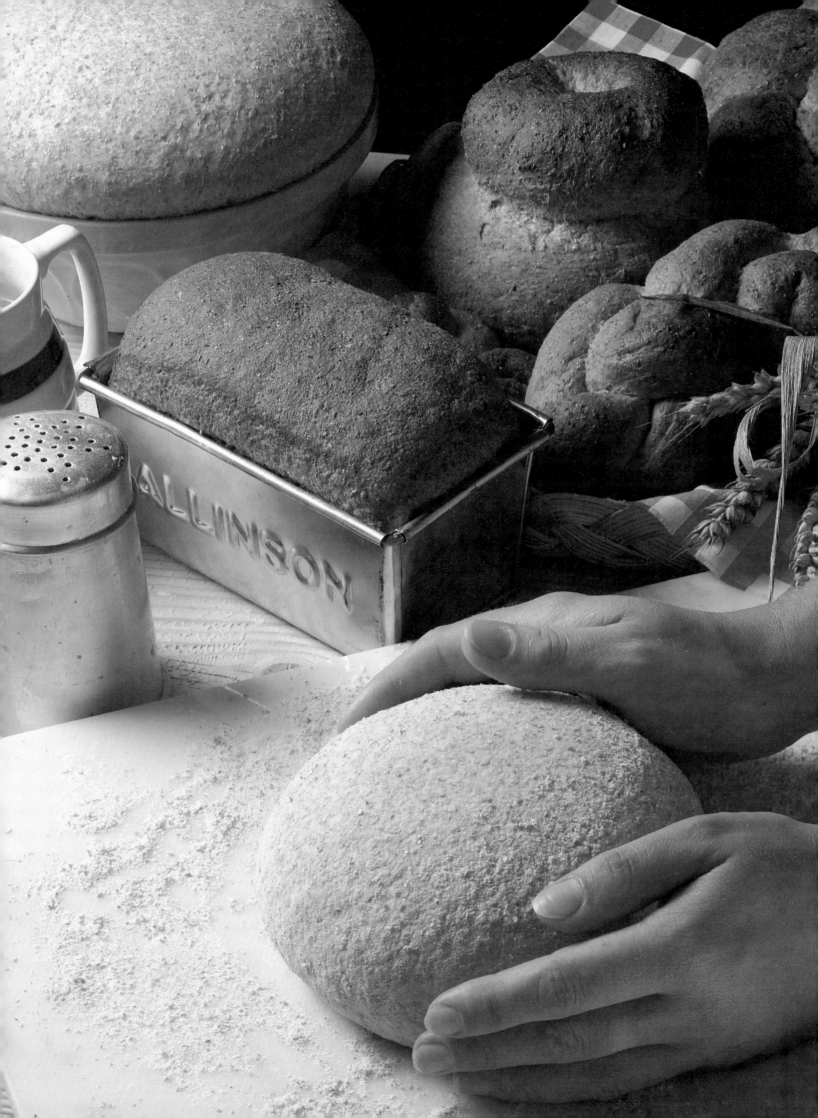

Breads, Pastries and Teatime Favourites

Rich original scones
(Illustrated on pages 122-123)

225 g/8 oz (U.S. 2 cups) wholewheat flour
5 teaspoons (U.S. 7 teaspoons) baking powder
100 g/4 oz (U.S. ½ cup) soft margarine
50 g/2 oz light muscovado sugar
(U.S. ¼ cup light brown sugar)
1 medium-sized cooking apple, peeled and grated
50 g/2 oz Original Crunchy breakfast cereal
(U.S. ½ cup toasted fruit, oat and nut breakfast cereal)
150 ml/¼ pint (U.S. ⅔ cup) milk
little milk to glaze

Heat the oven to 220°C/425°F, Gas Mark 7 and lightly grease a baking sheet (U.S. cookie sheet).

Stir the flour with the baking powder in a bowl and rub or cut in the margarine until the mixture resembles breadcrumbs. Stir in the sugar, apple and cereal, then add the milk and mix to a soft dough.

Turn on to a floured surface and pat out to a thickness of about 2 cm/¾ inch. Stamp out rounds using a plain 5-cm/2-inch cutter. Arrange the scones on the prepared sheet and brush with milk.

Bake for about 15 minutes, or until well risen and golden brown on top. Serve warm with butter or margarine. **Makes about 10**

Wholewheat bread chain
(Illustrated opposite)

1 (50-mg) tablet Vitamin C, crushed
1 tablespoon light muscovado sugar (U.S. light brown sugar)
600 ml/1 pint (U.S. 2½ cups) cold water
450 ml/¾ pint (U.S. scant 2 cups) boiling water
25 g/1 oz dried yeast (U.S. 2 packages active dried yeast)
1.4 kg/3 lb wholewheat flour
1 tablespoon salt
25 g/1 oz (U.S. 2 tablespoons) lard or vegetable fat
extra flour for dusting

Put the vitamin tablet and 1 teaspoon of the sugar into a bowl. Mix together 200 ml/7 fl oz (U.S. scant 1 cup) of the cold water and 150 ml/¼ pint (U.S. ⅔ cup) of the boiling water and add to the bowl. Whisk in the yeast and leave in a warm place for about 10 minutes, or until frothy. Meanwhile, warm and grease the chosen tins or baking sheets (U.S. cookie sheets.

Put the flour and salt into a large bowl and rub or cut in the lard. Stir in the remaining sugar. Combine the rest of the cold and boiling water and add to the bowl with the yeast liquid. Mix to a dough.

Turn out on a floured surface and knead for at least 10 minutes. This dough is sufficient to make 4×450-g/1-lb loaves or 3 loaves and 8 rolls. Divide the dough into 4 equal portions and shape as follows:

Tin loaf
Flatten one portion of dough into a rectangle about 30 cm/12 inches by 17.5 cm/7 inches. Fold into three and place in a greased 450-g/1-lb loaf tin with the fold underneath.

Cottage loaf
Shape two-thirds of the dough into a ball, then the remainder into a smaller ball. Place the larger ball on a greased baking sheet and brush with water. Put the smaller ball on top. Flour the handle of a wooden spoon and press this down through the 2 balls of dough to touch the tin.

Plait (U.S. Braid)
Divide the portion of dough into 3 equal pieces and shape each into a strip about 30 cm/12 inches long. Lay the strips side by side and plait them (U.S. braid them) from the centre to each end. Place on a greased baking sheet, tucking the ends under neatly.

Coburg
Shape the portion of dough into a ball and place on a greased baking sheet. Cut a deep cross in the top with a sharp knife.

Rolls
Divide one portion of dough into 8 pieces and shape each into a strip. Tie this in a loose single knot. Arrange the rolls on a greased baking sheet, allowing room for spreading. Miniature Cottage loaves and Coburgs can be made.

Rising
Cover the shaped dough loosely with greased cling film and leave in a warm place until double in size. Tin loaves should rise about 1.25 cm/½ inch above the sides of the tin. Meanwhile, arrange the oven shelves as needed and heat oven to highest temperature.

Toppings
If wished, brush the risen dough with milk, melted butter or beaten egg and sprinkle with more flour, poppy seeds or cracked wheat before baking.

Baking
Put the loaves or rolls into the oven then immediately reduce the oven temperature to 230°C/450°F, Gas Mark 8. Bake rolls for about 12 minutes and loaves for 30-35 minutes. Reduce the oven temperature to 220°C/425°F, Gas Mark 7 if the loaves brown too quickly. They are cooked if they sound hollow when tapped on base with knuckles.

129

Lemon
and almond flan

(Illustrated on page 6)

100 g/4 oz wholemeal flour
(U.S. 1 cup wholewheat flour)
pinch of salt
50 g/2 oz (U.S. $\frac{1}{4}$ cup) block margarine
1-2 tablespoons (U.S. 2-3 tablespoons) water
Filling
4 lemons
100 g/4 oz (U.S. $\frac{1}{2}$ cup) granulated sugar
50 g/2 oz (U.S. $\frac{1}{4}$ cup) butter or margarine
50 g/2 oz light muscovado sugar
(U.S. $\frac{1}{4}$ cup light brown sugar)
1 egg
25 g/1 oz wholemeal flour (U.S. $\frac{1}{4}$ cup wholewheat flour)
50 g/2 oz (U.S. $\frac{1}{2}$ cup) ground almonds

Heat the oven to 200°C/400°F, Gas Mark 6, and have ready a 20-cm/8-inch flan tin or shallow cake tin.

Put the flour and salt in a bowl and rub or cut in the margarine until the mixture resembles breadcrumbs. Add enough water to make a firm dough and knead lightly until smooth. Roll out on a floured surface and use to line the flan tin. Put in a sheet of greaseproof paper (U.S. waxed paper) and half-fill with baking beans. Bake blind for 5 minutes, remove the lining paper and beans and bake for a further 3 minutes. Leave to cool. Reduce the oven temperature to 190°C/375°F, Gas Mark 5.

Meanwhile, grate the rind from 1 lemon and set aside. Remove the skin and pips from the other 3 lemons and slice them thinly. Keep any juice and put it in a pan with the juice from the fourth lemon. Add the granulated sugar and heat gently, stirring, until the sugar has dissolved. Boil rapidly for 5 minutes. Put in the lemon slices and simmer for 5 minutes. Leave to cool.

Cream the butter and brown sugar together in a bowl until light and fluffy. Beat in the egg and fold in the flour, almonds and reserved lemon rind. Spread this mixture in the pastry case.

Bake for 30 minutes, or until the filling is golden brown. Leave until cold, then transfer to a serving plate. Arrange the lemon slices attractively in the flan and spoon the syrup over. Chill well. **Serves 6**

Date bread

(Illustrated opposite)

225 g/8 oz wholemeal flour (U.S. 2 cups wholewheat flour)
225 g/8 oz plain flour (U.S. 2 cups all-purpose flour)
65 g/2$\frac{1}{2}$ oz (U.S. generous $\frac{1}{4}$ cup) soft margarine
115 g/4$\frac{1}{4}$ oz light muscovado sugar (U.S. generous $\frac{1}{2}$ cup light brown sugar)
1$\frac{1}{2}$ teaspoons salt
15 g/$\frac{1}{2}$ oz fresh yeast (U.S. 3/5-oz cake compressed yeast)
300 ml/$\frac{1}{2}$ pint (U.S. 1$\frac{1}{4}$ cups) luke-warm water
225 g/8 oz stoned dates (U.S. $\frac{1}{2}$ lb pitted dates), chopped
1-2 tablespoons clear honey

Put the flours in a bowl and rub or cut in 15 g/$\frac{1}{2}$ oz (U.S. 1 tablespoon) of the margarine. Stir in 1 tablespoon of the sugar and the salt. Cream the yeast until smooth and gradually blend in the water. Add to the dry ingredients and mix to a dough. Turn out on a floured surface and knead for 10 minutes. Grease the mixing bowl, return the ball of dough to it and turn once to coat. Cover and leave in a warm place until double in bulk.

Turn the dough out on a floured surface and knead for 2 minutes until firm. Melt the rest of the margarine and stir in the dates and sugar. Knead this mixture into the dough until it is no longer streaky. Shape into a round and place in a greased 20-cm/8-inch cake tin. Cover and leave in a warm place for 30 minutes. Meanwhile, heat the oven to 220°C/425°F, Gas Mark 7.

Uncover the bread and bake for 30 minutes, or until well risen and golden brown. Turn out of the tin. The bread is cooked if it sounds hollow when tapped on the base with the knuckles. Return to the oven for a further few minutes on a baking sheet (U.S. cookie sheet) if necessary. Cool on a wire rack and brush the top with honey.
Makes 1 (20-cm/8-inch) loaf

Above: Date bread. Centre: Granary teacakes (recipe page 132).
Below: Cheesy corn scones (recipe page 138)

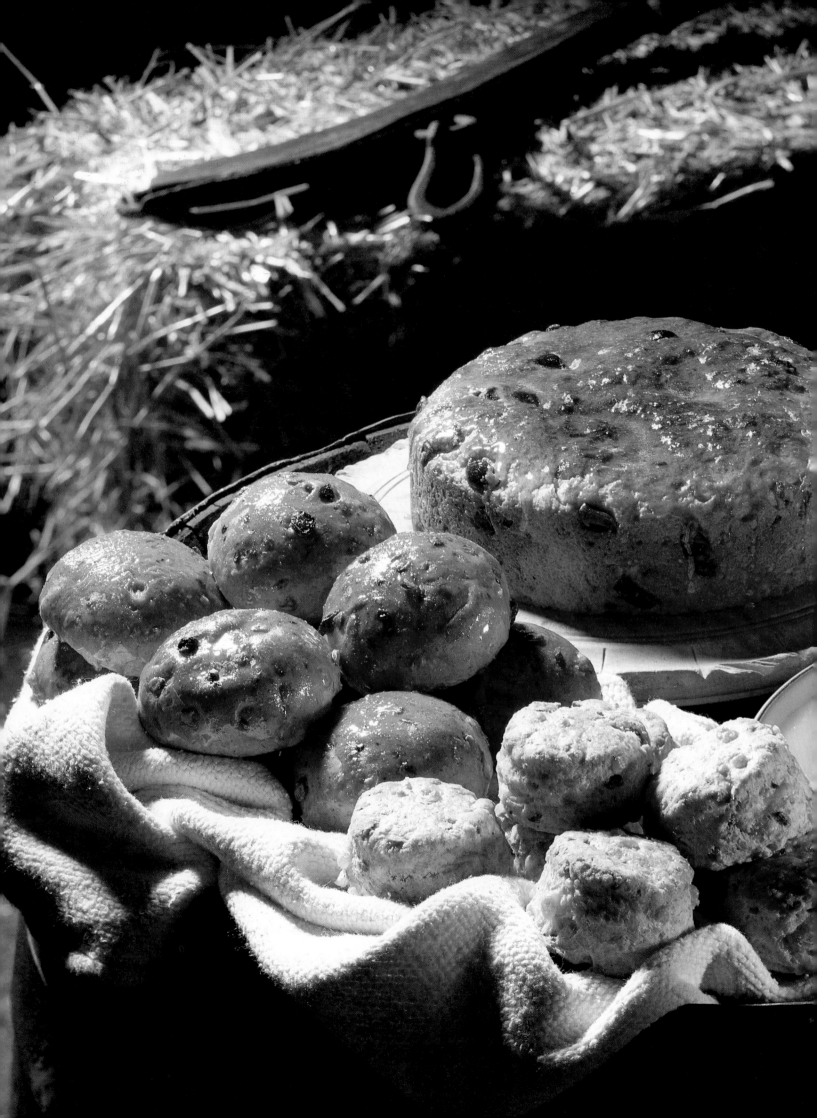

Spicy sultana squares

(Illustrated opposite)

175 g/6 oz plain flour (U.S. 1½ cups all-purpose flour)
1 tablespoon (U.S. 4 teaspoons) baking powder
pinch of salt
½ teaspoon ground cinnamon
175 g/6 oz wholemeal flour
(U.S. 1½ cups wholewheat flour)
175 g/6 oz (U.S. ¾ cup) margarine
175 g/6 oz light muscovado sugar
(U.S. ¾ cup light brown sugar)
75 g/3 oz sultanas (U.S. ½ cup seedless white raisins)
2 eggs
4 tablespoons (U.S. 6 tablespoons) milk

Heat the oven to 180°C/350°F, Gas Mark 4. Grease a 15-cm/6-inch square cake tin and line with grease-proof paper (U.S. waxed paper).

Sift the white flour, baking powder, salt and cinnamon into a bowl. Stir in the brown flour and rub or cut in the margarine until the mixture resembles breadcrumbs. Stir in the sugar and sultanas. Add the eggs and milk and beat to form a stiff dough. Transfer to the prepared tin and level the top.

Bake for 1½ hours, until brown and firm to the touch. Cut the cake into 9 squares and leave to cool in the tin. **Makes 9**

Granary teacakes

(Illustrated on page 131)

450 g/1 lb granary flour
(U.S. 4 cups fancy wholewheat flour)
1 teaspoon ground mixed spices
50 g/2 oz (U.S. ¼ cup) soft margarine
25 g/1 oz light muscovado sugar
(U.S. ⅛ cup light brown sugar)
50 g/2 oz sultanas (U.S. ⅓ cup seedless white raisins)
15 g/½ oz fresh yeast (U.S. 3/5-oz cake compressed yeast)
300 ml/½ pint (U.S. 1¼ cups) lukewarm water
Glaze
1 tablespoon light muscovado sugar (U.S. light brown sugar)
2 tablespoons (U.S. 3 tablespoons) hot water

Put the flour and spices in a bowl and rub or cut in the margarine. Add the sugar and dried fruit. Cream the yeast until smooth and gradually blend in the water. Add to the dry ingredients and mix to a dough. Turn out on a floured surface and knead for 10 minutes. Grease the mixing bowl, return the ball of dough to it and turn once to coat. Cover and leave in a warm place until double in bulk.

Turn the dough out on a floured surface and knead for 2 minutes until firm. Divide into 12 portions and shape each into a round. Place on a greased baking sheet (U.S. cookie sheet). Cover lightly with greased cling film and leave in a warm place until almost double in size. Meanwhile, heat the oven to 230°C/450°F, Gas Mark 8.

Uncover the teacakes and bake for about 15 minutes, or until golden brown. The teacakes are cooked if they sound hollow when tapped on the base with the knuckles. Dissolve the sugar in the water and boil for 1 minute. Brush the teacakes with glaze and cool on a wire rack. Serve freshly baked with butter or margarine. **Makes 12**

Apple and ginger squares

(Illustrated opposite)

175 g/6 oz (U.S. ¾ cup) margarine
175 g/6 oz light muscovado sugar
(U.S. ¾ cup light brown sugar)
3 eggs, beaten
1 tablespoon honey
100 g/4 oz plain flour (U.S. 1 cup all-purpose flour)
2 teaspoons (U.S. 3 teaspoons) baking powder
1½ teaspoons ground ginger
½ teaspoon ground cinnamon
100 g/4 oz wholemeal flour (U.S. 1 cup wholewheat flour)
450 g/1 lb cooking apples, peeled, cored and chopped

Heat the oven to 180°C/350°F, Gas Mark 4. Grease a 20-cm/8-inch square tin and line it with greaseproof paper (U.S. waxed paper).

Cream the margarine and sugar in a bowl until light. Gradually add the eggs, beating well after each addition. Beat in the honey. Sift the white flour with the baking powder and spices. Add to the creamed mixture with the brown flour and mix well. Stir in the chopped apple. Transfer to the prepared tin and level the top.

Bake for 1½ hours, until brown and firm to the touch. Turn out to cool on a wire rack, strip off the lining paper and cut into 9 squares. **Makes 9**

Above: Spicy sultana squares. Below: Apple and ginger squares

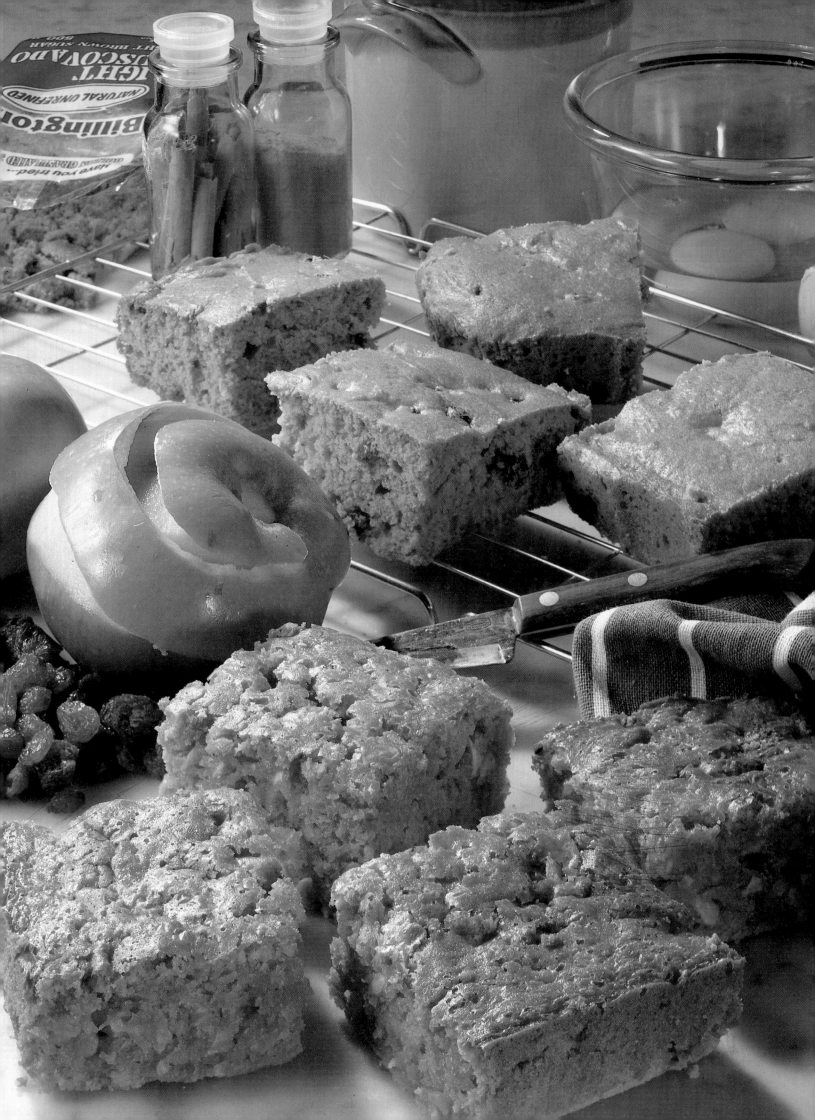

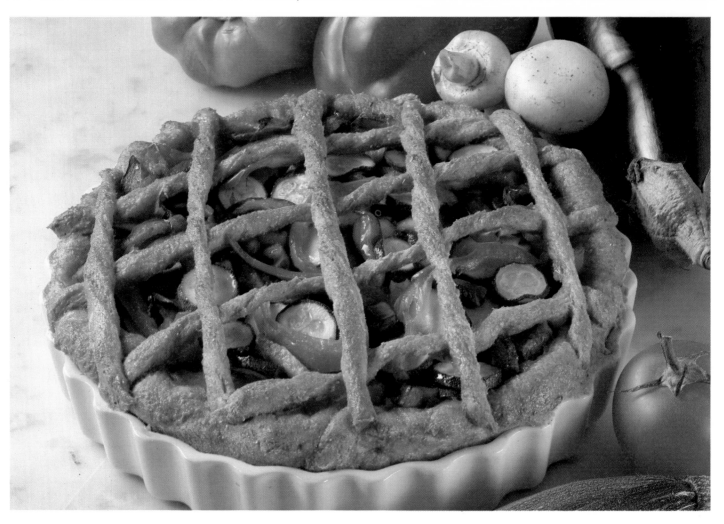

Savoury lattice flan

(Illustrated above)

450 g/1 lb wholewheat bread dough, kneaded
(about $\frac{1}{5}$ recipe page 129)
2 tablespoons (U.S. 3 tablespoons) oil
1 small onion, peeled and chopped
1 clove garlic, finely chopped
1 small green pepper, seeds removed and sliced
1 (175-g/6-oz) aubergine (U.S. 1 (6-oz) eggplant),
sliced
50 g/2 oz (U.S. $\frac{1}{2}$ cup) sliced mushrooms
3 medium-sized tomatoes, peeled and chopped
1 medium-sized courgette (U.S. 1 small zucchini),
sliced
salt and freshly ground black pepper
1 egg, beaten

Grease a 20-cm/8-inch flan tin with a loose base or a
flan ring standing on a baking sheet (U.S. cookie
sheet). Roll out three-quarters of the bread dough to
fit the chosen tin. Roll out the remaining dough
thinly and cut into strips about 1.25-cm/$\frac{1}{2}$-inch wide.
Cover all the dough with greased cling film and leave
in a warm place for about 30 minutes, or until puffy.

Meanwhile, heat the oil in a large pan and gently
fry the onion and garlic until soft. Add the remaining
vegetables and stir well. Simmer for about 15
minutes, stirring occasionally, or until soft but not
pulpy. Heat the oven to 200°C/400°F, Gas Mark 6.

Season the vegetable mixture and spoon into the
bread case. Twist the dough strips and lay them in a
lattice pattern over the filling. Trim to fit, brush the
ends with egg and press to seal them to the bread
case. Brush all exposed bread dough with egg.

Bake for 20 minutes, or until golden brown on top.
Serve hot or cold with salad. **Serves 4-5**

Variation

Sausage and spinach flan Omit the vegetable
filling. Thinly slice 225 g/8 oz pork sausages (U.S. $\frac{1}{2}$
lb pork links) and fry in 1 tablespoon oil for about 10
minutes, stirring frequently, until brown. Defrost and
drain a 225-g/8-oz (U.S. $\frac{1}{2}$-lb) pack chopped spinach,
mix with the sausage, 2 beaten eggs and 175 g/6 oz
(U.S. 1$\frac{1}{2}$ cups) grated mozzarella cheese. Season with
garlic salt and pepper and transfer to the bread case.
Decorate with the bread strips and bake as above.
Serve hot or cold.

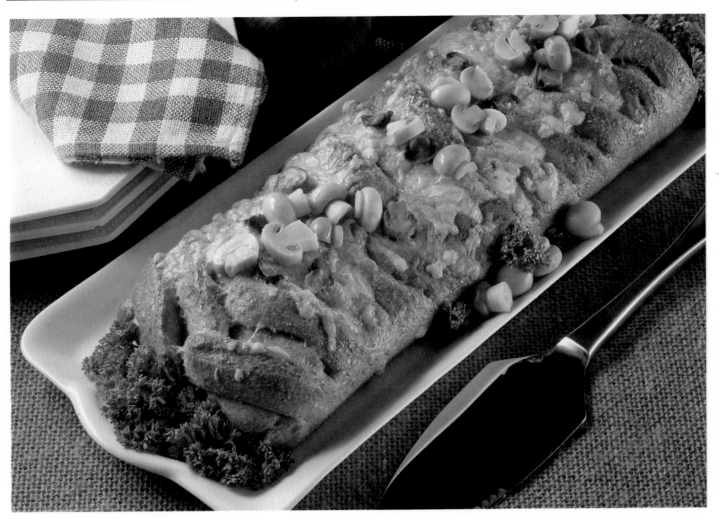

Cheese and mushroom plait

(Illustrated above)

450 g/1 lb wholewheat bread dough, kneaded
(about ⅕ recipe page 129)
100 g/4 oz (U.S. 1 cup) grated Cheddar cheese
1 (212-g/7.5-oz) can button mushrooms, drained
1 red pepper, seeds removed and chopped
1 teaspoon dried mixed herbs
freshly ground black pepper
1 egg, beaten
sprigs of parsley to garnish

Roll out the dough on a floured surface to a rectangle measuring about 30 cm/12 inches by 15 cm/6 inches. Transfer to a greased baking sheet (U.S. cookie sheet), cover with greased cling film and leave in a warm place for about 30 minutes, or until puffy. Meanwhile, heat the oven to 200°C/400°F, Gas Mark 6.

Reserve a quarter of the cheese and a third of the mushrooms for topping the plait. Sprinkle half the remaining cheese down the centre of the dough,

leaving a border of 5 cm/2 inches either side. Top this with the mushrooms and chopped pepper and sprinkle with the herbs and ground pepper to taste. Scatter over the remaining cheese.

Make diagonal cuts every 2.5 cm/1 inch along the uncovered sides of the rectangle and fold these alternately over the filling to make a plait. Tuck in the ends neatly and brush the plait with egg. Sprinkle over the remaining mushrooms and the rest of the cheese.

Bake for 20 minutes, or until crisp and golden brown. Serve hot or cold, garnished with parsley sprigs. **Serves 4**

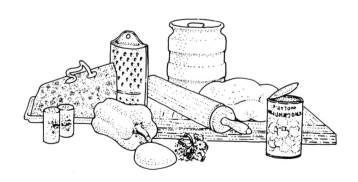

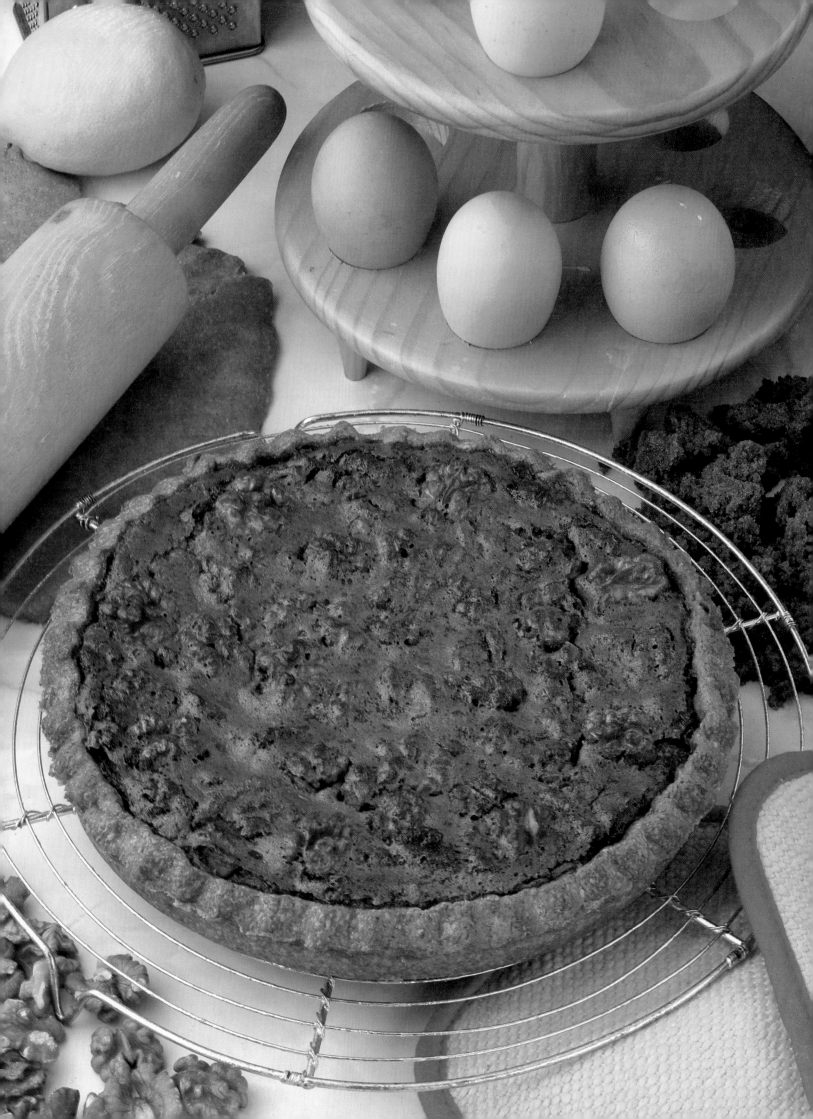

Wholewheat pecan pie

(Illustrated opposite)

Pastry
150 g/5 oz wholemeal flour
(U.S. 1¼ cups wholewheat flour)
pinch of salt
65 g/2½ oz (U.S. generous ¼ cup) block margarine
1–2 tablespoons (U.S. 2–3 tablespoons) water
Filling
175 g/6 oz (U.S. ¾ cup) butter or margarine
225 g/8 oz muscovado sugar (U.S. 1 cup brown sugar)
3 eggs
finely grated rind of 2 lemons
juice of 1½ lemons
175 g/6 oz (U.S. 1½ cups) pecan or walnut halves

Heat the oven to 180°C/350°F, Gas Mark 4 and have ready a 20-cm/8-inch flan tin or shallow cake tin.

Mix the flour and salt in a bowl and rub or cut in the margarine until the mixture resembles breadcrumbs. Add enough water to make a firm dough and knead briefly until smooth. Roll out on a lightly floured surface to line the tin. Line with a sheet of greaseproof paper (U.S. waxed paper) and half-fill with baking beans. Bake blind for 10 minutes.

Meanwhile, make the filling. Cream the butter with the sugar in a bowl until light and fluffy. Add the eggs, one at a time, beating well after each addition. Beat in the lemon rind and juice, then fold in the nuts. Transfer to the pastry case. Bake for 45 minutes, or until well risen. Serve warm. **Serves 6**

Wholewheat drop pancakes

(Illustrated on pages 122-123)

100 g/4 oz (U.S. 1 cup) wholewheat flour
1 teaspoon baking powder
25 g/1 oz light muscovado sugar
(U.S. ⅛ cup light brown sugar)
1 egg
200 ml/7 fl oz (U.S. ⅞ cup) milk
50 g/2 oz Original Crunchy breakfast cereal
(U.S. ½ cup toasted fruit, oat and nut breakfast cereal)
little oil for cooking

Put the flour, baking powder and sugar in a bowl and make a well in the centre. Drop in the egg and add half the milk. Whisk until the batter is smooth then gradually add the remaining milk. Stir in the cereal and leave the batter to stand for 10 minutes.

Wholewheat pecan pie

Heat a griddle or heavy frying pan (U.S. skillet) over moderate heat and brush lightly with oil. Beat the batter and using scant 2 tablespoons for each pancake, spoon on to the hot surface to make rounds measuring about 6.5 cm/2½ inches in diameter. When bubbles start to rise to the surface, turn the pancakes and cook on until golden underneath.

Stack the pancakes on a warm plate and cover with a clean cloth until all the batter is used. Serve warm with butter or margarine. **Makes about 16**

Muesli bumpy loaves

(Illustrated on pages 122-123)

350 ml/12 fl oz (U.S. 1½ cups) cold water
225 ml/8 fl oz (U.S. 1 cup) boiling water
1 teaspoon sugar
1 tablespoon dried yeast
(U.S. 4 teaspoons active dried yeast)
800 g/1¾ lb strong white flour
(U.S. 7 cups white bread flour)
1½ teaspoons (U.S. 2 teaspoons) salt
25 g/1 oz (U.S. 2 tablespoons) butter or margarine
175 g/6 oz country muesli (U.S. 2 cups dried fruit, oats and nut breakfast cereal)
Topping
little milk
25 g/1 oz country muesli (U.S. ⅓ cup dried fruit, oats and nut breakfast cereal)

Mix together half the cold and half the boiling water and stir in the sugar. Sprinkle on the yeast and leave to stand in a warm place for about 10 minutes, or until frothy.

Sift the flour and salt into a bowl and rub or cut in the butter. Stir in the muesli and make a well in the centre. Combine the remaining cold and boiling water and add to the bowl with the yeast liquid. Mix to a dough. Turn out on a floured surface and knead for 10 minutes. Grease the bowl, return the ball of dough to it and turn once to coat. Cover and leave in a warm place until double in bulk.

Grease two 450-g/1-lb loaf-shaped tins. Turn the dough out again on a floured surface and knead for 2 minutes. Divide in half, then cut each portion into 4 equal pieces. Shape these into oblongs the width of the tin. Place 4 oblongs, side by side, in each prepared tin. Cover with greased cling film and leave in a warm place until the dough has risen and is about 1.25 cm/½ inch above the edge of the tin. Meanwhile, heat the oven to 200°C/400°F, Gas Mark 6.

Uncover the loaves, brush them with milk and sprinkle with muesli. Bake for about 30 minutes, or until golden brown. The loaves are cooked if they sound hollow when tapped on the base with the knuckles. **Makes 2 medium-sized loaves**

Coconut cookies

(Illustrated opposite)

2 tablespoons (U.S. 3 tablespoons) set honey
100 g/4 oz (U.S. ½ cup) margarine
175 g/6 oz plain flour (U.S. 1½ cups all-purpose flour)
1½ teaspoons (U.S. 2 teaspoons) baking powder
100 g/4 oz (U.S. generous 1 cup) rolled oats
100 g/4 oz desiccated coconut
(U.S. 1⅓ cups shredded coconut)
50 g/2 oz muscovado sugar
(U.S. ¼ cup brown sugar)
pinch of salt
1 egg, beaten

Heat the oven to 150°C/300°F, Gas Mark 2 and grease 2 baking sheets (U.S. cookie sheets).

Melt the honey and margarine together in a large pan. Remove from the heat and stir in the remaining ingredients. Mix well. Shape into small balls, using about 2 teaspoons (U.S. scant 1 tablespoon) of the mixture for each one, and arrange on the prepared sheets, keeping them 4 cm/1½ inches apart.

Bake for about 15 minutes, or until brown. Cool on a wire rack. **Makes about 30**

Cheesy corn scones

(Illustrated on page 131)

225 g/8 oz granary flour (U.S. 2 cups fancy
wholewheat flour)
1 tablespoon (U.S. 4 teaspoons) baking powder
50 g/2 oz (U.S. ¼ cup) margarine
100 g/4 oz (U.S. 1 cup) grated Cheddar cheese
50 g/2 oz (U.S. ½ cup) cooked or canned corn kernels
1 teaspoon mild continental mustard
7 tablespoons (U.S. generous ½ cup) milk

Heat the oven to 220°C/425°F, Gas Mark 7 and grease a baking sheet (U.S. cookie sheet).

Combine the flour and baking powder in a bowl. Rub or cut in the margarine until the mixture resembles breadcrumbs. Add the cheese and corn. Stir the mustard into the milk, add to the bowl and mix to a soft dough. Pat out on a floured surface to a thickness of about 2 cm/¾ inch. Stamp out rounds with a 4-cm/1½-inch cutter and arrange on the prepared sheet.

Bake for about 10 minutes, or until well risen and golden brown. **Makes about 8**

Left: Honey and ginger nuts (recipe page 127). Right: Coconut cookies

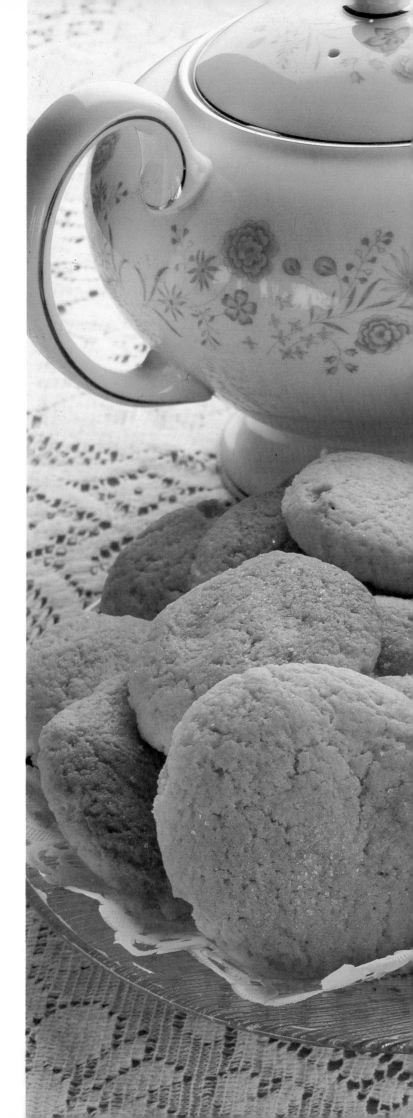

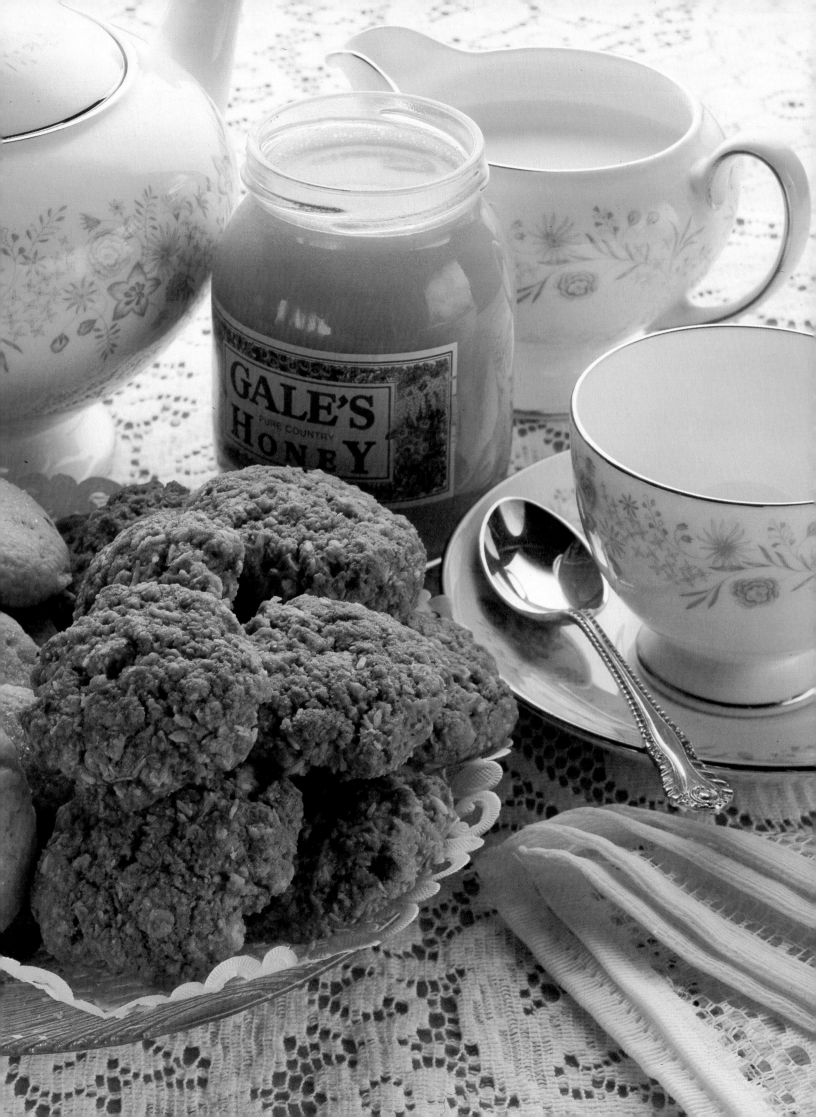

Cheesy bean quiche

(Illustrated opposite)

225 g/8 oz wholewheat shortcrust pastry
(U.S. ½ lb wholewheat pastry)
(see page 137)
2 eggs
150 ml/¼ pint (U.S. ⅔ cup) milk
1 tablespoon chopped parsley
salt and freshly ground black pepper
1 (425-g/15-oz) can butter beans
(U.S. lima beans), drained
100 g/4 oz (U.S. 1 cup) grated Cheddar cheese
sprig of parsley to garnish

Heat the oven to 190°C/375°F, Gas Mark 5 and have ready a 20-cm/8-inch flan dish or a pie plate.

Roll out the pastry on a lightly floured surface and use to line the chosen dish. Line with greaseproof paper (U.S. waxed paper) and half-fill with baking beans. Bake blind for 15 minutes. Remove the beans and lining paper and return the pastry case to the oven for a further 5 minutes.

Meanwhile, whisk together the eggs, milk, chopped parsley and seasoning to taste. Add the beans and most of the cheese. Pour into the pastry case and sprinkle with the remaining cheese.

Bake for about 45 minutes, or until the filling is firm and golden brown. Serve hot, garnished with the parsley sprig. **Serves 4**

Crusty soda-bread triangles

450 g/1 lb wholemeal flour
(U.S. 4 cups wholewheat flour)
1 teaspoon bicarbonate of soda (U.S. baking soda)
1 teaspoon cream of tartar
1 teaspoon salt
40 g/1½ oz (U.S. 3 tablespoons) butter or margarine
300 ml/½ pint (U.S. 1¼ cups) milk
little extra flour for sprinkling

Heat the oven to 200°C/400°F, Gas Mark 6 and grease a baking sheet (U.S. cookie sheet).

Put half the flour in a bowl, add the bicarbonate of soda, cream of tartar and salt, and mix thoroughly. Add the remaining flour and mix again. Rub or cut in the butter until the mixture resembles breadcrumbs, then add the milk to make a fairly soft dough. Turn out on a floured surface and knead lightly until smooth. Shape into a 22.5-cm/9-inch round and place on the prepared sheet. Using a sharp knife, cut a cross half-way through the dough, to make 4 triangles, then sprinkle the bread with flour.

Bake for 40 minutes, or until well risen and golden brown. The loaf is cooked if it sounds hollow when tapped on the base with the knuckles. Cool briefly on a wire rack and break into the marked triangles for serving with butter or margarine. **Serves 4-6**

Apricot and almond teabread

225 g/8 oz (U.S. ½ lb) tender dried apricots
150 ml/¼ pint (U.S. ⅔ cup) milk
4 tablespoons (U.S. 6 tablespoons) water
½ teaspoon almond essence (U.S. almond extract)
175 g/6 oz plain flour
(U.S. 1½ cups all-purpose flour)
1 tablespoon (U.S. 4 teaspoons) baking powder
pinch of salt
175 g/6 oz wholemeal flour
(U.S. 1½ cups wholewheat flour)
100 g/4 oz light muscovado sugar
(U.S. ½ cup light brown sugar)
50 g/2 oz flaked almonds
(U.S. ½ cup slivered almonds), lightly toasted
75 g/3 oz (U.S. ⅓ cup) margarine, melted
2 eggs
2 teaspoons clear honey

Snip the apricots into small pieces, place in a bowl and pour over the milk, water and almond essence. Leave to stand for 30 minutes. Heat the oven to 160°C/325°F, Gas Mark 3 and line a 1-kg/2-lb loaf-shaped tin with greaseproof paper (U.S. waxed paper).

Sift the white flour with the baking powder and salt into a bowl and stir in the brown flour, sugar and nuts. Make a well in the centre, add the soaked apricots and any liquid, the margarine and eggs. Beat until well blended.

Transfer to the prepared tin and smooth the top. Bake for about 1¼-1½ hours, or until firm to the touch. Leave in the tin for 5 minutes, then turn out on a wire rack and brush the top with honey. Leave until cool before removing the lining paper. Serve thinly sliced and spread with butter or margarine.
Makes 1 loaf, about 16 slices

Cheesy bean quiche

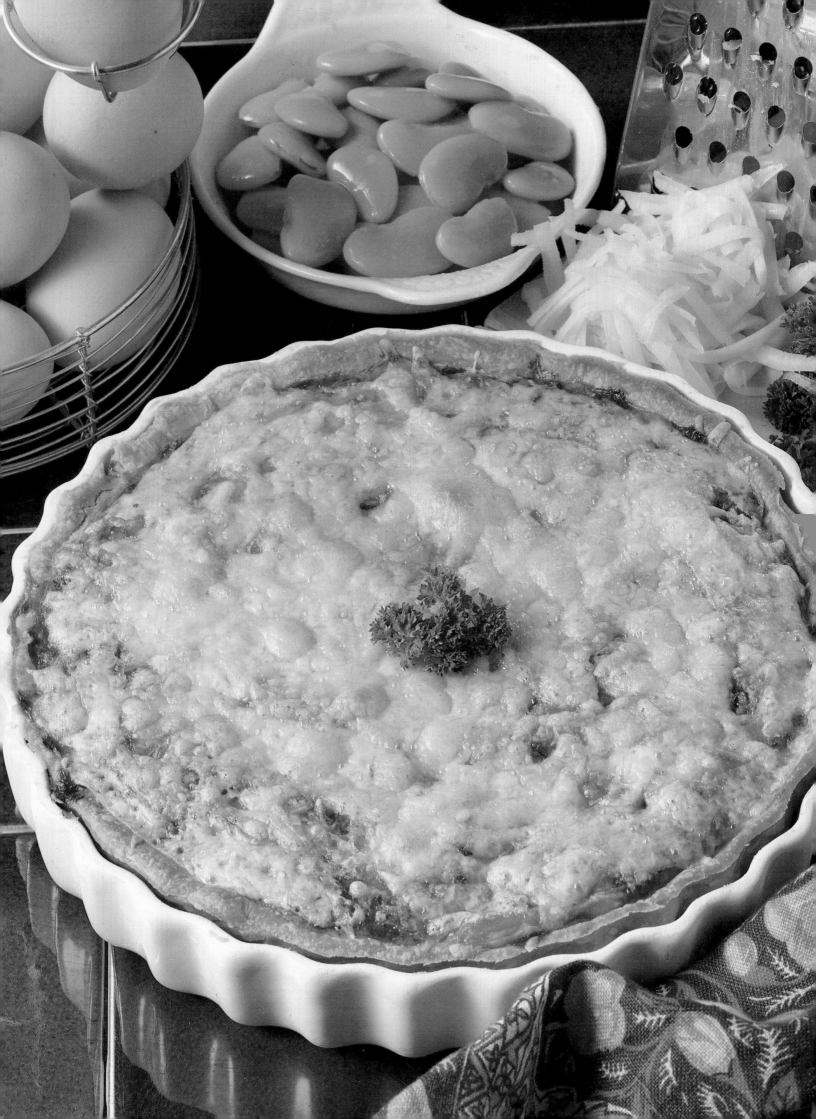

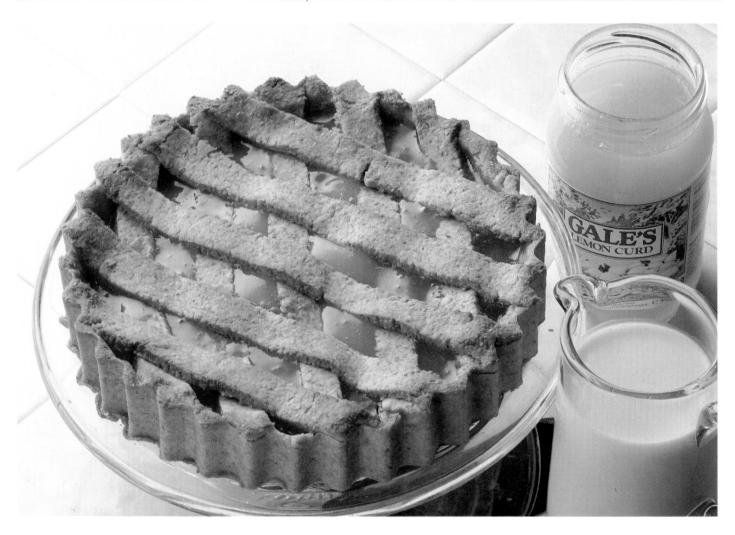

Lemon linzertorte

(Illustrated above)

150 g/5 oz wholemeal flour
(U.S. 1¼ cups wholewheat flour)
½ teaspoon ground cinnamon
75 g/3 oz (U.S. ⅓ cup) butter or block margarine
50 g/2 oz light muscovado sugar
(U.S. ¼ cup light brown sugar)
50 g/2 oz (U.S. ½ cup) ground almonds
2 egg yolks
about 1 tablespoon water
350 g/12 oz (U.S. ¾ lb) cooking apples, peeled and
grated
350 g/12 oz (U.S. 1 cup) lemon curd

Heat the oven to 190°C/375°F, Gas Mark 5 and have ready a 20-cm/8-inch flan ring standing on a baking sheet (U.S. cookie sheet), or a shallow cake tin with a loose base.

Mix together the flour and cinnamon in a bowl and rub or cut in the butter until the mixture resembles breadcrumbs. Add the sugar, almonds and egg yolks and mix, adding just enough water to make a firm dough. Knead lightly until smooth. Roll out two-thirds of the pastry on a lightly floured surface and use to line the prepared ring or tin. Make a layer of the apple in the base and press lightly with the back of a spoon to flatten. Stir the lemon curd and spoon it over the apple.

Roll out the remaining pastry and cut into 1.25-cm/½-inch wide strips. Lay them over the filling in a lattice pattern, trim to fit, dampen the ends of the strips and press to the edge of the pastry case.

Bake for about 30 minutes, or until the pastry is pale golden. Leave until cold before moving the linzertorte to a serving plate. Serve with cream.
Serves 6

Variation

Banana and lime meringue pie Omit the almonds and substitute 2 tablespoons (U.S. 3 tablespoons) finely ground coffee. Use all the pastry to fit the prepared tin, line with paper and baking beans and bake for 12 minutes. Remove the paper and beans and bake for a further 5 minutes, or until cooked. Slice 2 bananas, mix with 225 g/8 oz (U.S. ⅔ cup) lime or orange curd and spread in the pastry case. Make a meringue with 2 egg whites and 100 g/4 oz light muscovado sugar (U.S. ½ cup light brown sugar), spread over the filling and bake for 15 minutes, or until the meringue is golden. Serve cold.

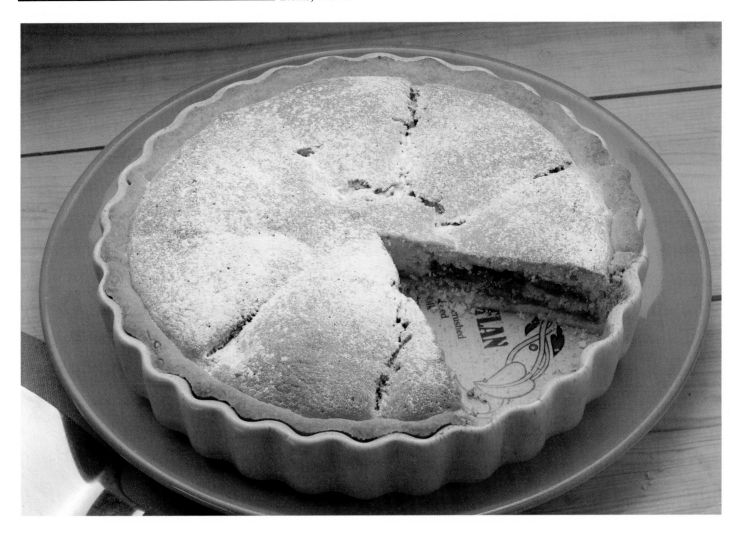

Flakewell tart

(Illustrated above)

75 g/3 oz plain flour (U.S. ¾ cup all-purpose flour)
1½ teaspoons (U.S. 2 teaspoons) baking powder
large pinch of salt
75 g/3 oz wholemeal flour
(U.S. ¾ cup wholewheat flour)
100 g/4 oz (U.S. ½ cup) block margarine
1 egg yolk
2 teaspoons caster sugar
(U.S. 1 tablespoon granulated sugar)
about 2 teaspoons (U.S. 1 tablespoon) water
little sifted icing sugar
(U.S. confectioners' sugar) for sprinkling
Filling
25 g/1 oz plain flour (U.S. ¼ cup all-purpose flour)
¾ teaspoon (U.S. 1 teaspoon) baking powder
50 g/2 oz wholemeal flour
(U.S. ½ cup wholewheat flour)
75 g/3 oz (U.S. ⅓ cup) margarine
75 g/3 oz caster sugar (U.S. ⅓ cup granulated sugar)
2 eggs, beaten
25 g/1 oz (U.S. ¼ cup) ground almonds
few drops of almond essence (U.S. almond extract)
5 tablespoons (U.S. 7 tablespoons) jam
8 small milk chocolate flakes

Sift the white flour with the baking powder and salt into a bowl. Stir in the brown flour and rub or cut in the margarine until the mixture resembles breadcrumbs. Add the egg yolk, sugar and enough water to make a firm dough. Knead lightly until smooth. Roll out on a floured surface and use to line a 25-cm/10-inch fluted flan dish or shallow cake tin. Prick the base and chill while making the filling. Heat the oven to 200°C/400°F, Gas Mark 6.

Sift the white flour with the baking powder and stir in the brown flour. Cream the margarine and sugar together in a bowl until light and fluffy. Gradually add the egg then fold in the dry ingredients, the almonds and almond essence.

Spread the jam in the pastry case and arrange the flakes on this like the spokes of a wheel. Spoon the almond mixture carefully over, disturbing the flakes as little as possible yet levelling the surface.

Bake for 15 minutes then reduce the oven temperature to 180°C/350°F, Gas Mark 4 and continue cooking for a further 20 minutes, or until the filling is firm to the touch. Serve hot or cold, sifted with sugar. **Serves 8**

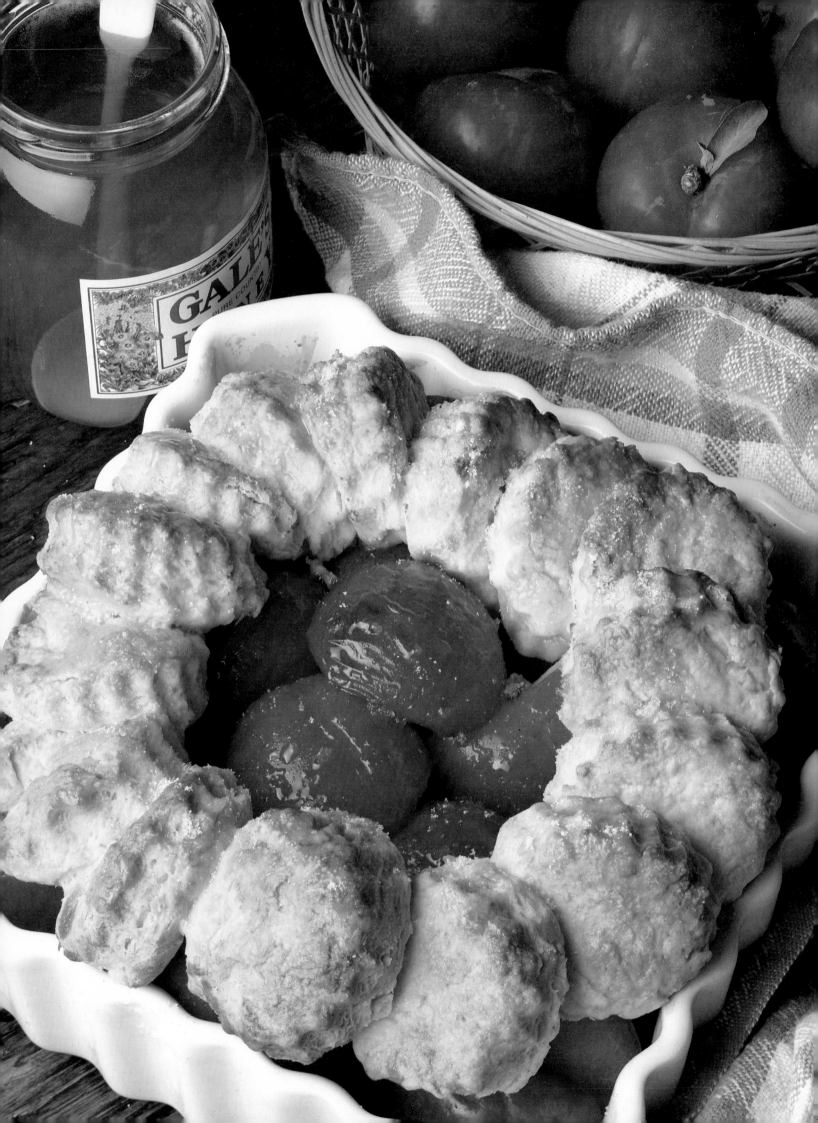

Bacon and pear flan

(Illustrated on page 147)

225 g/8 oz granary flour
(U.S. 2 cups fancy wholewheat flour)
pinch of salt
50 g/2 oz (U.S. ¼ cup) butter or block margarine
50 g/2 oz (U.S. ¼ cup) lard or white fat
2-3 tablespoons (U.S. 3-4 tablespoons) water
Filling
225 g/8 oz rashers streaky bacon
(U.S. ½ lb bacon slices), rind removed and chopped
1 large onion, peeled and thinly sliced
25 g/1 oz (U.S. 2 tablespoons) butter or margarine
25 g/1 oz plain flour
(U.S. ¼ cup all-purpose flour)
300 ml/½ pint (U.S. 1¼ cups) milk
salt and freshly ground black pepper
½ teaspoon ground coriander
2 tablespoons (U.S. 3 tablespoons) chopped parsley
Topping
2 Conference or small Comice pears, fairly firm
(U.S. 2 eating pears, fairly firm), peeled, quartered
and cored
4 whole cloves
3 tablespoons (U.S. 4 tablespoons) wine vinegar
50 g/2 oz (U.S. ¼ cup) sugar
7 bacon rolls
2 tablespoons (U.S. 3 tablespoons) wheat flakes
40 g/1½ oz mature Cheddar cheese, grated
(U.S. ⅓ cup grated sharp Cheddar cheese)
sprigs of parsley to garnish

Heat the oven to 200°C/400°F, Gas Mark 6 and have ready a 22.5-cm/9-inch flan tin or ring standing on a baking sheet (U.S. cookie sheet).

To make the pastry, mix the flour and salt together and rub or cut in the fats until the mixture resembles breadcrumbs. Add enough water to make a stiff dough. Roll out on a floured surface and use to line the chosen tin. Prick the base, line with greaseproof paper (U.S. waxed paper) and half-fill with baking beans. Bake blind for 20 minutes. Remove the paper and beans and return to the oven for a further 10 minutes, or until cooked through.

While the pastry case is cooking, make the filling. Put the bacon and onion into a pan with no added fat and cook over low heat, stirring frequently, until the onion is soft. Continue cooking until both the bacon and onion begin to brown, then drain well. Melt the butter in a clean pan, blend in the flour and cook for 1 minute, stirring. Gradually add the milk and bring to the boil, stirring constantly. Simmer for 2 minutes, season well with salt, pepper and coriander and stir in

Plums with coconut cobbler

the parsley and the bacon and onion mixture. Keep hot.

To make the topping, put the pear quarters in a pan with the minimum of water and add the cloves and vinegar. Poach the pears for about 5 minutes, or until just tender. Add the sugar and cook for a further 3 minutes. At the same time, grill (U.S. broil) the bacon rolls until golden and crisp.

Spoon the bacon filling into the pastry case. Drain the pear quarters and arrange on the filling. Mix together the wheat flakes and cheese and sprinkle over the pears.

Protect the pastry edges with foil and place the flan under a moderate grill (U.S. broiler) until lightly browned. Garnish with the bacon rolls and small parsley sprigs before serving hot. **Serves 7**

Plums with coconut cobbler

(Illustrated opposite)

1 kg/2 lb ripe plums, halved and stoned
(U.S. halved and pitted)
4-6 tablespoons (U.S. 6-9 tablespoons) clear honey
Cobbler topping
100 g/4 oz plain flour (U.S. 1 cup all-purpose flour)
2 teaspoons (U.S. 1 tablespoon) baking powder
100 g/4 oz wholemeal flour (U.S. 1 cup wholewheat
flour)
50 g/2 oz (U.S. ¼ cup) margarine
25 g/1 oz light muscovado sugar
(U.S. ⅛ cup light brown sugar)
2 tablespoons desiccated coconut
(U.S. 3 tablespoons shredded coconut)
1 egg, beaten
5-6 tablespoons (U.S. 7-9 tablespoons) milk

Heat the oven to 200°C/400°F, Gas Mark 6 and lightly grease an ovenproof pie dish.

Put the plums into the prepared dish and spoon over honey to taste (depending upon the sweetness of the fruit). Cover with foil and place in the oven for 15 minutes.

Meanwhile, sift the white flour with the baking powder into a bowl and stir in the brown flour. Rub or cut in the margarine, then stir in the sugar and coconut. Add the egg and enough milk to form a soft dough. Pat the dough out on a floured surface to a thickness of about 2 cm/¾ inch. Stamp out 5-cm/2-inch rounds using a fluted cutter.

Remove the foil from the plums and arrange the dough rounds, overlapping, in a ring on top. Brush the topping with milk and return the dish to the oven for about 30 minutes, or until the cobbler topping is golden brown. Serve hot with cream. **Serves 4-6**

English apple flan
(Illustrated opposite)

175 g/6 oz plain flour
(U.S. 1½ cups all-purpose flour)
pinch of salt
50 g/2 oz (U.S. ¼ cup) butter or margarine
50 g/2 oz (U.S. ¼ cup) lard or white fat
25 g/1 oz wheat flakes
(U.S. scant 1 cup wheat flakes), crushed
about 2 tablespoons (U.S. 3 tablespoons) water
Filling
675 g/1½ lb Bramley apples
(U.S. cooking apples)
about 75 g/3 oz (U.S. ⅓ cup) sugar
4 tablespoons (U.S. 6 tablespoons) jellied cranberry
sauce

Heat the oven to 200°C/400°F, Gas Mark 6 and have ready a 20-cm/8-inch flan tin or a ring standing on a baking sheet (U.S. cookie sheet).

To make the pastry, sift the flour and salt into a bowl and rub or cut in the fats until the mixture resembles breadcrumbs. Stir in the wheat flakes, then add enough water to make a stiff dough. Roll out on a floured surface and use to line the chosen tin. Prick the base, line with greaseproof paper (U.S. waxed paper) and half-fill with baking beans. Bake blind for 20 minutes. Remove the paper and beans and return the case to the oven for a further 10 minutes, or until cooked through. Cool.

Peel, core and roughly slice two-thirds of the apples and stew in the minimum of water until soft and pulpy. Beat in the sugar to taste and leave to cool.

Spoon most of the apple purée into the pastry case. Peel, core and thinly slice the remaining apple and arrange the slices, overlapping, in a circle on top of the apple purée, leaving a gap in the centre. Fill this with the rest of the apple purée. Melt the cranberry jelly and brush it liberally over the apple slices.

Protect the edges of the pastry with foil and put the flan under a moderate grill (U.S. broiler). Cook until the apple slices begin to turn golden. Remove from the heat and serve warm or cold with cream.
Serves 4-5

Above: Bacon and pear flan (recipe page 145). Below: English apple flan

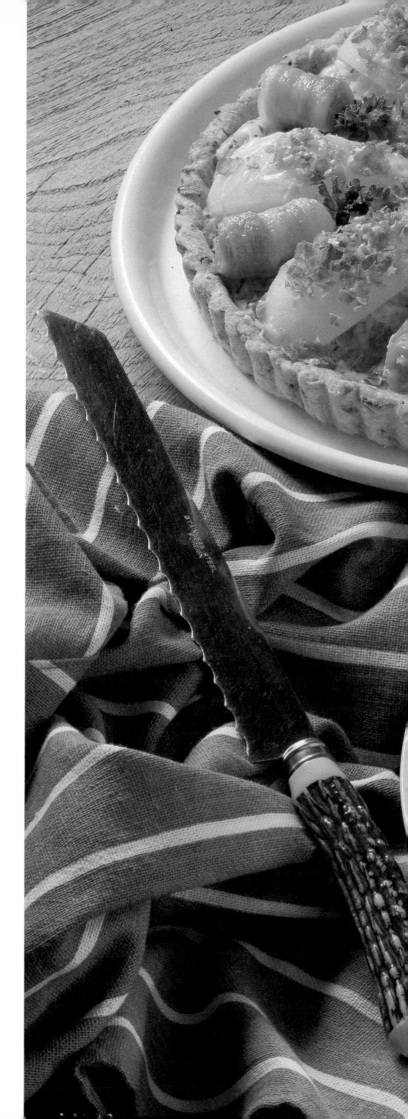

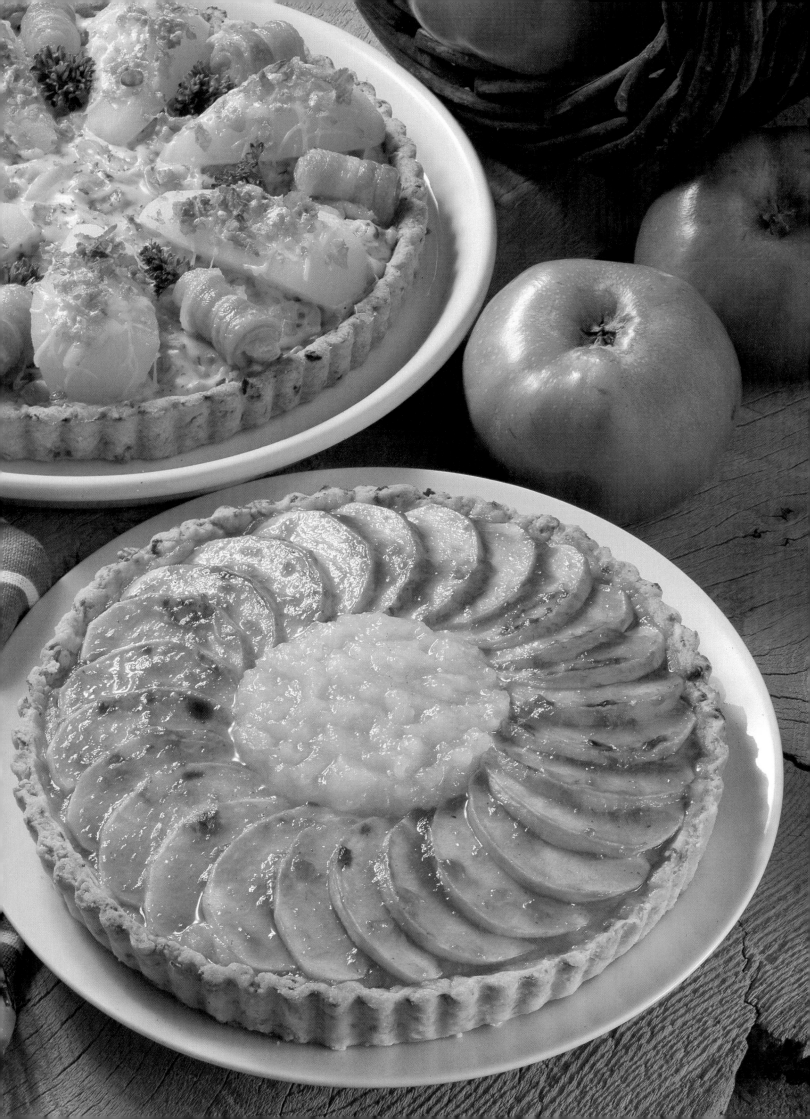

Bacon and bean plate pie

100 g/4 oz plain flour
(U.S. 1 cup all-purpose flour)
225 g/8 oz wholemeal flour
(U.S. 2 cups wholewheat flour)
75 g/3 oz (U.S. ⅓ cup) lard
75 g/3 oz (U.S. ⅓ cup) block margarine
1 egg yolk
3 tablespoons (U.S. 4 tablespoons) water
Filling
2 tablespoons (U.S. 3 tablespoons) oil
1 large onion, peeled and sliced
225 g/8 oz lean smoked bacon or gammon
(U.S. ½ lb uncooked smoked ham),
rind removed and diced
100 g/4 oz (U.S. ¼ lb) mushrooms, sliced
1 (425-g/15-oz) can baked beans in tomato sauce
1 teaspoon dried sage
salt and freshly ground black pepper

Heat the oven to 190°C/375°F, Gas Mark 5.

Sift the white flour into a bowl and stir in the brown flour. Rub or cut in the fats until the mixture resembles breadcrumbs. Add the egg yolk and water and mix to a firm dough. Knead lightly until smooth. Roll out half the pastry on a lightly floured surface and use to line a 20-cm/8-inch deep pie plate.

Heat the oil in a pan and fry the onion and bacon over moderate heat, stirring, until the onion is soft. Add the mushrooms and cook for a further 2 minutes, stirring occasionally. Mix in the beans, sage and add seasoning if desired.

Transfer to the pastry case. Brush the exposed pastry edges with water. Roll out the remaining pastry to make a lid and put it in place. Crimp the edges firmly together and flute them. Prick the top of the pie several times with a fork.

Bake for 45 minutes, or until golden brown on top. Serve hot. **Serves 4**

Apple and hazelnut flan

(Illustrated opposite)

100 g/4 oz wholemeal flour
(U.S. 1 cup wholewheat flour)
pinch of salt
50 g/2 oz (U.S. ¼ cup) block margarine
25 g/1 oz light muscovado sugar
(U.S. ⅛ cup light brown sugar)
25 g/1 oz finely chopped hazelnuts
(U.S. ¼ cup finely chopped filberts)
1 egg yolk
1-2 tablespoons (U.S. 2-3 tablespoons) milk
Filling
350 g/12 oz (U.S. ¾ lb) cooking apples, peeled, cored
and chopped
25 g/1 oz light muscovado sugar
(U.S. ⅛ cup light brown sugar)
2 tablespoons (U.S. 3 tablespoons) water
2 red-skinned eating apples, cored
2 tablespoons (U.S. 3 tablespoons) apricot jam,
sieved
Decoration
150 ml/¼ pint double cream
(U.S. ⅔ cup heavy cream), whipped
7 whole hazelnuts (U.S. filberts)

Heat the oven to 200°C/400°F, Gas Mark 6 and have ready a 17.5-cm/7-inch fluted flan ring standing on a baking sheet (U.S. cookie sheet), or a fluted flan tin.

Put the flour and salt in a bowl and rub or cut in the margarine until the mixture resembles breadcrumbs. Stir in the sugar and nuts, add the egg yolk and enough milk to make a firm dough. Knead briefly then roll out on a lightly floured surface and use to line the flan ring. Line with a sheet of greaseproof paper (U.S. waxed paper) and half-fill with baking beans. Bake blind for 15 minutes. Remove the lining paper and beans and return to the oven for a further 5-10 minutes, or until the base is just dry.

Meanwhile, put the chopped apple in a pan, add the sugar and 1 teaspoon of the water. Cook over very low heat for about 10 minutes, stirring very frequently, until the apples form a smooth purée. Leave to cool.

Spread the apple purée in the pastry case. Thinly slice the eating apples and immediately arrange the slices, overlapping, on the purée. Mix together the jam and remainder of the water in a small pan and heat gently, stirring, until smooth. Brush over the apple slices.

Bake for about 15 minutes, then leave to cool. Transfer to a serving plate and decorate with rosettes of cream, each topped with a nut. **Serves 4-6**

Apple and hazelnut flan

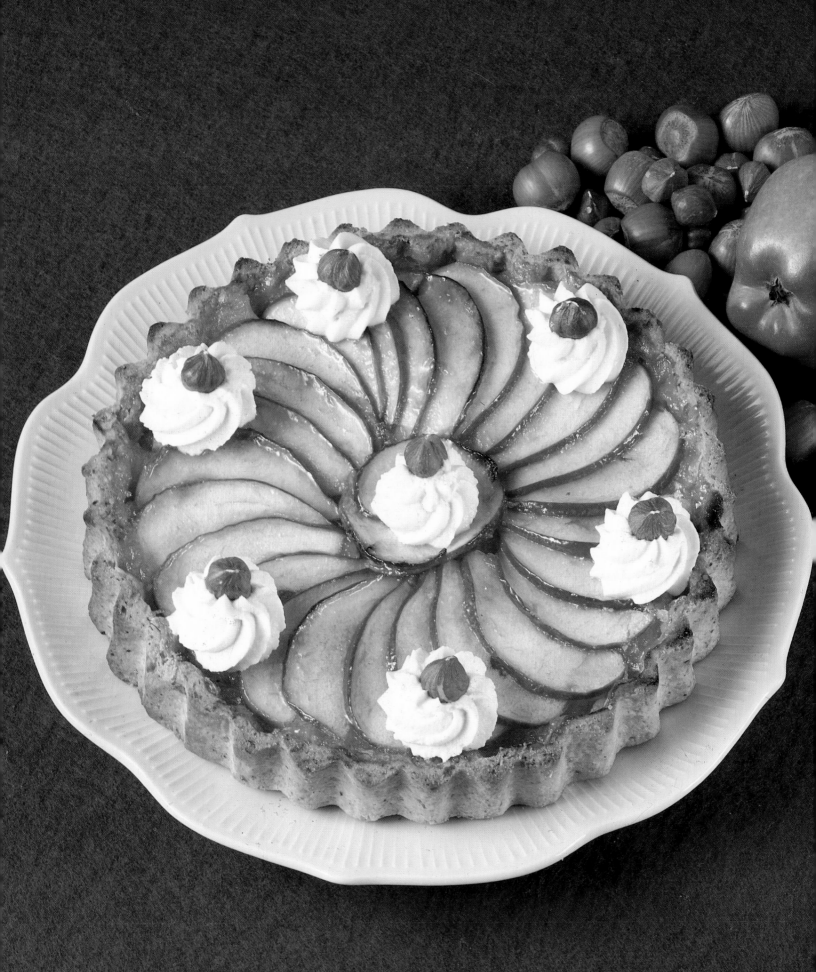

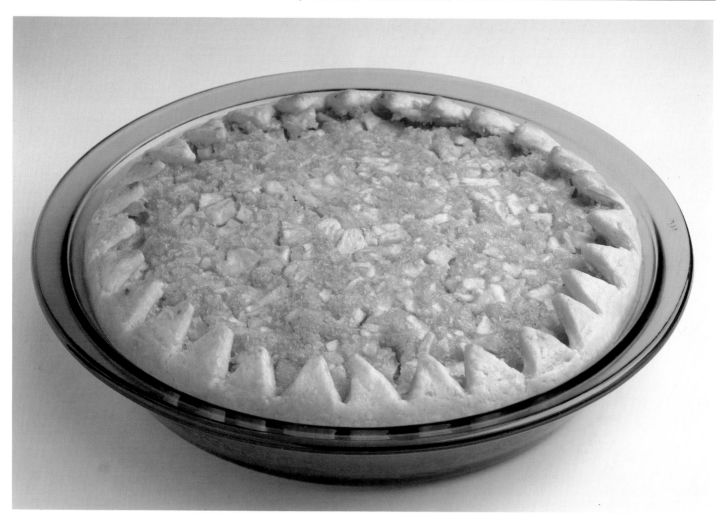

Apple syrup nut tart

(Illustrated above)

50 g/2 oz plain flour
(U.S. $\frac{1}{2}$ cup all-purpose flour)
50 g/2 oz wholemeal flour
(U.S. $\frac{1}{2}$ cup wholewheat flour)
50 g/2 oz (U.S. $\frac{1}{4}$ cup) butter or block margarine
1-2 tablespoons (U.S. 1-3 tablespoons) water
Filling
350 g/12 oz (U.S. $\frac{3}{4}$ lb) cooking apples, peeled, cored
and chopped
75 g/3 oz fresh wholemeal breadcrumbs
(U.S. 1$\frac{1}{2}$ cups fresh wholewheat bread crumbs)
1 tablespoon lemon juice
finely grated rind of $\frac{1}{2}$ lemon
175 g/6 oz golden syrup (U.S. $\frac{1}{2}$ cup light corn syrup)
25 g/1 oz (U.S. 2 tablespoons) butter or margarine,
melted
50 g/2 oz (U.S. $\frac{1}{2}$ cup) chopped almonds

Heat the oven to 180°C/350°F, Gas Mark 4 and have ready a 20-cm/8-inch deep ovenproof glass pie plate.

Sift the white flour into a bowl and stir in the brown flour. Rub or cut in the butter until the mixture resembles breadcrumbs. Add enough water to make a dough. Knead lightly until smooth. Roll out on a floured surface and use to line the chosen pie plate, trimming the edge level with the rim of the plate. Cut out triangles all round to form a vandyked effect.

Mix together all the ingredients for the filling and spoon into the pastry case. Fold the edges of the pastry in over the filling.

Bake for about 50 minutes, or until the filling is firm. If using an ovenproof glass plate, you can check that the pastry is cooked underneath. Serve hot with cream. **Serves 4-6**

Variation

Cherry walnut tart Omit the apples and substitute 350 g/12 oz (U.S. $\frac{3}{4}$ lb) cherries, halved and stones removed (U.S. pitted). Use chopped walnuts or pecans instead of the almonds and serve portions of the tart hot, sprinkled with a little sifted icing sugar (U.S. confectioners' sugar) and accompanied by vanilla ice cream.

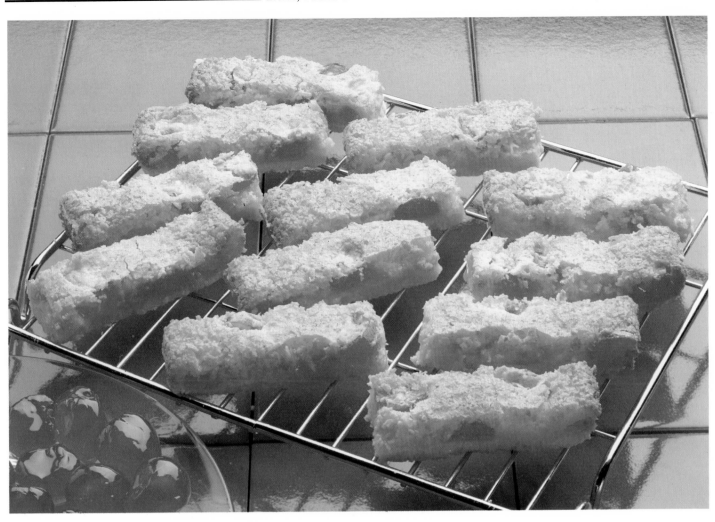

Cherry macaroon bars

(Illustrated above)

150 g/5 oz wholemeal flour
(U.S. 1¼ cups wholewheat flour)
75 g/3 oz (U.S. ⅓ cup) butter or margarine
1 tablespoon light muscovado sugar
(U.S. light brown sugar)
Topping
25 g/1 oz wholemeal flour
(U.S. ¼ cup wholewheat flour)
¼ teaspoon baking powder
50 g/2 oz desiccated coconut
(U.S. ⅔ cup shredded coconut)
175 g/6 oz light muscovado sugar
(U.S. ¾ cup light brown sugar)
75 g/3 oz glacé cherries
(U.S. scant ½ cup candied cherries), halved
2 eggs

Heat the oven to 150°C/300°F, Gas Mark 2 and have ready a 25-cm/9½-inch by 19-cm/7½-inch oblong ovenproof glass flan dish.

Put the flour in a bowl and rub or cut in the butter until the mixture resembles breadcrumbs. Stir in the sugar. Transfer the mixture to the chosen dish and press down firmly to make a flat base. Bake for 15 minutes, or until pale golden.

Meanwhile, make the topping. Mix the flour with the baking powder, coconut and sugar in a bowl. Stir in the cherries and eggs. Mix well and spread evenly over the base. Bake for 20-25 minutes, or until golden brown. Leave to cool in the dish, then cut into fingers. **Makes 12**

Variations

Ginger flapjack bars Omit the cherries and coconut and substitute 75 g/3 oz (U.S. ⅓ cup) chopped preserved ginger and 50 g/2 oz (U.S. scant ½ cup) rolled oats.

Pineapple crumb bars Omit the cherries and coconut and substitute 75 g/3 oz chopped glacé pineapple (U.S. ⅓ cup chopped candied pineapple) and 40 g/1½ oz wholemeal breadcrumbs (U.S. ¾ cup fresh wholewheat bread crumbs).

Raspberry bakewell bars Omit the cherries and coconut and substitute 75 g/3 oz flaked almonds (U.S. ¾ cup slivered almonds) for them both. Spread raspberry jam over the baked base before covering with the almond topping.

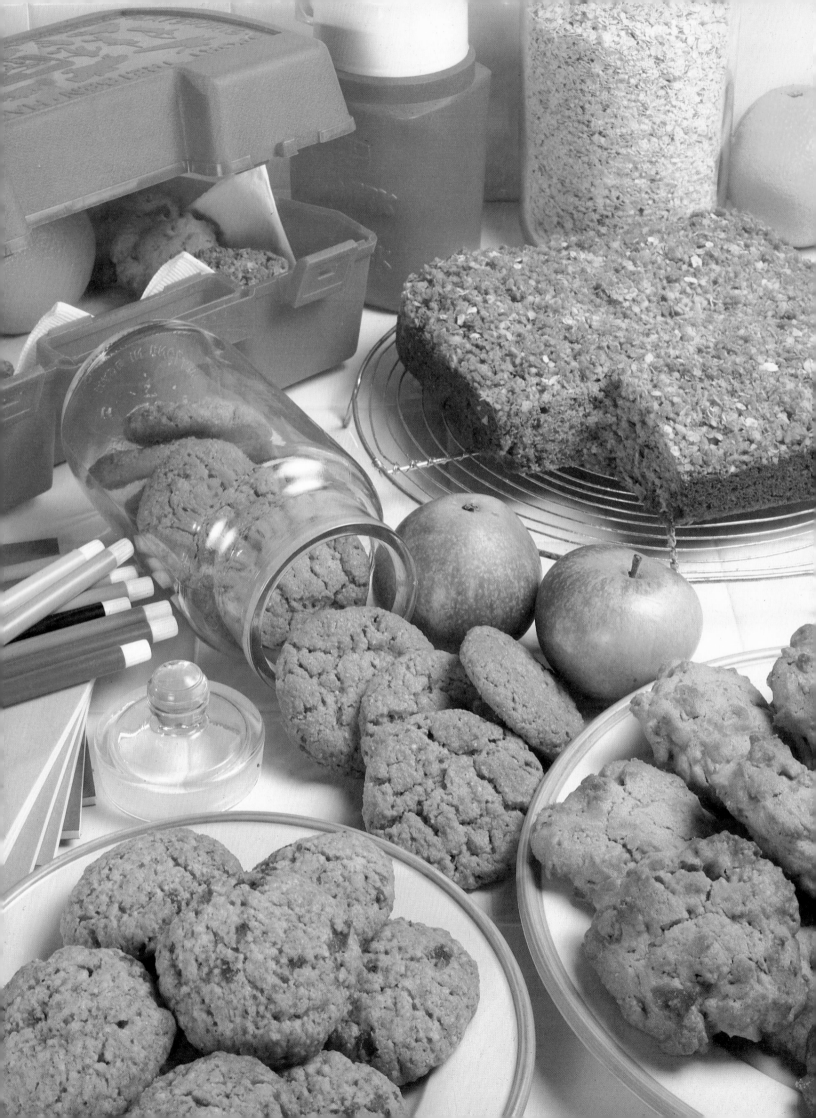

Bonus oat cakes

(Illustrated opposite)

190 g/6½ oz porage oats (U.S. 2 cups rolled oats)
1 teaspoon bicarbonate of soda (U.S. baking soda)
¼ teaspoon salt
175 g/6 oz (U.S. ¾ cup) butter or margarine
175 g/6 oz (U.S. ¾ cup) peanut butter
150 g/5 oz light muscovado sugar (U.S. generous
½ cup light brown sugar)
2 eggs, beaten
2 tablespoons (U.S. 3 tablespoons) water
75 g/3 oz Oat Krunchies (U.S. 1½ cups puffed oat
cereal), roughly crushed

Heat the oven to 180°C/350°F, Gas Mark 4 and have ready several baking sheets (U.S. cookie sheets).

Grind the oats in a food processor or blender until fine. Combine with the bicarbonate of soda and salt. Cream the butter with the peanut butter and sugar in a bowl until fluffy. Gradually beat in the egg and water. Stir in the flour mixture then the crushed cereal. Drop rounded tablespoons of the dough on to the ungreased tins, keeping them well apart.

Bake for 15 minutes, or until pale golden. Leave to cool on the tins for 2 minutes. **Makes about 35**

Banana crunch cake

(Illustrated opposite)

Topping
50 g/2 oz porage oats (U.S. generous ½ cup rolled
oats)
50 g/2 oz light muscovado sugar (U.S. ¼ cup light
brown sugar)
25 g/1 oz (U.S. 2 tablespoons) butter, melted
2 tablespoons (U.S. 3 tablespoons) chopped mixed
nuts
½ teaspoon ground cinnamon
Cake
100 g/4 oz porage oats (U.S. 1⅛ cups rolled oats)
100 g/4 oz plain flour (U.S. 1 cup all-purpose flour)
1 teaspoon salt
1 teaspoon bicarbonate of soda (U.S. baking soda)
50 g/2 oz (U.S. ½ cup) chopped mixed nuts
100 g/4 oz (U.S. ½ cup) butter or margarine
115 g/4½ oz light muscovado sugar (U.S. generous ½
cup light brown sugar)
1 medium-sized banana, peeled and mashed
2 eggs, beaten
1 teaspoon vanilla essence (U.S. vanilla extract)

Above: Banana crunch cake. Centre: Bonus oat cakes. Below left: Oat and nut cookies. Below right: Peanut butter dreams (recipe page 167)

Heat the oven to 180°C/350°F, Gas Mark 4 and grease a 20-cm/8-inch square cake tin.

Mix together all the ingredients for the topping and set aside. Grind the oats for the cake in a food processor or blender until fine. Combine with the flour, salt, bicarbonate of soda and nuts. Cream the butter and sugar together in a bowl until light and fluffy. Beat in the banana, egg and vanilla essence. Gradually add the dry ingredients, mixing well after each addition. Transfer to the prepared tin and sprinkle evenly with the topping.

Bake for about 1 hour, or until a fine skewer inserted in the centre of the cake comes out clean. Leave in the tin until cold, then cut into squares. **Makes 1 (20-cm/8-inch) cake, about 16 squares**

Oat and nut cookies

(Illustrated opposite)

175 g/6 oz (U.S. ¾ cup) butter or margarine
150 g/5 oz light muscovado sugar (U.S. ⅔ cup light
brown sugar)
1 egg
1 teaspoon vanilla essence (U.S. vanilla extract)
100 g/4 oz wholemeal flour
(U.S. 1 cup wholewheat flour)
½ teaspoon bicarbonate of soda (U.S. baking soda)
½ teaspoon salt
100 g/4 oz porage oats (U.S. generous 1 cup rolled
oats)
50 g/2 oz (U.S. 1 cup) wheatgerm
50 g/2 oz (U.S. ½ cup) chopped blanched peanuts
4 pieces preserved ginger, chopped

Heat the oven to 180°C/350°F, Gas Mark 4 and grease 2 baking sheets (U.S. cookie sheets).

Put the butter, sugar, egg and vanilla essence into a bowl and beat until well blended. Stir in the flour, bicarbonate of soda, salt, oats, wheatgerm, nuts and ginger. Mix well. Drop the mixture on to the prepared sheets, using about 1 rounded tablespoon each time and allowing room for spreading.

Bake for about 12 minutes, or until the edges are golden brown. Cool on the sheets for 2 minutes, then remove to a wire rack. Store in an airtight container. **Makes about 24**

Variation

Cheese and bacon cookies Omit the peanuts and ginger. Fry or grill (U.S. broil) 4 rashers streaky bacon (U.S. 4 bacon slices), rind removed, until crisp. Chop roughly and add to the cookie dough with 100 g/4 oz (U.S. 1 cup) grated Cheddar cheese. When cool, store, covered, in the refrigerator.

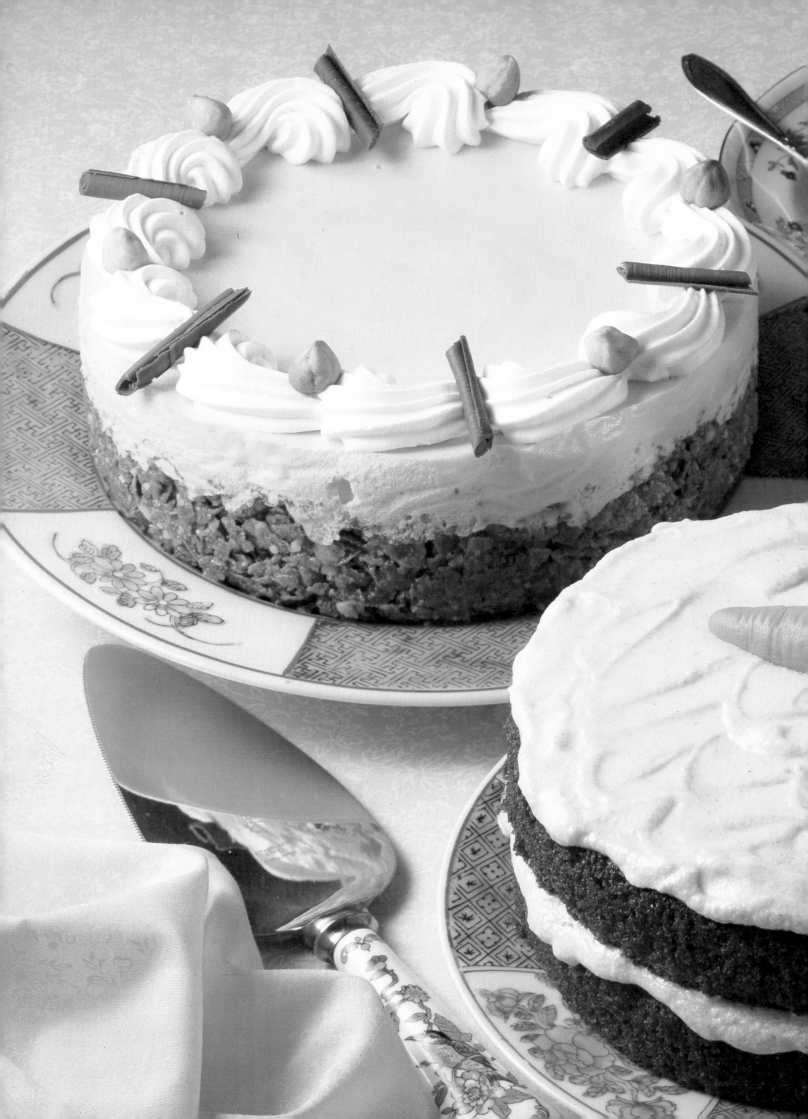

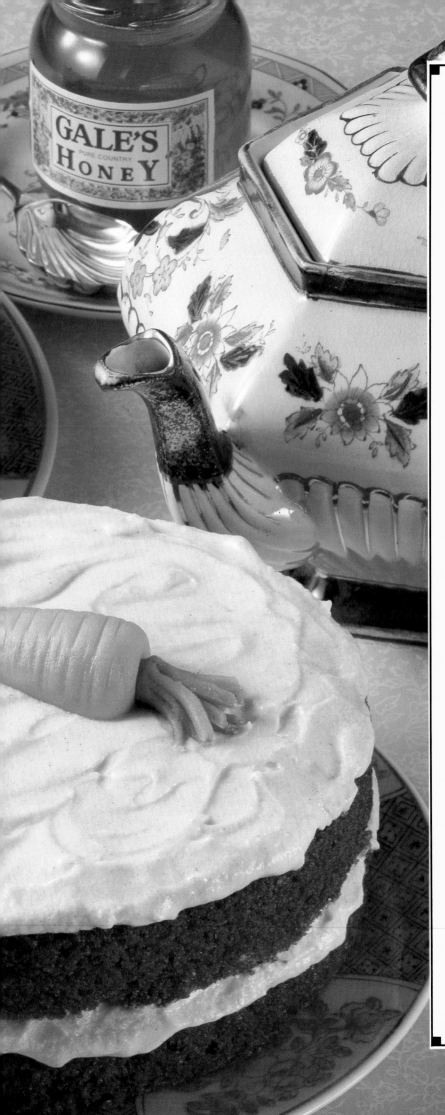

Cakes, Puddings and Cold Desserts

Here is the stage of the meal where you may feel it is difficult to include fibre-full ingredients. But this is not so; in fact it's easy when you know how.

Any basic mixture for a cake or pudding that requires flour can be adapted to use a proportion of brown flour, although the texture may be altered. Immediately this pushes up the fibre count. Fruit, particularly dried fruit, is the star of this section. You could sweeten with white sugar or a preserve made with white sugar, but why do this when the natural sugar in fruit can do the trick to such good effect? I have specified brown sugar in my recipes whenever suitable. There is no doubt that natural raw sugars have more flavour and are better for you than highly refined white sugar.

It may seem surprising that ingredients like oats and bran flakes can be incorporated in flan cases, cookies and puddings, but by experimenting with imagination and an adventurous spirit, it is possible to produce many new flavour treats. Crumble puddings, for instance, are easily up-dated by adding coconut or other nuts according to your fancy, to a simple half-and-half blend of white and wholemeal flour.

When your choice for a sweet is a sherbet or a fruit salad, boost the day's fibre count by serving on the side a few high-fibre cookies to be found in this and the previous section. Save pieces of brown bread to make crunchy diced toppings for fruit, as well as croûtons. The sweet course can still have a place in the healthiest of diets.

Above: Hazelnut honey cheesecake (recipe page 156). Below: Honey carrot cake (recipe page 161)

Hazelnut honey cheesecake

(Illustrated on page 154)

75 g/3 oz (U.S. ⅓ cup) butter or margarine
3 tablespoons (U.S. 4 tablespoons) clear honey
175 g/6 oz (U.S. 5 cups) bran flakes, lightly crushed
25 g/1 oz hazelnuts, finely chopped (U.S. ¼ cup finely chopped filberts)
Topping
1 tablespoon gelatine (U.S. 1 envelope unflavored gelatin)
2 tablespoons (U.S. 3 tablespoons) water
225 g/8 oz (U.S. ½ lb) cream cheese
1 tablespoon vanilla essence (U.S. vanilla extract)
2 tablespoons (U.S. 3 tablespoons) clear honey
2 eggs, separated
25 g/1 oz light muscovado sugar (U.S. ⅛ cup light brown sugar)
150 ml/¼ pint double cream (U.S. ⅔ cup heavy cream), whipped
Decoration
150 ml/¼ pint double cream (U.S. ⅔ cup heavy cream), whipped
few whole hazelnuts (U.S. filberts)
few chocolate curls made from dark plain chocolate (U.S. semi-sweet chocolate)

Heat the oven to 180°C/350°F, Gas Mark 4 and generously grease a 20-cm/8-inch spring release flan tin with a loose base.

Melt the butter and stir in the honey, flakes and nuts. Mix well and press into the prepared tin, raising the sides slightly all round. Bake for 10 minutes. Leave to cool.

To make the topping, sprinkle the gelatine over the water in a small bowl. Stand this over hot water until the gelatine has completely dissolved. Cool. Cream the cheese until absolutely smooth and gradually mix in the vanilla and honey. Put the egg yolks in a bowl and add the sugar. Whisk until thick. Gradually whisk in the cheese mixture and dissolved gelatine. Fold in the cream. Whisk the egg whites in a clean bowl until stiff and fold them in thoroughly. Pour into the tin and chill until set.

Carefully remove the tin and transfer the cheesecake, still on the metal base, to a serving plate. Pipe scrolls of cream round the top edge and decorate with hazelnuts and chocolate curls. **Serves 6**

Crunchy apple layer

(Illustrated opposite)

75 g/3 oz (U.S. ⅓ cup) butter or margarine
225 g/8 oz fresh wholemeal breadcrumbs
(U.S. 4 cups fresh wholewheat bread crumbs)
100 g/4 oz demerara sugar (U.S. ½ cup brown sugar)
1 medium-sized cooking apple (about 225 g/8 oz (U.S. ½ lb)), peeled, cored and sliced
25 g/1 oz sultanas (U.S. scant ¼ cup seedless white raisins)
2 tablespoons (U.S. 3 tablespoons) water
150 g/5 oz dark plain chocolate (U.S. scant 1 cup semi-sweet chocolate pieces)
300 ml/½ pint (U.S. 1¼ cups) whipping cream

Have ready a 20-cm/8-inch flan ring standing on a serving plate, or a flan tin with a loose base.

Melt the butter in a frying pan (U.S. skillet) and fry the breadcrumbs over moderately high heat, stirring, until golden. Stir in half the sugar.

Meanwhile, put the apple slices, sultanas, water and remaining sugar in a pan. Cook very gently until the apple is tender. Leave to cool.

Melt the chocolate in a bowl over a pan of hot water. Cool. Whip the cream, reserve about 2 tablespoons (U.S. 3 tablespoons) and fold the chocolate into the remainder.

Press half the crumb mixture into the flan ring and cover with half the chocolate cream. Reserve 4 apple slices and 1 sultana, and arrange the rest in the flan ring. Cover with the remaining chocolate cream. Spoon the last of the crumbs on top and press down gently. Chill for at least 4 hours.

At serving time, remove the flan ring. If using a tin, slip this off and serve the apple layer on the metal base. Arrange the reserved apple slices on top of the dessert. Pipe or spoon a rosette of cream close to the apple and top with the sultana. **Serves 6**

Crunchy apple layer

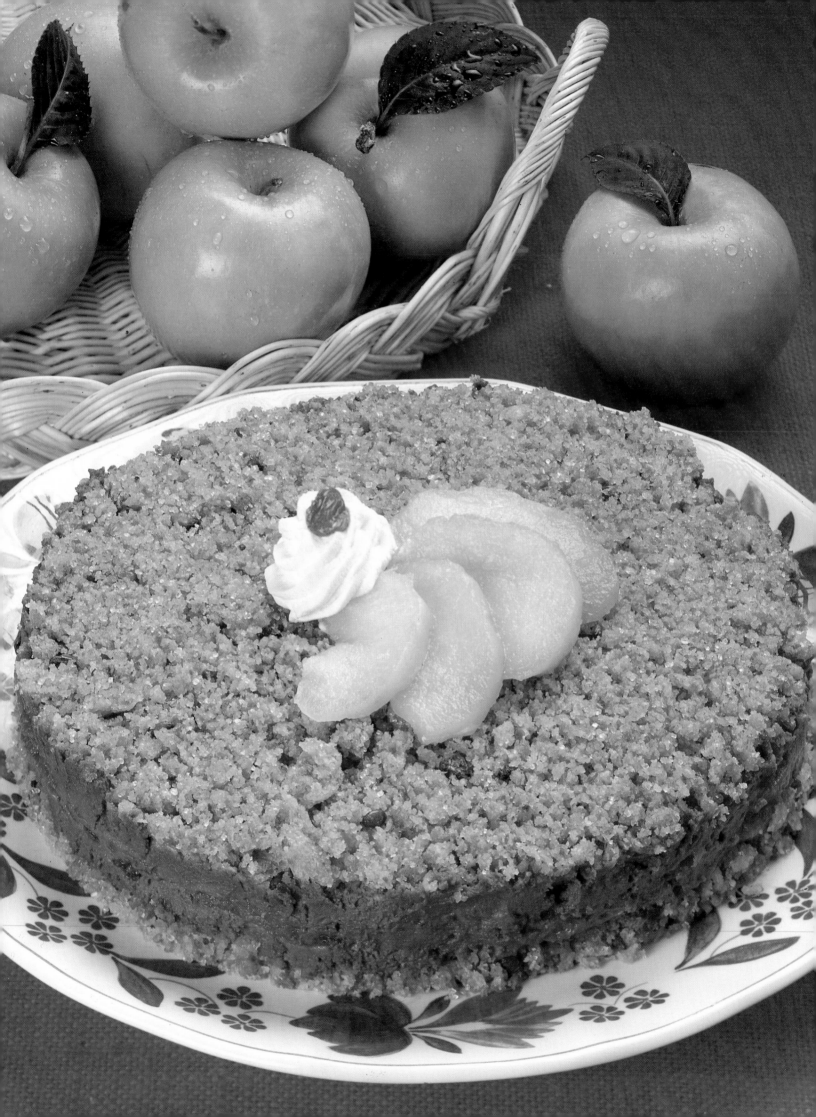

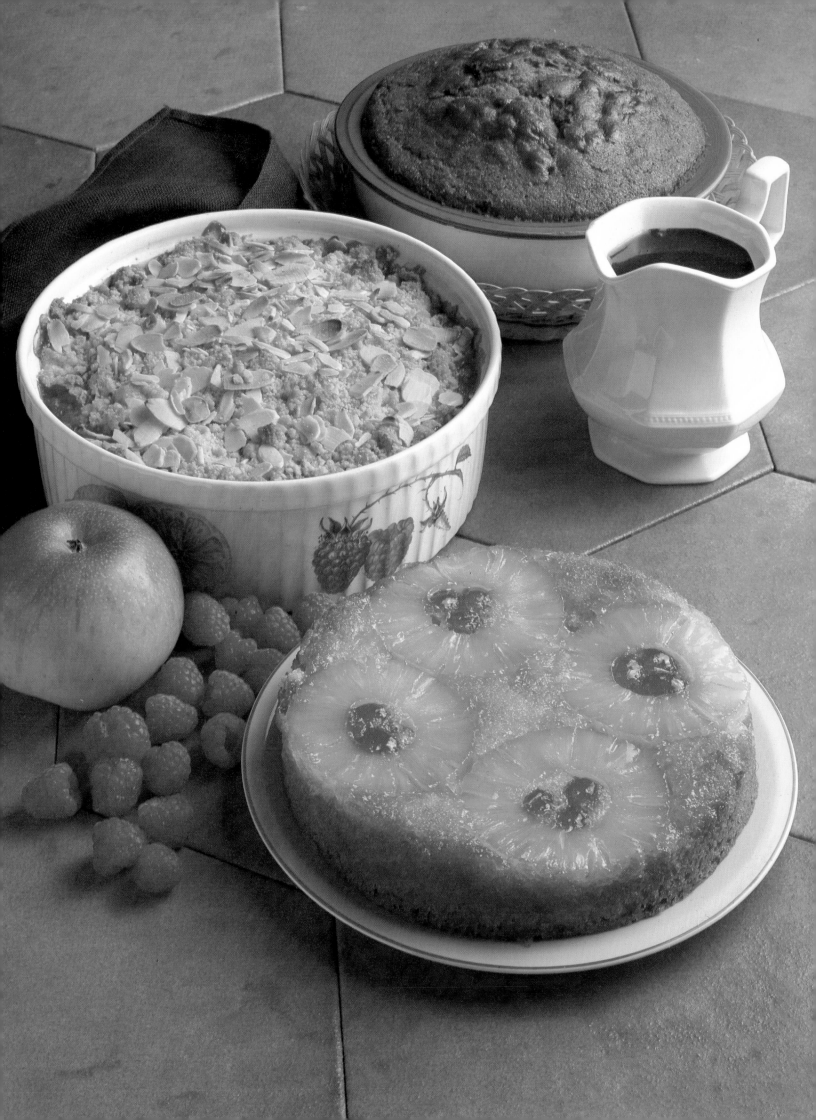

Butterscotch saucy pudding

(Illustrated opposite)

75 g/3 oz plain flour (U.S. $\frac{3}{4}$ cup all-purpose flour)
2$\frac{1}{2}$ teaspoons (U.S. 1 tablespoon) baking powder
75 g/3 oz wholemeal flour
(U.S. $\frac{3}{4}$ cup wholewheat flour)
100 g/4 oz light muscovado sugar (U.S. $\frac{1}{2}$ cup light brown sugar)
100 g/4 oz (U.S. $\frac{1}{2}$ cup) soft margarine
2 eggs
5 tablespoons (U.S. 7 tablespoons) milk
Sauce
75 g/3 oz (U.S. $\frac{1}{3}$ cup) butter or margarine
150 g/5 oz light muscovado sugar
(U.S. $\frac{2}{3}$ cup light brown sugar)
4 tablespoons double cream
(U.S. 6 tablespoons heavy cream)

Heat the oven to 180°C/350°F, Gas Mark 4 and lightly grease a shallow 1.5-litre/2$\frac{1}{2}$-pint (U.S. 6$\frac{1}{4}$-cup) ovenproof dish.

Sift the white flour with the baking powder into a bowl. Add the brown flour, sugar, margarine, eggs and milk, and beat for about 2 minutes, or until smooth. Transfer to the prepared dish and level the top.

Bake for about 1 hour, or until well risen and golden brown. Meanwhile, make the sauce. Melt the butter in a pan, add the sugar and cream and stir over low heat, until boiling. Simmer for 3 minutes, stirring occasionally. The sauce should be thick and glossy. Transfer to a warm serving jug and hand separately with the hot pudding. **Serves 6**

Pineapple upside-down pudding

(Illustrated opposite)

1 (225-g/8-oz) can pineapple slices in natural juice
2-6 glacé cherries (U.S. 2-6 candied cherries), halved
150 g/5 oz light muscovado sugar (U.S. scant $\frac{2}{3}$ cup light brown sugar)
50 g/2 oz wholemeal flour (U.S. $\frac{1}{2}$ cup wholewheat flour)
25 g/1 oz plain flour (U.S. $\frac{1}{4}$ cup all-purpose flour)
1$\frac{1}{4}$ teaspoons (U.S. 1$\frac{1}{2}$ teaspoons) baking powder
75 g/3 oz (U.S. $\frac{1}{3}$ cup) soft margarine
1 egg, beaten

Heat the oven to 190°C/375°F, Gas Mark 5 and generously grease a 17.5-cm/7-inch cake tin.

Drain 4 slices of pineapple (reserving the juice) and arrange in the base of the prepared tin. Press cherry halves in the centre of each, cut surface uppermost. Sprinkle 50 g/2 oz (U.S. $\frac{1}{4}$ cup) of the sugar evenly over the fruit.

Put the remaining ingredients in a bowl with 2 tablespoons (U.S. 3 tablespoons) of the pineapple juice from the can. Beat with a wooden spoon for about 2 minutes, or until well blended. Transfer the mixture to the tin and level the surface.

Bake for about 25 minutes, or until well risen and firm to the touch in the centre. Leave in the tin for 10 minutes, then turn out on a plate. Serve warm. **Serves 4**

Raspberry almond crumble

(Illustrated opposite)

50 g/2 oz plain flour (U.S. $\frac{1}{2}$ cup all-purpose flour)
50 g/2 oz wholemeal flour (U.S. $\frac{1}{2}$ cup wholewheat flour)
50 g/2 oz (U.S. $\frac{1}{2}$ cup) ground almonds
75 g/3 oz (U.S. $\frac{1}{3}$ cup) block margarine, diced
50 g/2 oz light muscovado sugar (U.S. $\frac{1}{4}$ cup light brown sugar)
25 g/1 oz flaked almonds (U.S. $\frac{1}{4}$ cup slivered almonds)
Filling
350 g/12 oz (U.S. $\frac{3}{4}$ lb) cooking apples, peeled, cored and sliced
350 g/12 oz (U.S. $\frac{3}{4}$ lb) raspberries
100 g/4 oz light muscovado sugar (U.S. $\frac{1}{2}$ cup light brown sugar)
2 tablespoons (U.S. 3 tablespoons) water

Heat the oven to 200°C/400°F, Gas Mark 6 and grease a pie dish.

To make the crumble, put the flours into a bowl with the ground almonds. Rub or cut in the margarine until the mixture resembles breadcrumbs. Stir in the sugar. For the filling, put the apples into the prepared dish and sprinkle with the raspberries, sugar and water. Spoon the crumble mixture over the fruit and sprinkle with the almonds.

Bake for 40 minutes, or until the crumble is golden brown. Serve hot. **Serves 6**

Above: Butterscotch saucy pudding. Centre: Raspberry almond crumble. Below: Pineapple upside-down pudding

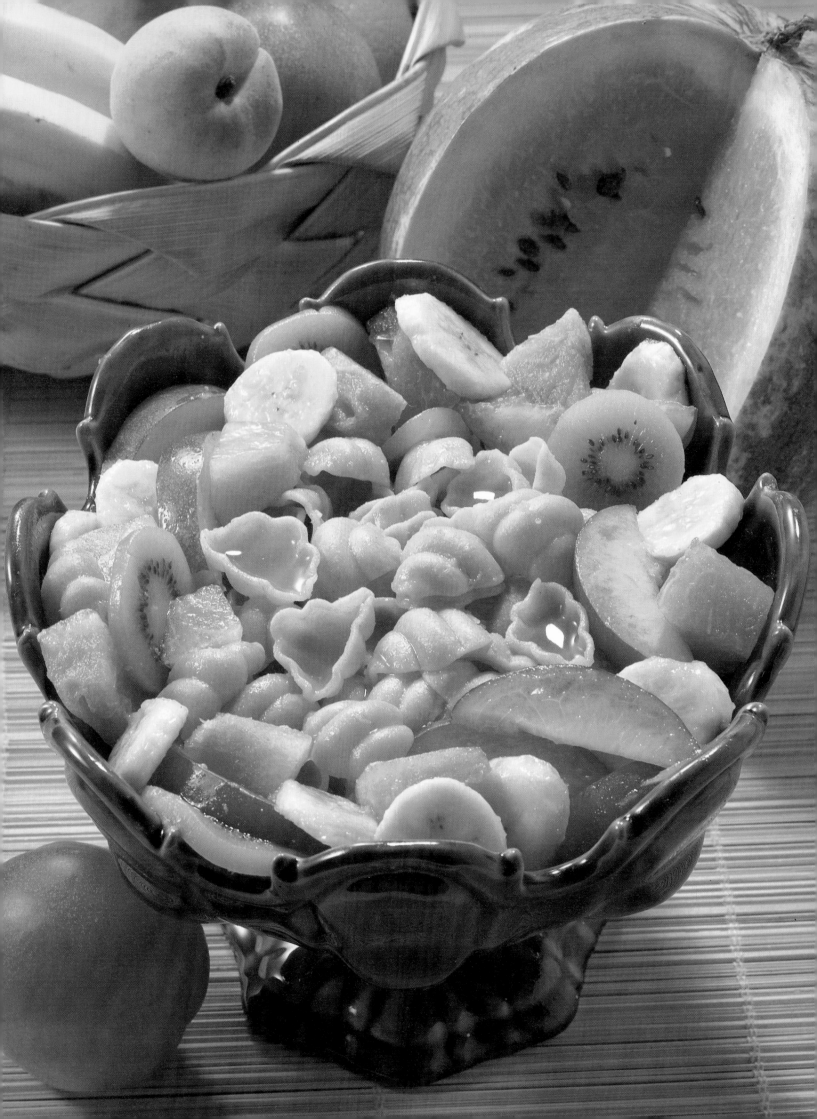

Honey carrot cake

(Illustrated on pages 154-155)

100 g/4 oz wholemeal flour
(U.S. 1 cup wholewheat flour)
$\frac{3}{4}$ teaspoon baking powder
$\frac{1}{2}$ teaspoon bicarbonate of soda (U.S. baking soda)
$\frac{1}{2}$ teaspoon ground cinnamon
pinch of salt
175 ml/6 fl oz (U.S. $\frac{3}{4}$ cup) oil
75 ml/3 fl oz (U.S. $\frac{1}{3}$ cup) clear honey
150 g/5 oz light muscovado sugar (U.S. $\frac{2}{3}$ cup light
brown sugar)
2 eggs
175 g/6 oz (U.S. 1$\frac{1}{2}$ cups) peeled and grated carrot
Frosting
50 g/2 oz (U.S. $\frac{1}{4}$ cup) butter or margarine
50 g/2 oz (U.S. $\frac{1}{4}$ cup) cream cheese
1 tablespoon clear honey
175 g/6 oz icing sugar (U.S. 1$\frac{1}{3}$ cups sifted confectioners' sugar)
$\frac{1}{4}$ teaspoon ground cinnamon

Heat the oven to 180°C/350°F, Gas Mark 4 and well grease two 17.5-cm/7-inch shallow cake tins.

Mix together the flour, baking powder, bicarbonate of soda, cinnamon and salt. Whisk the oil with the honey and sugar in a bowl until well blended. Beat in the eggs, one at a time. Fold in the dry ingredients. Lightly stir in the carrot. Divide the mixture between the tins and level the surface.

Bake for 40 minutes, or until well risen and firm to the touch. Leave in the tins for 5 minutes, then turn out and cool on a wire rack.

Beat together all the ingredients for the frosting until smooth. Use half to sandwich the cakes together. Place on a serving dish. Swirl the remaining frosting over the top of the cake and decorate with a moulded carrot. **Makes 1 (17.5-cm/7-inch) cake**

Decoration To make the marzipan carrot which decorates the cake, take 100 g/4 oz almond paste (U.S. $\frac{1}{4}$ lb almond marzipan) and pinch off one quarter of this. Knead in sufficient orange food colouring to tint the larger piece the colour of a carrot. Tint the smaller piece bright green with food colouring in the same way. Roll the larger piece into the shape of a carrot about 7.5 cm/3 inches long. Using a sharp knife, mark crosswise lines along the length. Roll the green paste to an oblong about 5 cm/2 inches by 2 cm/$\frac{3}{4}$ inch and snip along one long edge with scissors, leaving a small border on the other long edge unsnipped. Roll up, starting from one short side and pinch the uncut edges together. Place the carrot in the centre of the cake and press the 'stalk' into the top of it.

Tropical fruit dish

Tropical fruit dish

(Illustrated opposite)

175 g/6 oz (U.S. 2 cups) wholewheat pasta shells
1 large ripe banana, peeled and sliced
finely grated rind and juice of 1 orange
50 ml/2 fl oz golden syrup (U.S. $\frac{1}{4}$ cup light corn
syrup)
1 (225-g/8-oz) wedge watermelon, rind removed
2 ripe nectarines, halved and stoned
(U.S. pits removed)
1 kiwi fruit (optional)

Cook the pasta in a pan in boiling water as directed.

Meanwhile, put the banana slices in a bowl, pour the orange juice over and turn until the slices are coated. Drain the orange juice into the golden syrup in a small pan. Add the orange rind and heat very gently, stirring, until just blended. Cut the melon into bite-sized chunks, removing any seeds. Cut the nectarines and kiwi fruit into small neat slices.

Drain the pasta well and return it to the hot pan. Pour the syrup over and toss lightly. Pile up in a warm serving dish and arrange the prepared fruit in a ring round the edge. Serve while the pasta is still warm. **Serves 4**

New England ring cake

100 g/4 oz plain flour (U.S. 1 cup all-purpose flour)
2 teaspoons baking powder
pinch of salt
$\frac{1}{2}$ teaspoon ground cinnamon
1 teaspoon ground mace
small pinch of ground cloves
100 g/4 oz wholemeal flour
(U.S. 1 cup wholewheat flour)
225 g/8 oz light muscovado sugar (U.S. 1 cup light
brown sugar)
100 g/4 oz (U.S. 1 cup) grated carrot
100 g/4 oz (U.S. $\frac{1}{3}$ cup) cranberry sauce
175 ml/6 fl oz (U.S. $\frac{3}{4}$ cup) oil
2 eggs

Heat the oven to 180°C/350°F, Gas Mark 4 and generously grease a 22.5-cm/9-inch ring tin.

Sift the white flour with the baking powder, salt and spices into a bowl. Add the remaining ingredients and beat with a wooden spoon until the mixture is well blended. Transfer to the prepared tin.

Bake for about 45 minutes, or until firm to the touch. Leave in the tin for 5 minutes, then turn out and cool on a wire rack.
Makes 1 (22.5-cm/9-inch) ring cake

Raisin pudding with lemon sauce

(Illustrated opposite)

25 g/1 oz plain flour (U.S. ¼ cup all-purpose flour)
¾ teaspoon baking powder
pinch of salt
50 g/2 oz wholemeal flour (U.S. ½ cup wholewheat
flour)
75 g/3 oz fresh wholemeal breadcrumbs
(U.S. 1½ cups fresh wholewheat bread crumbs)
75 g/3 oz shredded suet (U.S. generous ½ cup
chopped beef suet)
50 g/2 oz light muscovado sugar (U.S. ¼ cup light
brown sugar)
100 g/4 oz (U.S. ⅔ cup) seedless raisins or currants
1 egg
about 6 tablespoons (U.S. 9 tablespoons) milk
Sauce
2 tablespoons custard powder (U.S. 3 tablespoons
Bird's English dessert mix)
2 tablespoons light muscovado sugar (U.S. 3 tablespoons light brown sugar)
600 ml/1 pint (U.S. 2½ cups) milk
1 tablespoon lemon juice
finely grated rind of 1 lemon

Sift the white flour with the baking powder and salt into a bowl. Stir in the brown flour, breadcrumbs, suet, sugar and fruit. Make a well in the centre, add the egg and enough milk to make a dropping consistency.

Transfer to a well-greased 900-ml/1½-pint pudding basin (U.S. 3¾-cup pudding bowl). Cover with a double layer of foil, putting a pleat in the centre, and crimp well under the rim of the basin. Stand this in a large pan and pour in boiling water to come half-way up the sides. Cover the pan and keep the water boiling gently for 2 hours, adding more boiling water if necessary during cooking.

Meanwhile, make the sauce. Blend the custard powder and sugar to a cream with a little of the milk in a jug. Heat the remaining milk to boiling point, add to the jug and mix well. Return the sauce to the pan and bring back to the boil, stirring constantly. Simmer for 2 minutes and stir in the lemon juice and most of the lemon rind. Turn the pudding out on a warm dish and sprinkle with the remaining lemon rind. Serve hot with the sauce. **Serves 4-6**

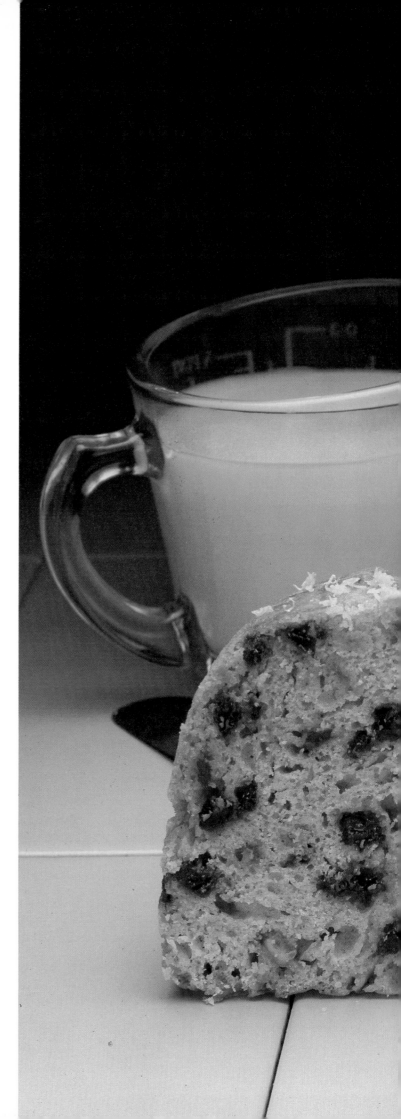

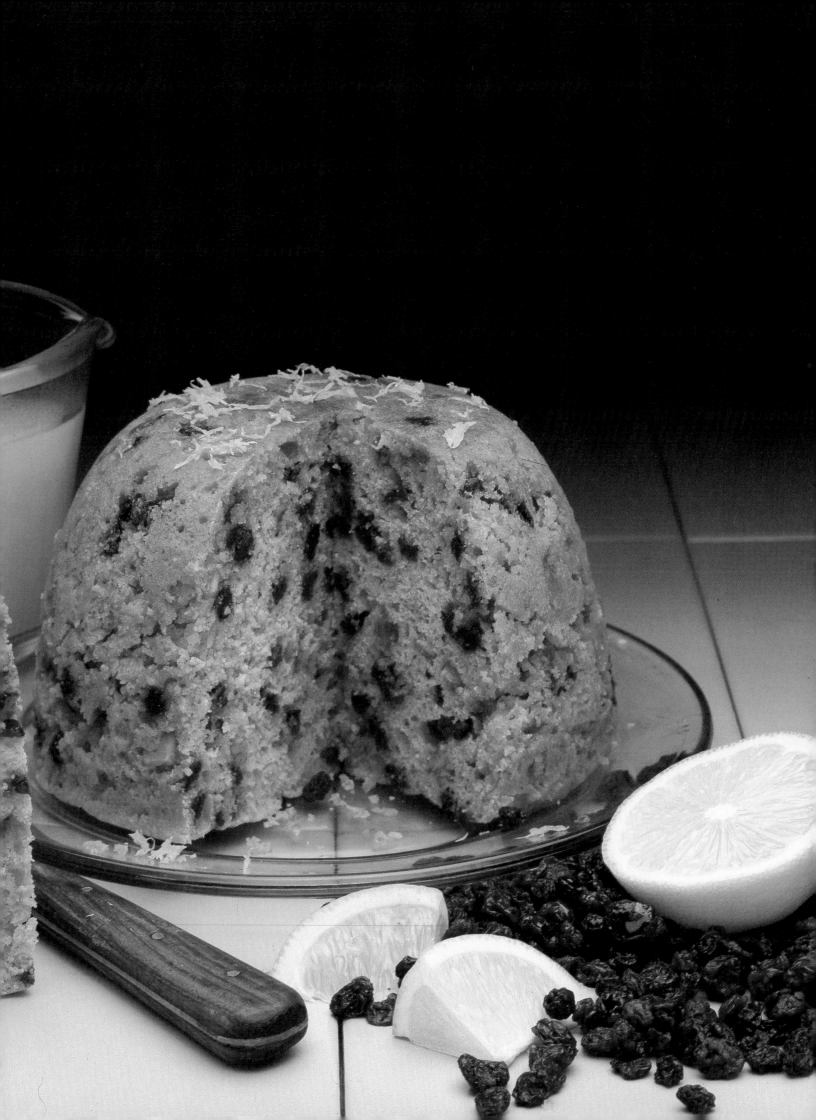

Grapefruit and pineapple sherbet

350 ml/12 fl oz (U.S. 1½ cups) water
2 teaspoons gelatine (U.S. ⅔ envelope unflavored gelatin)
150 g/5 oz (U.S. generous ½ cup) sugar
pinch of salt
1 large grapefruit
1 (425-g/15-oz) can pineapple in natural juice
2 egg whites

Take 4 tablespoons (U.S. 6 tablespoons) water from the measured quantity and place in a small bowl. Sprinkle the gelatine over and leave to stand. Place the remaining water in a pan with the sugar and salt. Bring to the boil, stirring, then simmer for 2 minutes. Stir in the softened gelatine until completely dissolved. Leave to cool, stirring occasionally.

Meanwhile, finely grate the rind from the grapefruit, then remove the pulp from the fruit, discarding all membranes and pith. Place the grapefruit flesh and rind in a blender or food processor, add the pineapple and juice from the can and process until smooth. When the syrup is cool, stir in the fruit mixture and transfer to a shallow container. Freeze until firm.

Turn out into a bowl and beat until mushy. Add the unbeaten egg whites and whisk with a rotary beater or electric mixer for about 1 minute, until fluffy. Return to the container, cover and freeze until required. Serve scooped into small glass dishes. **Serves 4-6**

Conference pear cake

100 g/4 oz plain flour (U.S. 1 cup all-purpose flour)
2 teaspoons (U.S. 1 tablespoon) baking powder
½ teaspoon salt
100 g/4 oz wholemeal flour
(U.S. 1 cup wholewheat flour)
225 g/8 oz (U.S. 1 cup) butter or margarine
225 g/8 oz light muscovado sugar (U.S. 1 cup light brown sugar)
4 eggs, beaten
2 firm Conference pears (U.S. firm eating pears), peeled and grated
finely grated rind of 1 lemon
50 g/2 oz desiccated coconut (U.S. ⅔ cup shredded coconut)

Heat the oven to 180°C/350°F, Gas Mark 4, line a rectangular roasting tin measuring about 30 cm/12 inches by 25 cm/10 inches and grease the lining paper.

Sift the white flour with the baking powder and salt. Stir in the brown flour. Cream the butter and sugar together in a bowl until light and fluffy. Gradually beat in the egg. Fold in the flour mixture, the pear, lemon rind and half the coconut. Transfer to the prepared tin and level the surface. Sprinkle with the remaining coconut.

Bake for about 45 minutes, or until firm to the touch. Leave in the tin for 5 minutes, then lift out and cool on a wire rack, using the lining paper to help you. Cut into squares. **Makes 30**

Note: Left-over Conference pear cake can be used to make Gingered pear trifle (see page 170).

Citrus soufflé

(Illustrated opposite)

1 grapefruit
finely grated rind and juice of 1 orange
3 eggs, separated
225 g/8 oz caster sugar (U.S. 1 cup granulated sugar)
1 tablespoon gelatine (U.S. 1 envelope unflavored gelatin)
4 tablespoons (U.S. 6 tablespoons) water
300 ml/½ pint double cream (U.S. 1¼ cups heavy cream)
40 g/1½ oz (U.S. ⅓ cup) chopped almonds, toasted
1 orange, peeled and divided into segments

Prepare a 15-cm/6-inch soufflé dish, by tying a double thickness of greaseproof paper (U.S. waxed paper) around the dish, to extend at least 10 cm/4 inches above the rim.

Finely grate the rind from the whole grapefruit and squeeze the juice from half of it. Place the grapefruit rind and juice and the orange rind and juice in a bowl with the egg yolks and sugar. Place over a pan containing simmering water to come about half-way up the sides of the bowl. Place the pan over low heat and whisk the mixture steadily until thick and mousse-like. Remove from the heat and continue whisking until the bowl is cold.

Dissolve the gelatine in the water in a small bowl over hot water. Cool slightly and whisk into the egg mousse. Whip the cream until just thick and fold in gently. Finally, whisk the egg whites and, when stiff, fold them in. Turn into the prepared dish and chill until firmly set.

Carefully peel off the paper and press almonds around the exposed sides. Remove any pith or membrane from the orange segments and use them to decorate the soufflé. **Serves 6**

Citrus soufflé

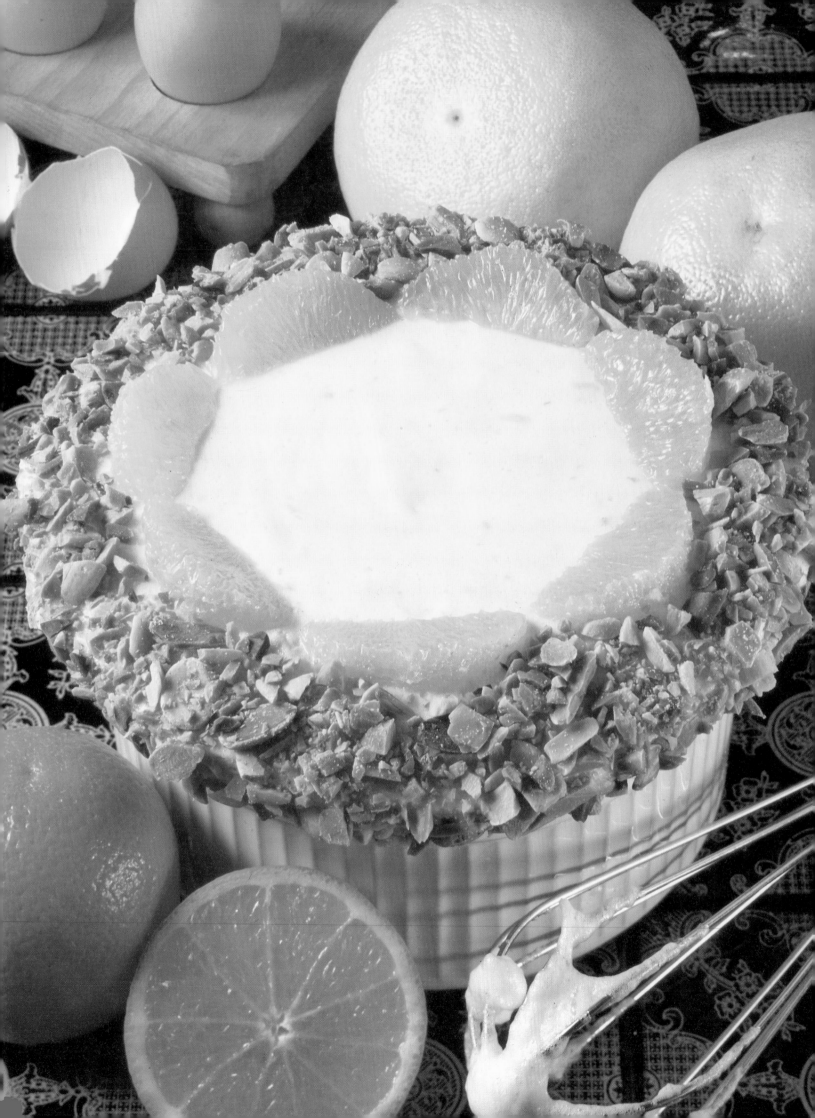

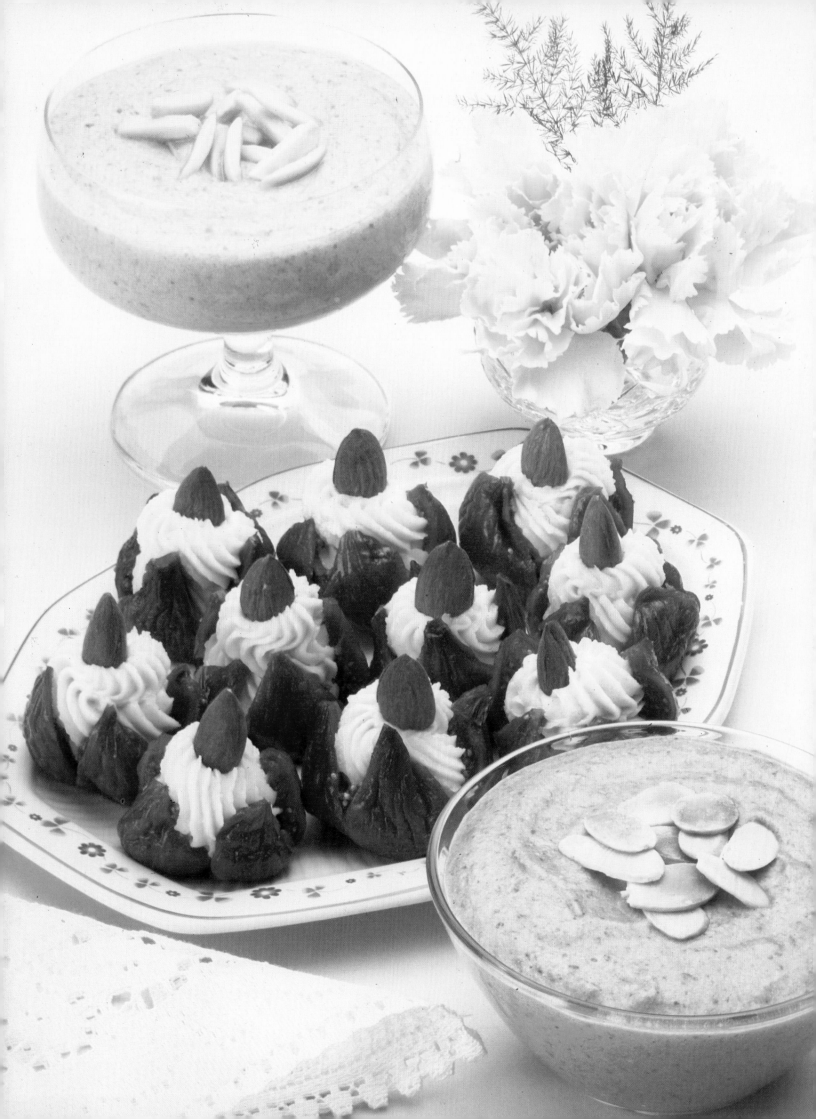

Fig mousse

(Illustrated opposite)

100 g/4 oz (U.S. $\frac{1}{4}$ lb) ready-to-eat figs
long strip of orange rind
300 ml/$\frac{1}{2}$ pint (U.S. 1$\frac{1}{4}$ cups) water
1 teaspoon ground cinnamon
300 ml/$\frac{1}{2}$ pint (U.S. 1$\frac{1}{4}$ cups) natural yogurt
about 2 teaspoons light muscovado sugar (U.S. about
1 tablespoon light brown sugar)
2 egg whites
2 tablespoons (U.S. 3 tablespoons) shredded almonds

Put the figs in a pan and add the orange rind and water. Bring to the boil and simmer for about 20 minutes, or until the figs are just soft. Discard the orange rind and purée the fruit with any liquid remaining in the pan and the cinnamon. Gradually add the yogurt and sweeten with sugar to taste. Whisk the egg whites until stiff and fold into the fig mixture.

Spoon into glass serving dishes and chill well. Serve sprinkled with almonds. **Serves 4**

Prune fool

(Illustrated opposite)

175 g/6 oz (U.S. 1 cup) no-need-to-soak prunes
300 ml/$\frac{1}{2}$ pint (U.S. 1$\frac{1}{4}$ cups) water
100 g/4 oz (U.S. $\frac{1}{2}$ cup) cottage cheese, sieved
150 ml/$\frac{1}{4}$ pint (U.S. $\frac{2}{3}$ cup) natural yogurt
2 tablespoons (U.S. 3 tablespoons) orange juice
about 25 g/1 oz light muscovado sugar (U.S. about
$\frac{1}{8}$ cup light brown sugar)
2 tablespoons desiccated coconut (U.S. 3 tablespoons
shredded coconut)
2 egg whites
2 tablespoons flaked almonds (U.S. 3 tablespoons
slivered almonds), lightly toasted

Put the prunes in a pan, pour the water over, bring to the boil and simmer for about 15 minutes, or until the fruit is tender. Stone (U.S. pit) the prunes and purée the flesh with any liquid remaining in the pan.

Beat together the cottage cheese, yogurt and orange juice. Sweeten with sugar to taste and stir in the prune purée and coconut. Whisk the egg whites until stiff and fold into the prune mixture.

Divide among glass serving dishes and chill. Serve sprinkled with almonds. **Serves 4**

Stuffed figs with almonds

(Illustrated opposite)

10 ready-to-eat figs
350 g/12 oz (U.S. 1$\frac{1}{2}$ cups) cream cheese
1 tablespoon clear honey
few drops of lemon juice
50 g/2 oz (U.S. $\frac{1}{2}$ cup) ground almonds
10 whole almonds

Trim off the stalk top from each fig then cut a cross almost through to the base. Open out the sections to form 'petals'.

Cream the cheese until softened. Add the honey, lemon juice and ground almonds and mix thoroughly. Pipe or spoon the mixture into the centre of each fig and gently press the 'petals' back into shape. Decorate with the whole almonds. **Serves 5**

Peanut butter dreams

(Illustrated on page 152)

250 g/9 oz porridge oats (U.S. 2$\frac{2}{3}$ cups rolled oats)
2 teaspoons bicarbonate of soda (U.S. 1 tablespoon
baking soda)
$\frac{1}{2}$ teaspoon salt
225 g/8 oz (U.S. 1 cup) butter or margarine
225 g/8 oz (U.S. 1 cup) peanut butter
200 g/7 oz light muscovado sugar (U.S. $\frac{7}{8}$ cup light
brown sugar)
90 g/3$\frac{1}{2}$ oz (U.S. scant $\frac{1}{2}$ cup) granulated sugar
2 eggs, beaten
1 teaspoon vanilla essence (U.S. vanilla extract)
150 g/5 oz (U.S. 1$\frac{1}{4}$ cups) chopped roasted peanuts

Grind the oats in a food processor or blender until fine. Combine with the bicarbonate of soda and salt. Cream the butter with the peanut butter and sugars in a bowl until fluffy. Gradually beat in the egg and vanilla essence. Mix in the dry ingredients and nuts. Chill for 1 hour.

Heat the oven to 180°C/350°F, Gas Mark 4 and have ready several baking sheets (U.S. cookie sheets).

Pinch off pieces of dough and shape into balls about 2.5 cm/1 inch in diameter. Arrange well apart on the ungreased tins and flatten each ball with a fork.

Bake for about 15 minutes, or until the edges are golden. Alternate the position of the baking sheets in the oven half-way through cooking. **Makes about 60**

Above: Fig mousse. Centre: Stuffed figs with almonds.
Below: Prune fool

Gooseberry custard pudding

225 g/8 oz (U.S. ½ lb) gooseberries
6 small slices wholemeal bread
(U.S. wholewheat bread)
40 g/1½ oz (U.S. 3 tablespoons) margarine
50 g/2 oz light muscovado sugar (U.S. ¼ cup light brown sugar)
½ teaspoon ground nutmeg
2 eggs
600 ml/1 pint (U.S. 2½ cups) milk

Top and tail the gooseberries and halve them if large. Trim the crusts from the bread slices if wished. Spread the bread with the margarine, then cut into 2.5-cm/1-inch squares. Reserve 2 teaspoons sugar. Layer up the bread squares and fruit in a well-greased ovenproof dish, sprinkling each layer lightly with some of the remaining sugar and the nutmeg, ending with a layer of bread squares, coated sides upwards. Beat the eggs with the milk, pour over the ingredients in the dish and leave to stand for 20 minutes. Meanwhile, heat the oven to 180°C/350°F, Gas Mark 4.

Sprinkle the pudding with the reserved sugar and bake for 30 minutes, or until the custard has set and the top is golden brown. Serve hot or warm. **Serves 4**

Fruit and oat crumble

450 g/1 lb ripe but firm plums
2 tablespoons (U.S. 3 tablespoons) water
75 g/3 oz demerara sugar (U.S. ⅓ cup brown sugar)
100 g/4 oz wholemeal flour
(U.S. 1 cup wholewheat flour)
1 teaspoon ground mace
75 g/3 oz (U.S. ⅓ cup) margarine
50 g/2 oz (U.S. ⅔ cup) rolled oats
25 g/1 oz (U.S. ⅓ cup) shredded coconut

Heat the oven to 190°C/375°F, Gas Mark 5 and grease a pie dish.

Halve the plums and remove the stones (U.S. pits). Place in the prepared dish and sprinkle with the water and one third of the sugar.

Put the flour and spice in a bowl and rub or cut in the margarine until the mixture resembles breadcrumbs. Stir in almost all the remaining sugar, the oats and coconut. Spoon this evenly over the fruit and press down lightly. Sprinkle the last of the sugar on top.

Bake for about 30 minutes, or until the top is golden brown. Serve hot. **Serves 4**

Variations

Greengage and walnut crumble Omit the plums and substitute greengages (U.S. greengage plums), using 2 tablespoons (U.S. 3 tablespoons) chopped walnuts or pecans instead of the coconut in the topping.

Gooseberry and coconut crumble Omit the plums and substitute topped and tailed gooseberries. Add an extra 25 g/1 oz (U.S. 2 tablespoons) sugar and use 1 teaspoon ground cinnamon instead of the mace.

Raisin crunch flan

(Illustrated opposite)

25 g/1 oz (U.S. 2 tablespoons) butter
1 tablespoon set honey
2 tablespoons golden syrup (U.S. 3 tablespoons light corn syrup)
150 g/5 oz (U.S. 1½ cups) rolled oats
25 g/1 oz (U.S. ¼ cup) finely chopped walnuts
Filling
350 g/12 oz (U.S. 2 cups) seedless raisins
finely grated rind and juice of 1 lemon
25 g/1 oz light muscovado sugar (U.S. ⅛ cup light brown sugar)
½ teaspoon ground mixed spices
150 ml/¼ pint (U.S. ⅔ cup) water
2 teaspoons cornflour (U.S. 1 tablespoon cornstarch)
1 egg white
25 g/1 oz desiccated coconut (U.S. ⅓ cup shredded coconut)

Melt the butter with the honey and syrup in a large pan. Remove from the heat and stir in the oats and walnuts until the mixture binds together. Press into a greased 20-cm/8-inch flan dish or shallow cake tin to make an even shell. Chill while making the filling. Heat the oven to 180°C/350°F, Gas Mark 4.

Put the raisins in a pan with the lemon rind and juice, the sugar, spice and water. Bring to the boil and simmer for 5 minutes. Moisten the cornflour with a little cold water, add to the pan and bring to the boil, stirring constantly. Simmer for 1 minute. Pour into the flan case. Whisk the egg white until stiff and spread lightly over the surface of the raisin mixture. Sprinkle with the coconut.

Bake for about 20 minutes, or until golden on top. **Serves 4-5**

Raisin crunch flan

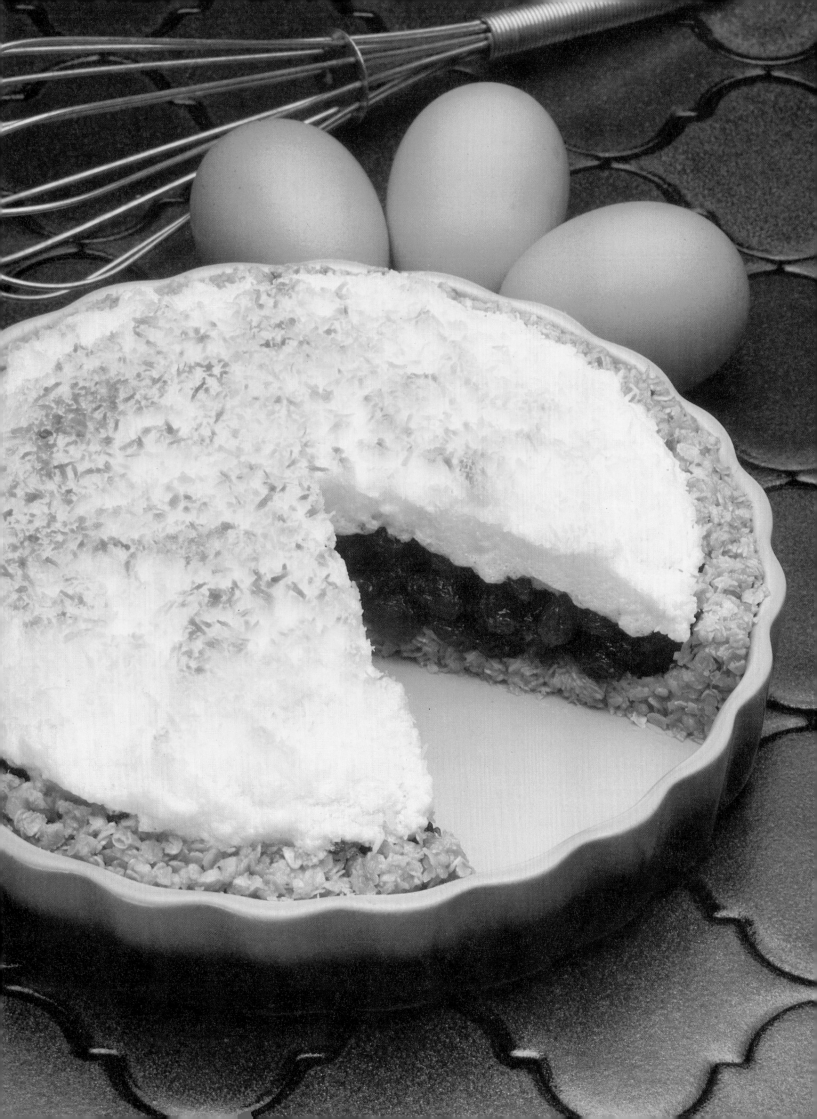

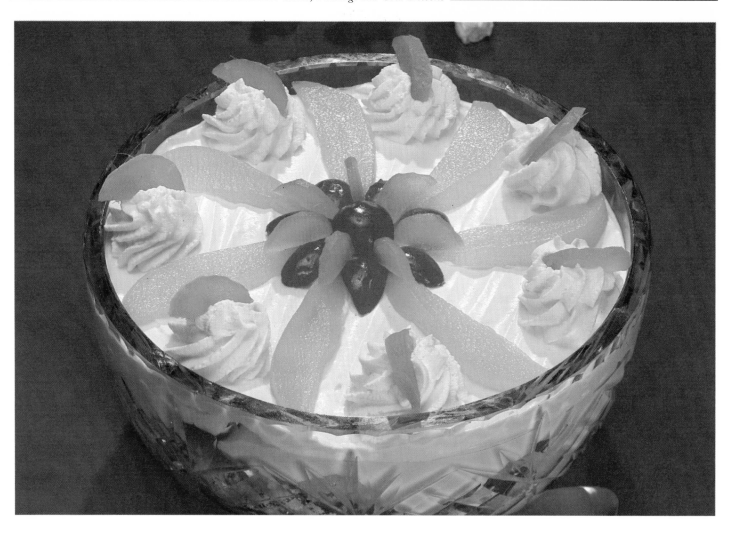

Gingered pear trifle

(Illustrated above)

4 ripe or firm Conference pears (U.S. 1 lb firm eating pears), peeled, cored and sliced
300 ml/½ pint medium cider (U.S. 1¼ cups hard cider)
2 tablespoons (U.S. 3 tablespoons) sugar
8 small slices Conference pear cake (see page 164)
4 tablespoons (U.S. 6 tablespoons) ginger marmalade
2 tablespoons (U.S. 3 tablespoons) syrup from jar of preserved ginger
450 ml/¾ pint pouring custard (U.S. 2 cups prepared Bird's English dessert mix)
300 ml/½ pint (U.S. 1¼ cups) whipping cream
Decoration
3 glacé (U.S. candied) cherries
2 pieces preserved ginger, sliced

Put the pear slices in a pan with the cider and sugar. Cover and simmer until just tender. Spread the cake slices with marmalade. Cut each into 2 or 3 pieces and place in a glass serving bowl.

Drain the pear slices, reserve 7 or 8 for the decoration and arrange the rest over the cake in the dish. Boil the syrup until reduced to about 150 ml/¼ pint (U.S. ⅔ cup), add the ginger syrup and allow to

cool. Spoon over the pears and leave for 10 minutes. Pour the custard into the dish and leave to set.

Whip the cream until stiff, spread about three-quarters over the trifle and use the remainder to pipe swirls around the edge of the dish. Decorate with the reserved pear slices, pieces of glacé cherry and preserved ginger. Chill before serving. **Serves 6-8**

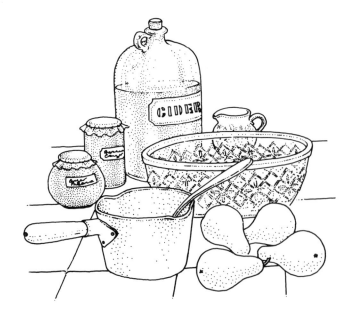

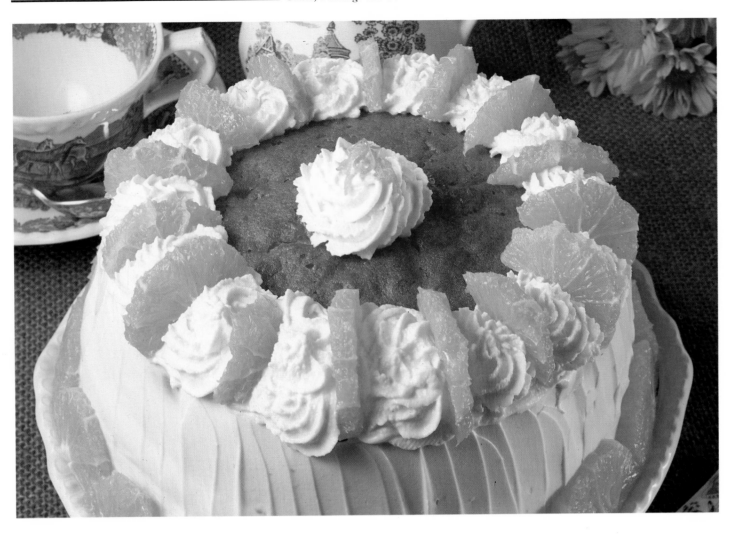

Orange delight cake

(Illustrated above)

50 g/2 oz plain flour (U.S. ½ cup all-purpose flour)
¾ teaspoon baking powder
75 g/3 oz wholemeal flour
(U.S. ¾ cup wholewheat flour)
150 g/5 oz (U.S. ⅔ cup) margarine
150 g/5 oz light muscovado sugar (U.S. ⅔ cup light
brown sugar)
finely grated rind and juice of 1 orange
3 eggs, beaten
Syrup
juice of 1 orange
50 g/2 oz light muscovado sugar (U.S. ¼ cup light
brown sugar)
Decoration
2 oranges
300 ml/½ pint (U.S. 1¼ cups) whipping cream,
whipped

Heat the oven to 180°C/350°F, Gas Mark 4 and
generously grease a 20-cm/8-inch deep loose-
bottomed cake tin.

Sift the white flour with the baking powder and stir
in the brown flour. Cream the margarine and sugar

together in a bowl until pale and fluffy. Add the
orange rind and gradually beat in the egg. Fold in the
flour mixture and the orange juice. Transfer to the
prepared tin.

Bake for about 50 minutes, or until golden brown
and firm to the touch. Remove the cake from the tin
and place on a serving dish.

Put the ingredients for the syrup in a small pan and
stir over low heat until the sugar has dissolved. Spoon
slowly over the hot cake and leave it to stand until
cold. Chill for 30 minutes.

Peel the oranges and cut them into thin slices,
trimming off all pith and discarding any pips. Cut
each slice in half. Spread the sides of the cake with
cream and mark in vertical lines with a round-bladed
knife. Pipe rosettes of cream around the top edge of
the cake and a single rosette in the centre. Decorate
with halved orange slices between the rosettes and
around the base of the cake.

Makes 1 (20-cm/8-inch) cake, about 10 servings

Cranberry family cake

(Illustrated opposite)

150 g/5 oz plain flour (U.S. 1¼ cups all-purpose flour)
2 teaspoons (U.S. 1 tablespoon) baking powder
pinch of salt
½ teaspoon ground cinnamon
75 g/3 oz wholemeal flour
(U.S. ¾ cup wholewheat flour)
75 g/3 oz (U.S. ⅓ cup) butter or margarine
100 g/4 oz light muscovado sugar
(U.S. ½ cup light brown sugar)
finely grated rind of ½ orange or lemon
100 g/4 oz (U.S. 1 cup) cranberries, roughly chopped
2 eggs, beaten
2 tablespoons (U.S. 3 tablespoons) milk
1 tablespoon demerara sugar (U.S. brown sugar)

Heat the oven to 180°C/350°F, Gas Mark 4, line a
450-g/1-lb loaf-shaped tin with greaseproof paper
(U.S. waxed paper) and grease the paper.

Sift the white flour with the baking powder, salt
and cinnamon into a bowl. Stir in the brown flour
and rub or cut in the butter until the mixture
resembles breadcrumbs. Stir in the sugar, fruit rind
and cranberries. Beat the eggs with the milk, add to
the bowl and mix to a soft dough. Transfer to the
prepared tin and sprinkle with sugar.

Bake for about 1 hour, or until well risen and a fine
skewer inserted in the centre comes out clean. Turn
out on a wire rack and do not remove the paper until
the loaf is cold. Serve cut into slices.

Makes 1 (450-g/1-lb) loaf, about 10 slices

Variation

Cranberry buns Use only sufficient milk to give a
stiff consistency. Put mounds of the mixture, using
about a tablespoon at a time, on greased baking sheets
(U.S. cookie sheets) or into well greased bun tins
(U.S. muffin or tartlet pans). Cook as above for
about 20 minutes, or until golden brown.

Cranberry family cake with Cranberry buns

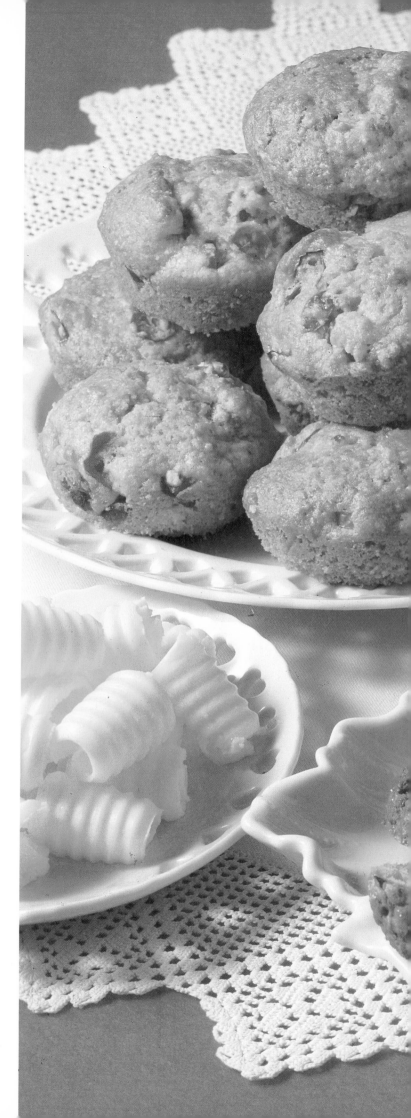

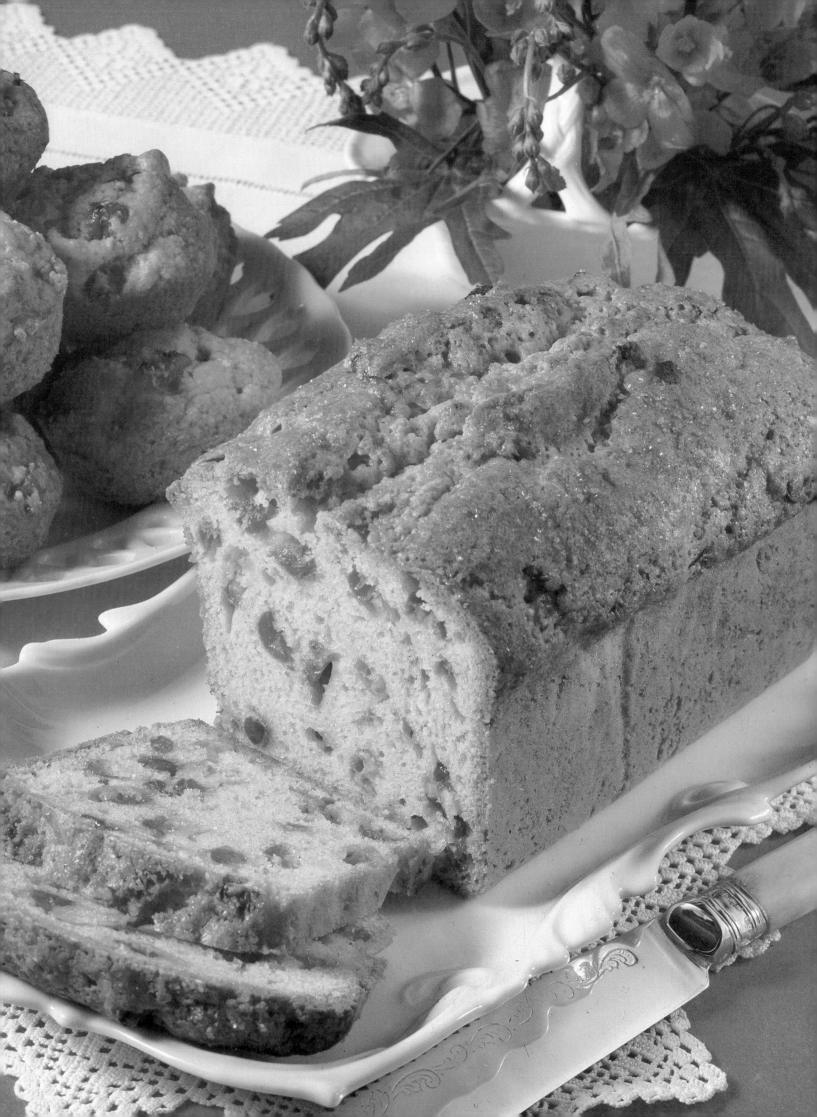

Semolina and fig pudding

2 dried figs
600 ml/1 pint (U.S. 2½ cups) milk
40 g/1½ oz semolina (U.S. ¼ cup semolina flour)
2 tablespoons light muscovado sugar
(U.S. 3 tablespoons light brown sugar)
1 egg
3 tablespoons (U.S. 4 tablespoons) apricot jam, sieved
1 tablespoon water

Trim away any hard pieces of stalk from the figs and chop the fruit roughly. Pour the milk into a heavy pan and heat gently until the surface is covered with bubbles. Sprinkle the semolina and sugar over the milk and stir constantly until the mixture boils. Reduce the temperature and allow to boil gently for 15 minutes, stirring occasionally. Beat in the egg, remove the pan from the heat and fold in the figs. Pour into a serving dish and leave until cold.

Warm the jam with the water in a small pan, stirring until smooth. Pour over the surface of the pudding and spread to cover it completely. Serve chilled. **Serves 4**

Nutty meringues

3 egg whites
pinch of cream of tartar
175 g/6 oz light muscovado sugar (U.S. ¾ cup light brown sugar)
50 g/2 oz toasted hazelnuts, chopped (U.S. ½ cup chopped toasted filberts)
2 rounded tablespoons desiccated coconut (U.S. 3 tablespoons shredded coconut)

Heat the oven to 130°C/250°F, Gas Mark ½ and line 2 baking sheets (U.S. cookie sheets) with non-stick baking parchment (U.S. waxed paper).

Whisk the egg whites until stiff, add the cream of tartar and continue whisking, adding the sugar, a tablespoon at a time, and whisking vigorously after each addition until the meringue is firm and glossy. Fold in the hazelnuts and coconut. Using 2 metal spoons, shape the meringue into 12 oval 'shells' on the prepared sheets.

Bake for about 1 hour, if necessary swapping the position of the 2 sheets half-way through cooking time. When ready, the meringues will lift easily from the lining paper. Cool on a wire rack. These meringues are delicious eaten plain but for a party they look very festive put together in pairs with whipped cream. **Makes 12**

Crusty-topped rhubarb and raisins

450 g/1 lb rhubarb, trimmed and sliced
50 g/2 oz (U.S. ⅓ cup) seedless raisins
75 g/3 oz demerara sugar (U.S. ⅓ cup brown sugar)
½ teaspoon ground allspice
4 thick slices wholemeal bread
(U.S. wholewheat bread)
50 g/2 oz (U.S. ¼ cup) margarine
1 tablespoon oil

Heat the oven to 190°C/375°F, Gas Mark 5 and grease a pie dish.

Arrange the fruit in the prepared dish. Reserve 2 tablespoons (U.S. 3 tablespoons) of the sugar and sprinkle the rest over the fruit with the spice.

Trim the crusts from the bread if wished, then cut the slices into neat cubes. Heat the margarine and oil in a shallow pan and toss the bread cubes over high heat, turning frequently, until just turning golden. Spoon over the fruit in the dish and sprinkle with the reserved sugar.

Bake for 30 minutes, or until the top is golden brown and crisp. Serve hot with pouring custard. **Serves 4**

Walnut ice cream with butterscotch sauce

(Illustrated opposite)

12 small scoops walnut supreme ice cream
8 walnut halves (optional)
Sauce
25 g/1 oz (U.S. 2 tablespoons) butter
2 tablespoons light muscovado sugar (U.S. 3 table-spoons light brown sugar)
1 tablespoon golden syrup (U.S. light corn syrup)
few drops of lemon juice

First make the sauce. Melt the butter in a small pan over low heat and stir in the sugar, syrup and lemon juice. When the sauce is smooth, bring to the boil and simmer for 1 minute. Remove from the heat and leave until warm.

Arrange the scoops of ice cream and the nuts on 4 small plates. Add a little of the sauce to each portion and serve at once. **Serves 4**

Walnut ice cream with butterscotch sauce

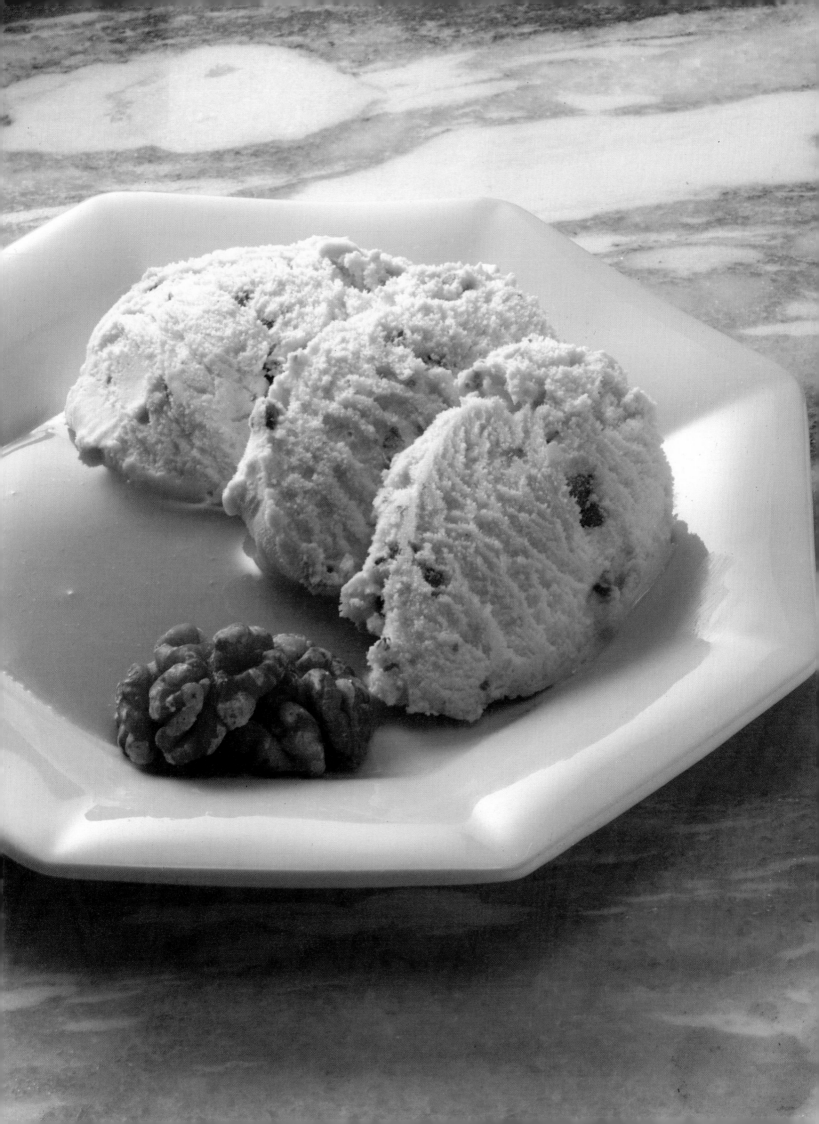

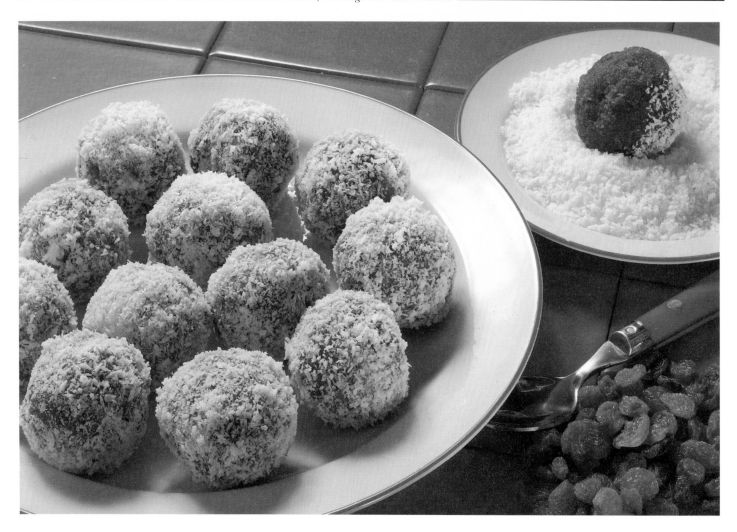

Snowballs

(Illustrated above)

25 g/1 oz (U.S. 2 tablespoons) butter or margarine
½ golden syrup cake, coarsely crumbled (U.S. 2 cups coarsely crumbled moist cake)
25 g/1 oz sultanas (U.S. scant ¼ cup seedless white raisins)
50 g/2 oz desiccated coconut (U.S. ⅔ cup shredded coconut)

Melt the butter in a pan, remove from the heat and add the cake and sultanas. Mix well and cool.

Divide the mixture into 12 equal portions and shape each into a ball. Place the coconut on a plate and roll the balls in this to coat them all over. Serve in small paper cases if wished. **Makes 12**

Cranberry and ginger yogurt freeze

1 (185-g/6½-oz) jar jellied cranberry sauce
2 pieces stem ginger (U.S. 2 pieces preserved ginger), chopped
300 ml/½ pint (U.S. 1¼ cups) fruit yogurt (such as apricot, strawberry or black cherry)
1 egg white
1 tablespoon light muscovado sugar (U.S. light brown sugar)

Mash the cranberry sauce and mix in the ginger. Stir in the yogurt and transfer to a shallow container. Cover and freeze until firm. Turn out into a bowl, break up with a fork and then beat until smooth.

Whisk the egg white in a clean bowl until stiff. Add the sugar and continue whisking until firm and glossy. Fold into the frozen mixture. Return to the shallow container, cover again and freeze until required. Scoop into stemmed glasses and serve with high-fibre cookies. **Serves 4-6**

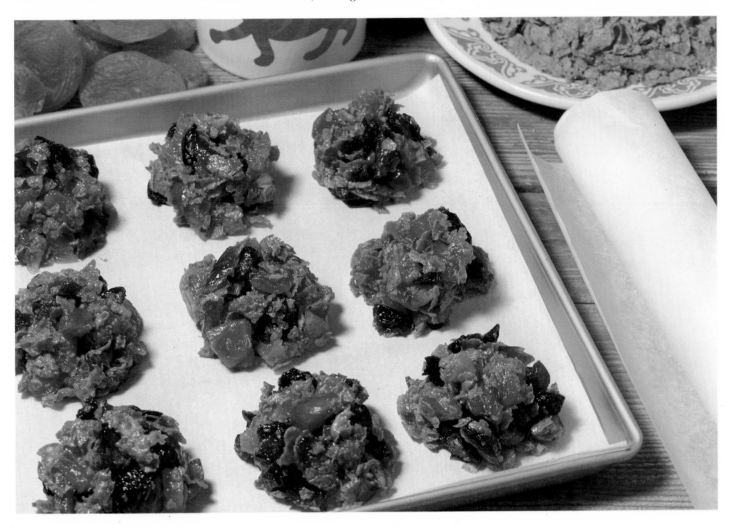

Fruit and flake nibbles

(Illustrated above)

40 g/1½ oz (U.S. 3 tablespoons) butter or margarine
40 g/1½ oz light muscovado sugar (U.S. scant ¼ cup
light brown sugar)
1 tablespoon golden syrup (U.S. light corn syrup)
50 g/2 oz no-need-to-soak prunes, stoned (U.S. ⅓
cup no-need-to-soak prunes, pitted), chopped
4 dried apricots, chopped
6 stoned dates (U.S. 6 pitted dates), chopped
50 g/2 oz (U.S. 1¾ cups) bran flakes

Line a baking sheet (U.S. cookie sheet) with non-stick cooking parchment.

Put the butter, sugar and syrup in a large pan and heat gently until the sugar has dissolved. Bring to boiling point and simmer for 4 minutes. Remove from the heat, add the chopped fruit and flakes and stir until coated with the syrup mixture. Spoon into 12 equal-sized clusters on the parchment and allow to set. **Makes 12**

Californian fruit salad

1 (225-g/8-oz) can peach slices in apple juice
1 (225-g/8-oz) can red cherries in syrup
150 ml/¼ pint (U.S. ⅔ cup) soured cream
100 g/4 oz (U.S. ¼ lb) strawberries
1 large banana, sliced
2 centre sticks celery, sliced

Drain the juice from the peach slices and the syrup from the cherries into a small bowl. Gradually whisk in the soured cream. Arrange the fruit and celery in a glass serving bowl and pour over the soured cream mixture. Stir lightly before serving. **Serves 4-6**

Variation

Exotic fruit salad Substitute canned apricots for the peaches and use 2 kiwi fruit (U.S. Chinese gooseberries), peeled and thinly sliced, for the strawberries.

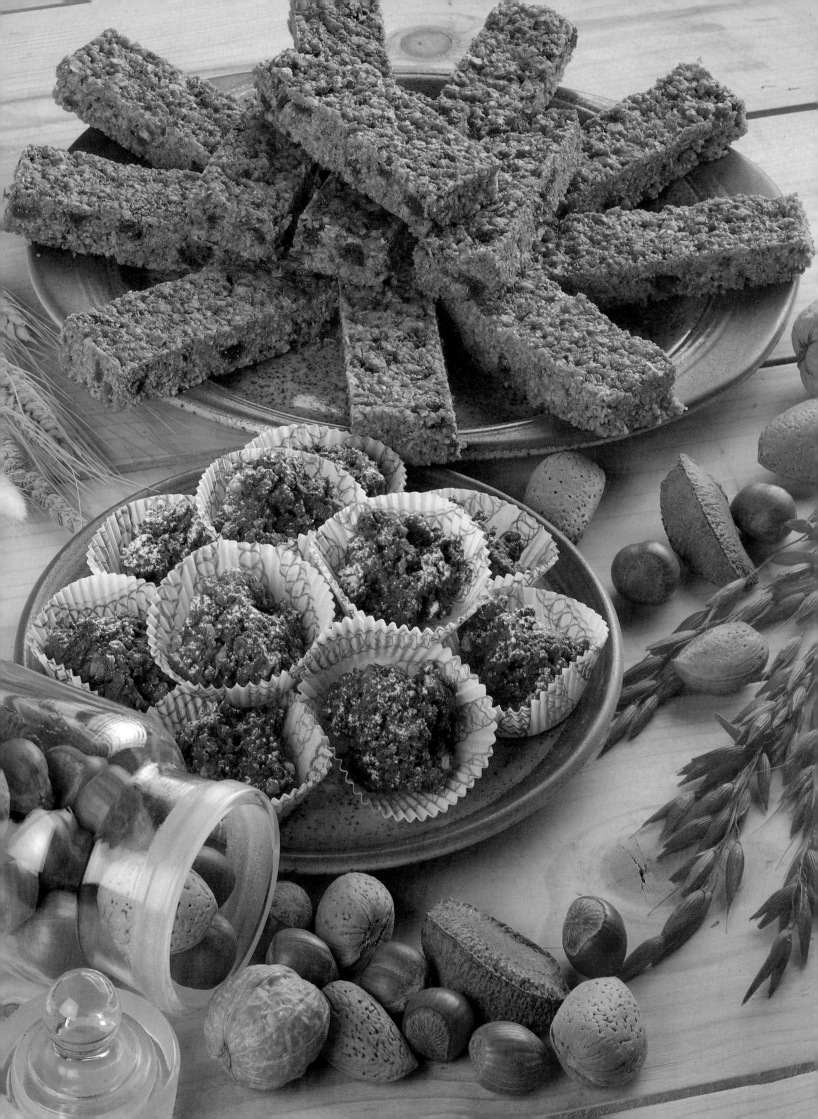

Chocolate and date fingers

(Illustrated opposite)

50 g/2 oz dark plain chocolate (U.S. ⅓ cup semi-sweet chocolate pieces)
175 g/6 oz (U.S. ¾ cup) margarine
50 g/2 oz light muscovado sugar (U.S. ¼ cup light brown sugar)
1 tablespoon golden syrup (U.S. light corn syrup)
100 g/4 oz stoned dates (U.S. ¼ lb pitted dates), chopped
225 g/8 oz (U.S. 2⅔ cups) rolled oats

Heat the oven to 180°C/350°F, Gas Mark 4 and grease a shallow tin measuring 27.5 cm/11 inches by 17.5 cm/7 inches.

Break up the chocolate and place in a medium-sized pan with the margarine, sugar and syrup. Heat very gently, stirring, until melted and smooth. Add the dates and oats, mix well then spread in the prepared tin.

Bake for 25 minutes. Cut into fingers and leave in the tin until cold. **Makes 18**

Nutty chocolate clusters

(Illustrated opposite)

150 g/5 oz dark plain chocolate (U.S. scant 1 cup semi-sweet chocolate pieces)
25 g/1 oz icing sugar, sifted (U.S. ¼ cup sifted confectioners' sugar)
50 g/2 oz ginger biscuits (U.S. 4 gingersnap cookies), crushed
50 g/2 oz (U.S. ½ cup) finely chopped walnuts or pecans
2 drops vanilla essence (U.S. vanilla extract)
little icing sugar (U.S. confectioners' sugar) for sprinkling

Break up the chocolate and place in a bowl. Stand this over a pan of hot water until the chocolate melts. Add the remaining ingredients and mix well.

Divide the mixture into 20 heaps, place each in a paper case and sprinkle lightly with sugar. Chill until firm. **Makes 20**

Lemon and coconut cake

4 eggs
finely grated rind of 1½ lemons
100 g/4 oz caster sugar (U.S. ½ cup granulated sugar)
50 g/2 oz plain flour (U.S. ½ cup all-purpose flour)
1 teaspoon baking powder
50 g/2 oz wholemeal flour
(U.S. ½ cup wholewheat flour)
100 g/4 oz desiccated coconut (U.S. 1⅓ cups shredded coconut)
100 g/4 oz (U.S. ½ cup) soft margarine
275 g/10 oz icing sugar, sifted (U.S. 2¼ cups sifted confectioners' sugar)
3 tablespoons (U.S. scant 5 tablespoons) lemon juice
few drops yellow food colouring (optional)

Heat the oven to 190°C/375°F, Gas Mark 5 and grease a 23-cm/9-inch round deep cake tin. Line the base with greaseproof paper (U.S. waxed paper) and grease the paper.

Put the eggs, lemon rind and sugar in a bowl and stand this over a pan half-filled with boiling water. Place over very low heat so that the water is kept just at simmering point. Whisk the mixture steadily until thick enough that when the beaters are lifted, the trail will hold its shape for about 30 seconds. Remove the bowl from the heat and whisk until the mixture is cool.

Sift the white flour with the baking powder and stir in the brown flour and one quarter of the coconut. Fold lightly but thoroughly into the whisked mixture. When evenly combined, transfer to the prepared tin.

Bake for about 30 minutes, or until firm in the centre. Remove from the tin, peel off the lining paper and cool on a wire rack. Meanwhile, spread the remaining coconut on a sheet of foil and toast lightly under a hot grill (U.S. broiler).

Cream the margarine with the icing sugar in a bowl until smooth. Gradually beat in the lemon juice. Tint pale yellow with food colouring if desired. Cut the cake into 2 layers and sandwich together with about one third of the icing. Use the remainder to cover the top and sides of the cake. Press the toasted coconut lightly around the sides. Mark the top surface into parallel lines with the prongs of a fork.
Makes 1 (23-cm/9-inch) cake, 8 servings

Above: Chocolate and date fingers. Below: Nutty chocolate clusters

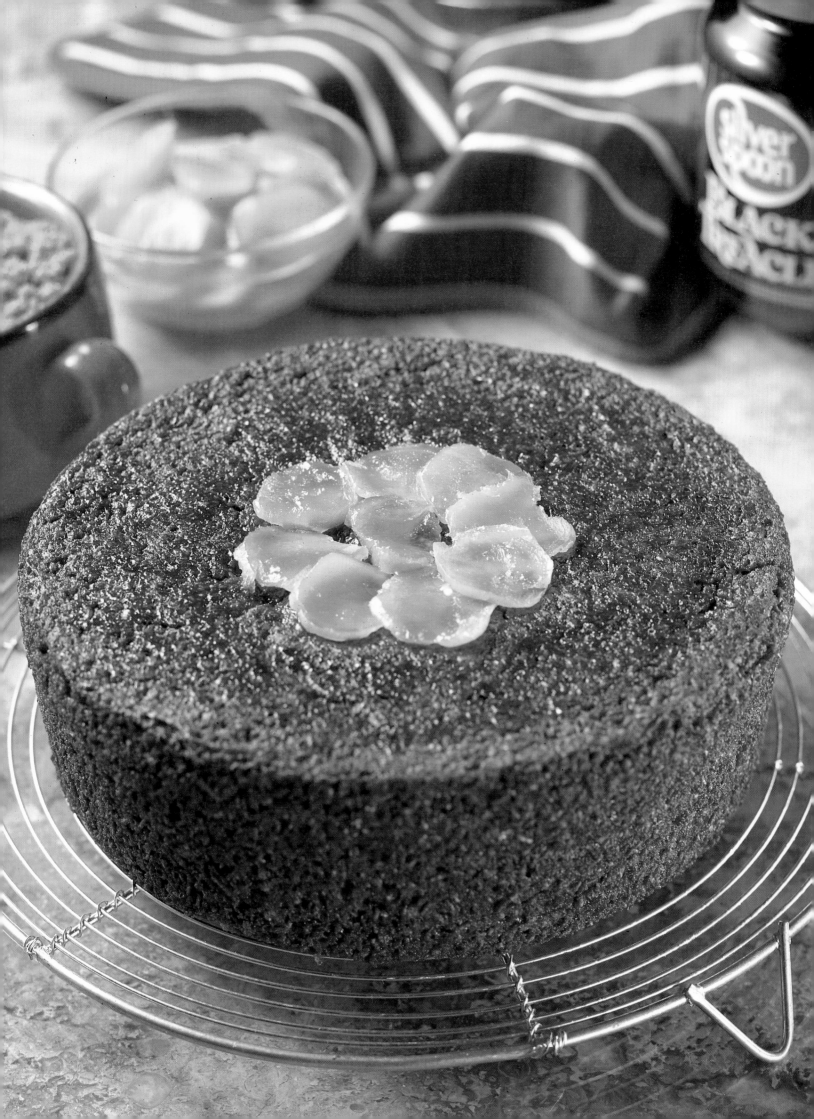

Treacle cake

(Illustrated opposite)

100 g/4 oz (U.S. ½ cup) margarine
100 g/4 oz rich dark soft sugar (U.S. ½ cup brown sugar)
75 ml/3 fl oz (U.S. ⅓ cup) thick-cut marmalade
3 tablespoons black treacle (U.S. 4 tablespoons molasses)
100 ml/4 fl oz (U.S. ½ cup) milk
175 g/6 oz plain flour (U.S. 1½ cups all-purpose flour)
4 teaspoons (U.S. 2 tablespoons) ground ginger
1½ teaspoons bicarbonate of soda (U.S. baking soda)
½ teaspoon baking powder
50 g/2 oz (U.S. 1 cup) natural unprocessed bran
1 egg, beaten
1 piece of preserved ginger, sliced

Heat the oven to 160°C/325°F, Gas Mark 3, line a deep 20-cm/8-inch cake tin with greaseproof paper (U.S. waxed paper) and grease the paper.

Put the margarine, sugar, marmalade, treacle and milk in a pan and heat gently, stirring, until the sugar has dissolved. Remove from the heat and leave to cool.

Sift the flour with the ginger, bicarbonate of soda and baking powder. Stir in the bran then add these ingredients to the pan with the egg. Mix with a wooden spoon until well blended then beat until shiny. Transfer to the prepared tin.

Bake for about 1¼ hours, or until firm to the touch in the centre. Leave in the tin for 5 minutes, then turn out on a wire rack and leave to cool. (This cake tends to sink a little in the centre even when fully cooked, but this is not noticeable when decorated with the ginger.) Remove the lining paper and store the cake in a sealed polythene bag for at least 2 days before cutting. Serve topped with the ginger slices.

Makes 1 (20-cm/8-inch) cake

Mulled fruit compôte

450 g/1 lb mixed dried fruits (such as apple rings, peach halves, apricot halves, prunes and pear halves)
4 tablespoons (U.S. 6 tablespoons) clear honey
150 ml/¼ pint (U.S. ⅔ cup) red wine
5-cm/2-inch stick cinnamon
4 whole cloves
¼ teaspoon allspice berries
pared rind of ½ lemon
150 ml/¼ pint double cream (U.S. ⅔ cup heavy cream), whipped

Put the fruit in a pan and pour over cold water to cover well. Put the lid on the pan and leave to stand for 8 hours.

Drain the fruit and return it to the pan with the honey and red wine. Tie the cinnamon stick, cloves, allspice and lemon rind in a piece of muslin (U.S. cheese cloth) and add to the pan. Bring to the boil and simmer for about 10 minutes, or until the fruit is soft. Leave to cool in the syrup, then chill well.

Serve in individual dishes and hand the whipped cream separately. **Serves 4**

Steamed prune and orange pudding

150 g/5 oz (U.S. scant 1 cup) tender dried prunes
75 g/3 oz plain flour (U.S. ¾ cup all-purpose flour)
1½ teaspoons baking powder
100 g/4 oz (U.S. ½ cup) margarine
100 g/4 oz light muscovado sugar (U.S. ½ cup light brown sugar)
2 eggs, beaten
finely grated rind and juice of 1 medium-sized orange
75 g/3 oz wholemeal flour (U.S. ¾ cup wholewheat flour)

Chop the flesh of the prunes, discarding the stones (U.S. pits). Sift the white flour with the baking powder. Cream the margarine and sugar together in a bowl until light and fluffy. Gradually add the egg, beating well after each addition. Beat in the orange rind. Fold in the dry ingredients with the orange juice and chopped prunes. Mix well and transfer to a well-greased 900-ml/1½-pint (U.S. 4-cup) pudding bowl. Cover with a double layer of greased foil, crimped securely under the rim of the bowl.

Stand the bowl in a large pan and pour in boiling water to come half-way up the side of the bowl. Cover the pan and, keeping the water boiling steadily all the time, cook for 1½ hours, adding more boiling water during cooking if necessary. Turn out, cut in wedges, and serve hot with vanilla ice cream.
Serves 4-6

Variation

Steamed date and lemon pudding Omit the prunes and orange and substitute 100 g/4 oz stoned dates (U.S. generous ½ cup pitted dates), chopped, and the finely grated rind and juice of 1 large lemon.

Treacle cake

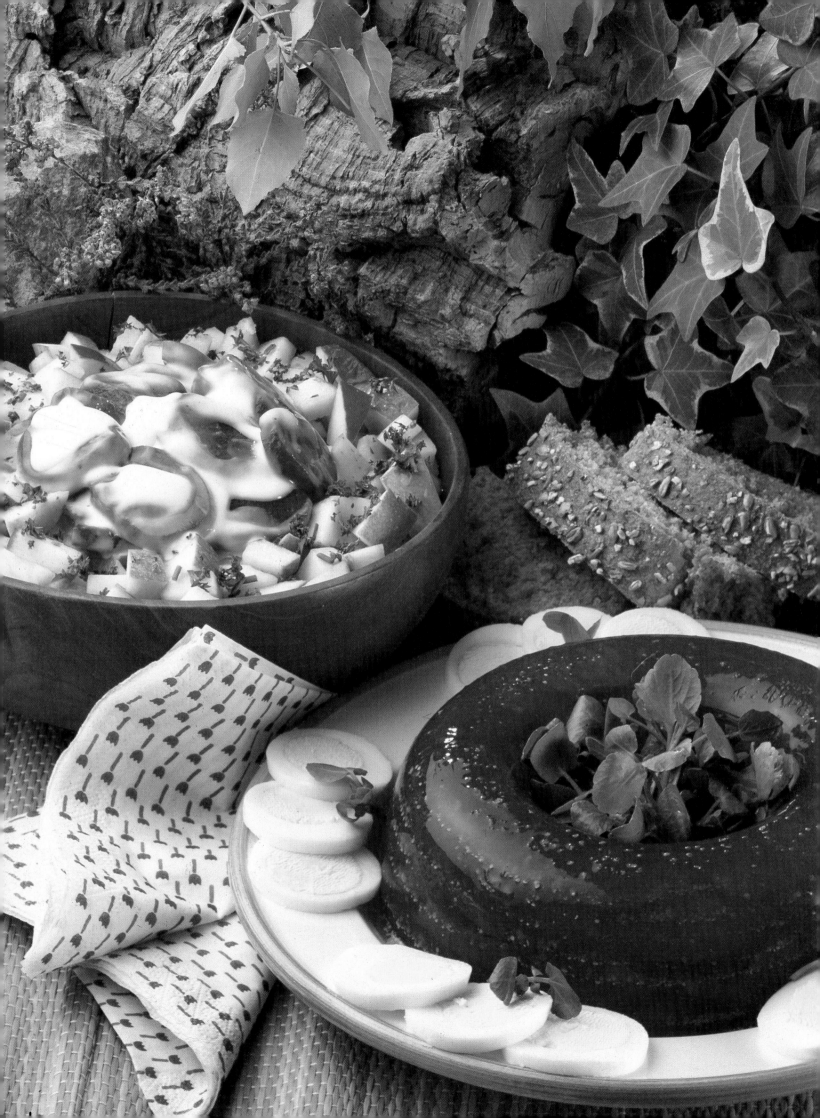

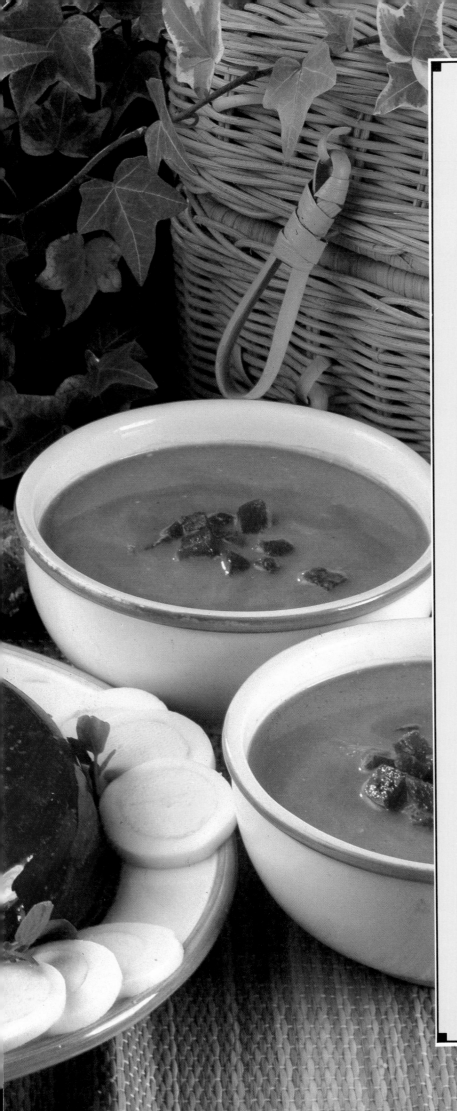

Picnics and Packed Meals

Many people still feel that a packed meal must consist of sandwiches. In these days when so much delicious food can be prepared ahead and stored in the freezer, or at least for several days in the refrigerator, there are lots of alternatives.

A small wide-mouthed insulated flask can be used in summer for a chilled drink that is still refreshingly cool at lunchtime, or for hot soup in winter. Turn to the soup section for ideas. My suggested menus are far from stodgy, but very satisfying and fibre-full. Although quantities are given for four, if there is only one member of the family taking a packed lunch, the rest of the batch can be consumed for a light meal, or in some cases stored for future reference. Eating in the garden is justly popular, and sometimes more is spent on patio furniture than replacements for the living room. If you really want to simplify, a three-decker sandwich made with toasted wholemeal bread is better for you than a hamburger clamped in a soft white bun. High-fibre white bread is already available and will become increasingly so. Ask at your supermarket for it if there is someone in the family who positively dislikes brown bread.

When a picnic is planned, make it easy to cater for and enjoy. Begin with an equipment checklist of all you will need and cross off the items as you pack them into your hamper or insulated coolbox. Picnicking is thirsty work. As well as the exciting drink recipes you'll find in this section, take mineral water and refreshing fruit beverages. Things you may forget: damp cloths in a sealed waterproof bag for sticky fingers, paper napkins, plastic cutlery and perhaps just one sharp knife (safely wrapped); a bin liner to contain all the rubbish after the picnic is over.

From the left – Beetroot and apple salad (recipe page 189). Beetroot salad ring (recipe page 186). Chilled borscht (recipe page 184)

Chilled borscht

(Illustrated on pages 182-183)

2 medium-sized carrots, peeled and sliced
2 medium-sized parsnips, peeled and sliced
3 stalks celery, chopped
1 litre/1¾ pints chicken stock (U.S. 4¼ cups chicken bouillon)
25 g/1 oz (U.S. ½ cup) natural unprocessed bran
salt and fresh ground black pepper
1 (340-g/12-oz) jar baby beets in sweet vinegar
150 ml/¼ pint (U.S. ⅔ cup) soured cream

Put the carrot, parsnip, celery, stock and bran into a pan and bring to the boil. Season to taste, cover and simmer for 25 minutes.

Strain the stock into a bowl and stir in the vinegar from the beetroot and the cream. Ladle into bowls or into containers for transport. Finely dice the beetroot and add to the borscht. Chill well. **Serves 4-5**

All-Bran picnic pasties

Filling

1 ripe but firm pear, peeled, cored and chopped
50 g/2 oz (U.S. ⅓ cup) finely diced potato
50 g/2 oz (U.S. ½ cup) cooked or canned corn kernels
1 small onion, peeled and chopped
1 small carrot, peeled and chopped
100 g/4 oz braising steak (U.S. ¼ lb chuck steak), cut into small dice
4 rashers streaky bacon (U.S. 4 bacon slices), rind removed and chopped
salt and freshly ground black pepper
25 g/1 oz wholemeal flour
(U.S. ¼ cup wholewheat flour)
4 tablespoons beef stock (U.S. ⅓ cup beef bouillon)
Pastry
250 g/9 oz plain flour (U.S. 2¼ cups all-purpose flour)
25 g/1 oz (U.S. ½ cup) All-Bran cereal
pinch of salt
150 g/5 oz (U.S. ⅔ cup) margarine
cold water for mixing
beaten egg for glazing

Mix together the pear, potato, corn, onion, carrot, steak and bacon. Season well, sprinkle over the flour and toss the ingredients until coated. Pour in the stock and leave to stand for 30 minutes, until the liquid has been absorbed.

Meanwhile, make the pastry. Mix together the flour, All-Bran and salt in a bowl. Rub or cut in the margarine until the mixture resembles breadcrumbs, then add enough water to give a firm dough.

Heat the oven to 200°C/400°F, Gas Mark 6. Roll out the pastry on a lightly floured surface and cut out 8×15-cm/6-inch squares. Divide the filling among the squares and brush the pastry edges with beaten egg. Bring the 2 opposite corners together over the filling, seal and flute the edges. Stand the pasties on a baking sheet (U.S. cookie sheet) and brush with egg.

Bake for 15 minutes. Reduce the oven temperature to 180°C/350°F, Gas Mark 4 and continue cooking for a further 30 minutes, or until the pasties are golden brown. Serve hot or cold. **Makes 8**

Figgy flapjacks

2 whole dried figs
225 g/8 oz (U.S. 2¼ cups) rolled oats
pinch of ground allspice or ground nutmeg
100 g/4 oz (U.S. ½ cup) margarine
2 tablespoons light muscovado sugar
(U.S. 3 tablespoons light brown sugar)
2 tablespoons golden syrup (U.S. 3 tablespoons light corn syrup)

Heat the oven to 190°C/375°F, Gas Mark 5 and grease a shallow tin measuring about 17.5 cm/7 inches by 27.5 cm/11 inches and 2.5 cm/1 inch deep.

Trim off any hard pieces of stalk from the figs and chop the fruit finely. Place the figs, oats and spice in a bowl and mix lightly. Put the margarine, sugar and syrup in a large pan and heat gently, stirring, until the fat melts. Remove from the heat, add the oats mixture and stir thoroughly. Transfer to the prepared tin and level the top.

Bake for about 30 minutes, or until golden brown. Remove from the oven, leave to stand for 3 minutes then cut into 16 bars. Leave in the tin until cold. **Makes 16**

— MENU —

Chilled borscht
All-Bran picnic pasties
Figgy flapjacks
Banana smoothie dessert
Fresh pears

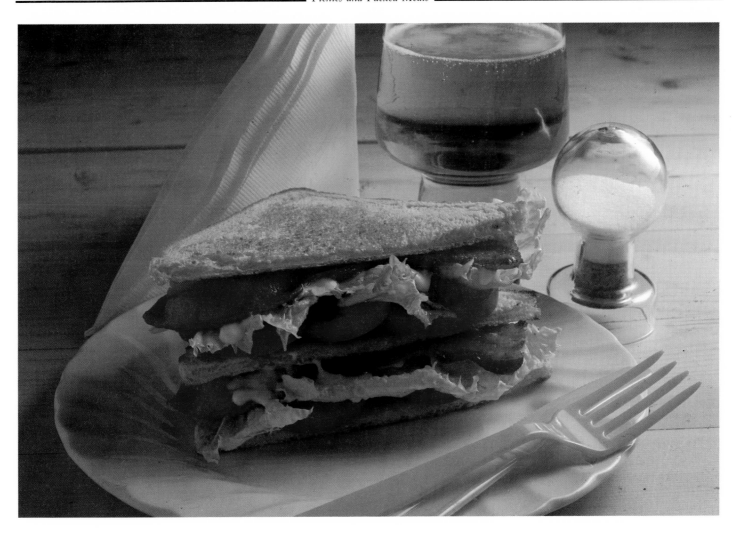

Banana smoothie dessert

150 ml/¼ pint (U.S. ⅔ cup) orange juice
2 tablespoons light muscovado sugar
(U.S. 3 tablespoons light brown sugar)
1½ teaspoons powdered gelatine
(U.S. 2 teaspoons unflavored gelatin)
2 large bananas, peeled and sliced
2 eggs, separated

Put the orange juice and sugar in a small pan. Sprinkle the gelatine over the surface and leave to stand for 5 minutes. Heat very gently until the gelatine and sugar have completely dissolved. Leave to cool.

Liquidise the banana with the egg yolks and gradually add the orange juice mixture. Leave until just on the point of setting. Whisk the egg whites in a clean bowl and fold lightly into the banana mixture. Pour into plastic containers and seal. Chill until set. **Serves 4**

BLT sandwich

(Illustrated above)

4 rashers streaky bacon (U.S. 4 bacon slices), rind removed
3 large slices wholemeal
(U.S. wholewheat) bread
butter or margarine for spreading
1 tablespoon mayonnaise
crisp lettuce leaves
1 medium-sized tomato, sliced

Grill (U.S. broil) the bacon until just crisp. Toast the bread slices and butter them lightly. Spread 2 slices with mayonnaise and arrange the lettuce, tomato and bacon on top. Stack up the toast and filling to make a double-decker sandwich. Cut in half diagonally and serve at once. **Serves 1**

Liver sausage and pickled cucumber sandwich
Omit the bacon, lettuce and tomato. Substitute thinly sliced smooth liver suasage and chopped sweet pickled cucumber (U.S. dill pickles) to fill the toast layers.

— MENU —

Vegetable and pineapple cocktail
Wholemeal pitta pockets
Beetroot salad ring
Brown sugar shortbread
Fresh apples

Vegetable and pineapple cocktail

10-cm/4-inch length of cucumber, peeled and roughly chopped
1 stalk of celery, roughly chopped
1 medium-sized carrot, peeled and roughly chopped
2 teaspoons lemon juice
600 ml/1 pint (U.S. $2\frac{1}{2}$ cups) pineapple juice

Put the vegetables and lemon juice into a blender or food processor and process until very finely chopped. With the machine switched on, gradually add the pineapple juice and continue processing until the mixture is smooth.

Divide among plastic tumblers and seal. Chill until required and shake well before opening. **Serves 4**

Variations

Fruity vegetable cocktail Add a sliced banana and large pinch of ground mace to the blender with the vegetables then top up with orange juice instead of pineapple. Omit the lemon juice unless you prefer a sharp flavour.

Savoury vegetable cocktail Omit the fruit juices and when the vegetables are chopped, make up with tomato juice and season the drink lightly before processing.

Wholemeal pitta pockets

Wholemeal pitta pockets

(Illustrated opposite)

4 wholemeal (U.S. wholewheat) pitta breads, halved
Filling
2 teaspoons chive mustard
50 ml/2 fl oz (U.S. $\frac{1}{4}$ cup) hummous
225 g/8 oz (U.S. 2 cups) shredded cooked chicken
8 black olives, stoned and halved (U.S. 8 ripe olives, pitted and halved)
50 g/2 oz (U.S. 1 cup) beansprouts
shredded lettuce
Garnish
few spring onions (U.S. scallions)
lemon wedges

First make the filling. Combine the mustard with the hummous. Put the chicken, olives and beansprouts in a bowl, pour over the mustard hummous and toss lightly.

Put a little lettuce in the base of each pitta pocket and top with the dressed chicken mixture. Pack each pair of filled pockets together in cling film. Serve garnished with onion 'curls' and lemon wedges, packed separately. **Serves 4**

Beetroot salad ring

(Illustrated on pages 182-183)

1 (135-g/$4\frac{3}{4}$-oz) packet lemon jelly tablet (U.S. 4-oz package lemon-flavored gelatin)
150 ml/$\frac{1}{4}$ pint (U.S. $\frac{2}{3}$ cup) boiling water
1 (340-g/12-oz) jar crinkle cut beets in sweet vinegar
1 tablespoon strong continental mustard
salt and freshly ground black pepper
Garnish
1 bunch of watercress
2 eggs, hard-boiled (U.S. hard-cooked), sliced

Dissolve the jelly in the hot water. Drain the vinegar from the beetroot into a measuring jug and make up to 300 ml/$\frac{1}{2}$ pint (U.S. $1\frac{1}{4}$ cups) with water. Whisk in the mustard and lemon jelly, then season to taste.

Put 4 tablespoons (U.S. 6 tablespoons) jelly into a lightly oiled 900-ml/$1\frac{1}{2}$-pint (U.S. $3\frac{3}{4}$-cup) ring mould. Chill until set. Arrange a few of the smaller beetroot slices on the jelly, spoon more liquid jelly on top and chill again until set. Repeat the layers until all the beetroot and jelly have been used. Chill.

Dip the mould into hot water for a few seconds and turn out on a plate. Garnish with watercress and slices of egg, or pack in containers with seals. **Serves 6**

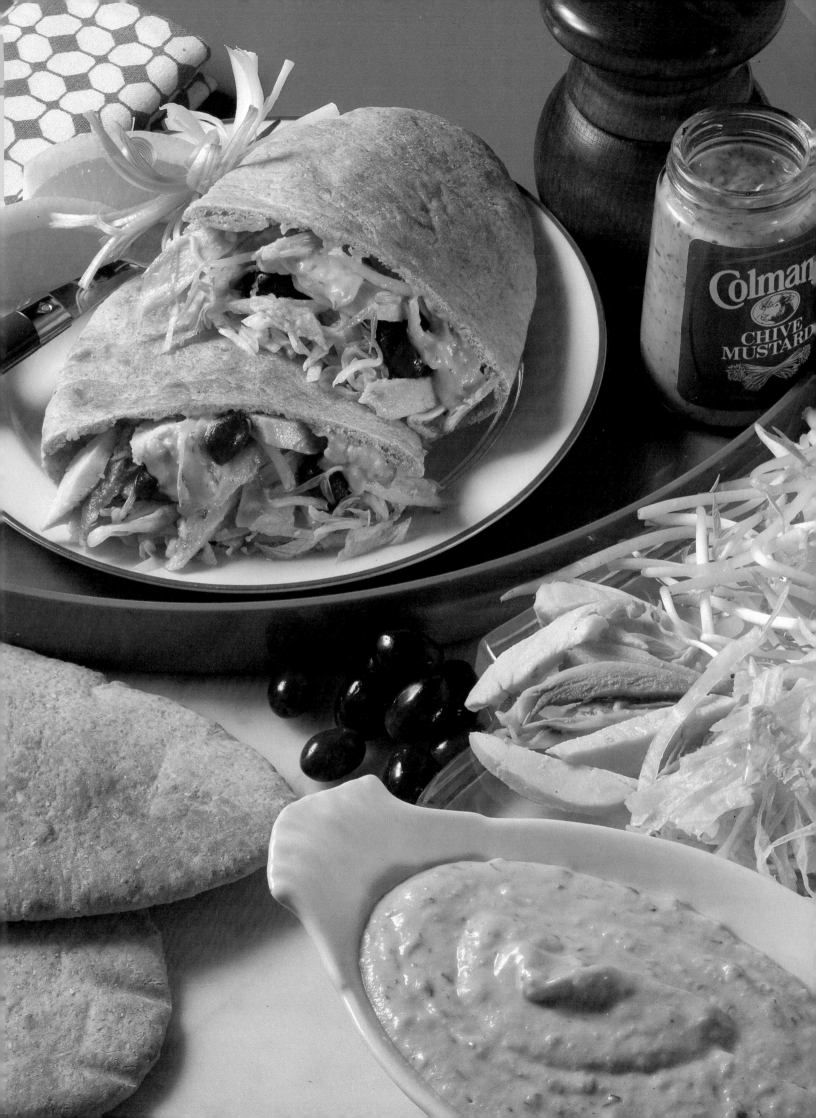

Brown sugar shortbread

100 g/4 oz wholemeal flour (U.S. 1 cup wholewheat flour)
100 g/4 oz plain flour (U.S. 1 cup all-purpose flour)
175 g/6 oz (U.S. ¾ cup) butter or margarine, or a mixture of both
50 g/2 oz light muscovado sugar (U.S. ¼ cup light brown sugar)
finely grated rind of 1 orange

Heat the oven to 180°C/350°F, Gas Mark 4 and grease a shallow tin about 17.5 cm/7 inches by 27.5 cm/11 inches.

Put the flours in a bowl and rub or cut in the butter until the mixture resembles breadcrumbs. Add the sugar and orange rind and work the ingredients by hand until a dough forms.

Press this into the prepared tin, smooth the top and prick the shortbread all over with a fork. Mark into 20 bars with a sharp knife.

Bake for 30 minutes, then reduce the oven temperature to 150°C/300°F, Gas Mark 2 and continue cooking for a further 15 minutes, or until very pale golden. Leave to stand for about 3 minutes, then cut into the marked bars. Cool in the tin and store in an airtight container. **Makes 20 bars**

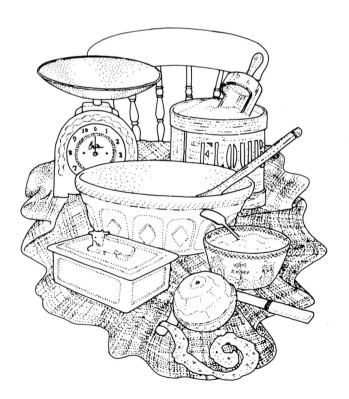

— MENU —

Cucumber snow
Curried rice and pork patties
Beetroot and apple salad
Wholemeal cheese scones
Fresh orange segments

Cucumber snow

15-cm/6-inch length of cucumber, peeled and roughly chopped
4 tablespoons (U.S. 6 tablespoons) roughly chopped watercress leaves
1 teaspoon salt
225 ml/8 fl oz (U.S. 1 cup) lemon-flavoured yogurt
225 ml/8 fl oz (U.S. 1 cup) water

Put the cucumber and watercress into a blender or food processor and add the salt and half the yogurt. Process until the mixture is smooth then, with the machine switched on, gradually add the remainder of the yogurt and the water.

Divide among plastic tumblers and seal. Chill until required and shake well before opening. **Serves 4**

Curried rice and pork patties

75 g/3 oz (U.S. scant ½ cup) long grain brown rice, cooked
175 g/6 oz (U.S. 1½ cups) chopped cooked pork
50 g/2 oz (U.S. ⅓ cup) chopped dried apricots
1½ teaspoons medium curry powder
150 ml/¼ pint (U.S. ⅔ cup) basic whisked sauce (see page 54)
2 egg yolks
salt
1 egg, beaten
about 100 g/4 oz fresh wholemeal breadcrumbs (U.S. about 2 cups fresh wholewheat bread crumbs)
oil for shallow frying

Mix together the rice, pork and apricots in a bowl. Sprinkle the curry powder over and toss the ingredients lightly. Mix in the sauce and egg yolks. When evenly combined, season with salt to taste. Chill for 20 minutes.

Divide the mixture into 8 equal portions and shape each into a round flat cake with floured hands. Place the egg in a shallow dish and put the breadcrumbs on a plate. Dip the patties in egg, then coat all over with breadcrumbs. Repeat if necessary so that they are completely covered. Chill again for at least 20 minutes.

Heat a little oil in a large frying pan (U.S. skillet) and cook the patties over moderate heat for about 6 minutes on each side, until crisp and golden brown. Serve cold with a crisp coleslaw.

Beetroot and apple salad

(Illustrated on page 182)

1 (340-g/12-oz) jar sliced beets in vinegar, drained
1 clove garlic, very finely chopped
150 ml/¼ pint (U.S. ⅔ cup) natural yogurt
salt and pepper
450 g/1 lb crisp eating apples, cored and diced
2 tablespoons (U.S. 3 tablespoons) lemon juice
1 tablespoon chopped parsley
1 tablespoon chopped chives
4 tablespoons (U.S. 6 tablespoons) olive oil

Place the beetroot in a bowl. Mix the garlic into the yogurt and season with salt and pepper. Pour over the beetroot, stir and pile up in the centre of a shallow dish.

Place the apple in a bowl, add the lemon juice and turn until coated. Add the herbs and oil and toss lightly. Add seasoning and spoon the apple mixture round the beetroot to make a border. Chill before serving or packing in containers with seals. **Serves 4**

Variation

Beetroot with mixed fruit salad Substitute soured cream for the yogurt and use part apple, part fresh melon dice and a little sliced banana for the salad.

Wholemeal cheese scones

100 g/4 oz plain flour (U.S. 1 cup all-purpose flour)
1 tablespoon (U.S. 4 teaspoons) baking powder
¼ teaspoon salt
good pinch of cayenne pepper
½ teaspoon dry mustard powder
100 g/4 oz wholemeal flour (U.S. 1 cup wholewheat flour)
50 g/2 oz (U.S. ¼ cup) block margarine, diced
100 g/4 oz (U.S. 1 cup) grated Cheddar cheese
150 ml/¼ pint (U.S. ⅔ cup) milk
beaten egg for glazing

Heat the oven to 220°C/425°F, Gas Mark 7 and lightly flour a baking sheet (U.S. cookie sheet).

Sift the white flour with the baking powder, salt, pepper and mustard into a bowl. Add the brown flour and rub or cut in the margarine until the mixture resembles breadcrumbs. Add the cheese and milk and mix to a soft dough.

Turn on to a floured surface and pat out to a thickness of about 2 cm/¾ inch. Stamp out 6.5-cm/2½-inch) rounds and place on the prepared sheet. Gather up the trimmings and use to make further rounds. You should get about 12 in all. Brush with beaten egg.

Bake for about 15 minutes, or until well risen and golden brown. These scones are delicious in a packed lunch, split and spread with butter or peanut butter, accompanied by crisp apples. **Makes 12**

Variations

Peanut and cheese scones Substitute 50 g/2 oz (U.S. ¼ cup) crunchy peanut butter for half the margarine and sprinkle the glazed scones with very finely chopped roasted peanuts before baking.

Cheese and raisin scones Omit half the cheese and add 50 g/2 oz (U.S. ⅓ cup) seedless raisins and ½ teaspoon ground cinnamon to the dough before mixing. If a sweeter scone is desired, omit the salt, pepper and mustard and add 1 teaspoon light muscovado sugar (U.S. light brown sugar) with the cheese.

Index